OCT and OCTA
in Retinal
Disorders

OCT and OCTA in Retinal Disorders

Editors-in-Chief:

Justis P. Ehlers, MD
The Norman C. and Donna L. Harbert
Endowed Chair for Ophthalmic Research
Director, The Tony and Leona Campane
Center for Excellence in Image-Guided
Surgery and Advanced Imaging Research
Cole Eye Institute, Cleveland Clinic
Cleveland, Ohio

Yasha Modi, MD
Assistant Professor, Department of
Ophthalmology
NYU Langone Eye Center
New York, New York

Sunil K. Srivastava, MD
Staff Physician, Vitreoretinal Service
Cole Eye Institute at Cleveland Clinic
Cleveland, Ohio

Peter K. Kaiser, MD
Chaney Family Endowed Chair for
Ophthalmology Research,
Vitreoretinal Service
Cole Eye Institute at Cleveland Clinic
Cleveland, Ohio

Assistant Editors:

Nitish Mehta, MD
Clinical Assistant Professor
Department of Ophthalmology
New York University
New York, New York

Joseph Abraham, MD
Cole Eye Institute at Cleveland Clinic
Cleveland, Ohio

Thuy K. Le, BA
Cole Eye Institute at Cleveland Clinic
Cleveland, Ohio

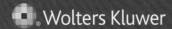

Wolters Kluwer

Philadelphia • Baltimore • New York • London
Buenos Aires • Hong Kong • Sydney • Tokyo

Acquisitions Editor: Chris Teja
Development Editor: Eric McDermott
Editorial Coordinator: Vinoth Ezhumalai
Marketing Manager: Kristin Ciotto
Production Project Manager: Barton Dudlick
Manager, Graphic Arts & Design: Stephen Druding
Manufacturing Coordinator: Beth Welsh
Prepress Vendor: TNQ Technologies
First edition

9 8 7 6 5 4 3 2 1

Printed in China

Library of Congress Cataloging-in-Publication

ISBN-13: 978-1-975144-22-7

Cataloging in Publication data available on request from publisher.

shop.lww.com

CCS0920

To our families who have sacrificed endlessly to allow us to pursue our dreams. Your love and support have enriched every day of our lives.

To our mentors who selflessly provided us an invaluable foundation and opened countless doors for our careers. You have collectively made us better thinkers, better observers, and better doctors.

ACKNOWLEDGMENTS

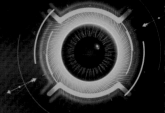

This project would not have been possible without an outstanding team of individuals supporting it along the way. We want to thank all of the authors that contributed to this project. Your time and dedication are what ultimately brought this project together and elevated this book to a new level. The opportunity to work with such an amazing network of friends, residents, fellows, mentors, and colleagues made the project even more rewarding.

Our assistant editors, Nitish Mehta, Joseph Abraham, and Thuy Le, deserve special attention for the hundreds of hours logged critically editing and evaluating each chapter.

Finally, we want to thank our families for supporting us through this process and tolerating our countless hours spent on this project.

PREFACE

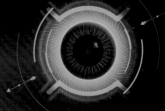

Optical coherence tomography (OCT) and most recently, optical coherence tomography angiography (OCTA), have revolutionized the way that we practice. Since the early 2000s when OCT entered our clinics, our understanding of retinal disease has evolved exponentially. We are now evaluating the retina in three dimensions, visualizing which layers are affected, and understanding how the retina responds to therapy. Through this wealth of information, we are able to diagnose patients sometimes exclusively based on OCT and OCTA imaging. This provides an opportunity to prognosticate visual outcomes and, occasionally, response to treatment. These imaging systems provide not only confirmation of many routine clinical diagnoses, but also are the only way to make many diagnoses that are not clinically apparent (eg, paracentral acute middle maculopathy [PAMM]).

Additionally, we are learning about OCT features that portend a good or poor prognosis. Disruption of the ellipsoid zone (EZ), external limiting membrane (ELM), disorganization of the retinal inner layers (DRIL), and intraretinal hyperreflective foci all provide prognostic information that apply to a host of different disease states. Recognition of these alterations allows us to better communicate with our patients and provide realistic expectations regarding the status of the disease.

In this handbook, we provide OCT and OCTA examples that are representative of each disease state, highlight OCT driven prognostic factors, and demonstrate responses to therapy where applicable. This is a synthesis of the most recently described imaging features on each disease state and we present it in a brief and digestible fashion. We all learned a tremendous amount putting this book together, and we hope this resource will be as valuable to you as it is to us.

Happy reading!

CONTRIBUTORS

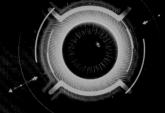

Aliaa Abdelhakim, MD, PhD
Vitreoretinal Fellow
Edward Harkness Eye Institute, Columbia
    University
New York University Department of
    Ophthalmology
New York, New York
Vitreoretinal Fellow
Ophthalmology
New York Presbyterial Hospital, Columbia
    University/New York University Langone
    Medical Center
New York, New York

Joseph Abraham, MD
Research Fellow
The Tony and Leona Campane Center for
    Excellence in Image-Guided Surgery and
    Advanced Imaging Research
Cole Eye Institute, Cleveland Clinic
Cleveland, Ohio

Sruthi Arepalli, MD
Vitreoretinal Fellow
Cole Eye Institute, Cleveland Clinic
Cleveland, Ohio

Amy S. Babiuch, MD
Assistant Professor
Cole Eye Institute, Cleveland Clinic
Cleveland, Ohio

Abhilasha Baharani, DNB, FRCS, FICO
Consultant Ophthalmologist
Uvea and Ocular Immunology
Neoretina Eyecare Institute
Hyderabad, Telangana, India

Irina Belinsky, MD
Clinical Assistant Professor of Oculoplastics
Ophthamalogy
NYU Langone Health
New York, New York

Audina M. Berrocal, MD
Professor of Clinical Ophthamology
Department of Ophthamalogy
Bascom Palmer Eye Institute, University of
    Miami, School of Medicine
Miami, Florida

Randy C. Bowen, MD, MS
Ophthalmic Oncology Fellow
Department of Ophthalmology
Cole Eye Institute, Cleveland Clinic
Cleveland, Ohio

Carmen Calabrise
The Tony and Leona Campane Center for
    Excellence in Image-Guided Surgery and
    Advanced Imaging Research
Cole Eye Institute, Cleveland Clinic
Cleveland, Ohio

Jessica L. Cao, MD
Cole Eye Institute, Cleveland Clinic
Cleveland, Ohio

Nicole Cardwell
The Tony and Leona Campane Center for
    Excellence in Image-Guided Surgery and
    Advanced Imaging Research
Cole Eye Institute, Cleveland Clinic
Cleveland, Ohio

Jay Chhablani, MD
Associate Professor
Ophthalmology
University of Pittsburgh
Pittsburgh, Pennsylvania
Faculty Physician
Ophthalmology
University of Pittsburgh Medical Center
Pittsburgh, Pennsylvania

Andrew X. Chen, BSE
Medical Student
School of Medicine
Case Western Reserve University
Cleveland, Ohio
Research Fellow
Center for Ophthalmic Bioinformatics
Cole Eye Institute, Cleveland Clinic
Cleveland, Ohio

Dinah K. Chen, MD
Resident
Department of Ophthalmology
New York University
New York, New York

Royce W. S. Chen, MD
Helen and Martin Kimmel Assistant Professor
Ophthamalogy
Columbia University Irving Medical Center
New York, New York

Netan Choudhry, MD, FRCSC
Vitreous Retina Macula Specialists of Toronto
Co-Founder & Medical Director
Toronto, Ontario, Canada
Vitreoretinal Surgeon
Ophthalmology
Cleveland Clinic Canada
Toronto, Ontario, Canada

Sara J. Coulon, MD
Resident Physician
Department of Ophthalmology
New York University
New York, New York

Jordan D. Deaner, MD
Uveitis Fellow
Department of Ophthalmology
Cole Eye Institute, Cleveland Clinic
Cleveland, Ohio

Meghan J. DeBenedictis, MS, LCGC, Med
Licensed, Certified Genetic Counselor
Department of Ophthalmology
Cleveland Clinic
Cleveland, Ohio

Vaidehi S. Dedania, MD
Assistant Professor
Department of Ophthalmology
New York University School of Medicine
New York, New York

Vlad Diaconita, MD, FRCSC
Vitreoretinal Fellow
Department of Ophthalmology
Columbia University
New York, New York

Anna T. Do, MD
Glaucoma Fellow
Ophthalmology
New York University
New York, New York

Eliot R. Dow, MD, PhD
Resident physician
Department of Ophthalmology
University of California
Los Angeles, California

Justis P. Ehlers, MD
The Norman C. and Donna L. Harbert
  Endowed Chair for Ophthalmic Research
Director, The Tony and Leona Campane Center
  for Excellence in Image-Guided Surgery and
  Advanced Imaging Research
Cole Eye Institute, Cleveland Clinic
Cleveland, Ohio

Natalia Figueiredo, MD
The Tony and Leona Campane Center for
  Excellence in Image-Guided Surgery and
  Advanced Imaging Research
Cole Eye Institute, Cleveland Clinic
Cleveland, Ohio

Rod Foroozan, MD
Associate Professor
Ophthmalogy
Baylor College of Medicine
Houstan, Texas

John Gabriel
The Tony and Leona Campane Center for
  Excellence in Image-Guided Surgery and
  Advanced Imaging Research
Cole Eye Institute, Cleveland Clinic
Cleveland, Ohio

Lediana Goduni, MD
Resident
Ophthalmology
NYU Langone Health
New York, New York

Doria M. Gold, MD
Clinical Assistant Professor
Department of Neurology
NYU Grossman School of Medicine
New York, New York

Vishal Govindahari, DNB
Consultant
Vitreoretina and Uveitis services
LV Prasad Eye Institute
Bhubaneswar, Odisha, India

Jenna M. Hach, BA
Research Coordinator
The Tony and Leona Campane Center for
  Excellence in Image-Guided Surgery and
  Advanced Imaging Research
Cole Eye Institute, Cleveland Clinic
Cleveland, Ohio

Christopher R. Henry, MD
Clinical Assistant Professor
Ophthmalogy
Houston Methodist Institute for Academic
  Medicine
Retina Consultants at Houston
Houston, Texas

Heidi J. Huang, BA
The Tony and Leona Campane Center for
  Excellence in Image-Guided Surgery and
  Advanced Imaging Research
Cole Eye Institute, Cleveland Clinic
Cleveland, Ohio

Yuji Itoh, MD, PhD
Assistant Professor
Ophthalmology
Kyorin University Hospital
Mitaka-Shi, Tokyo

Alice Jiang, MD
The Tony and Leona Campane Center for
  Excellence in Image-Guided Surgery and
  Advanced Imaging Research,
Cole Eye Institute, Cleveland Clinic
Cleveland, Ohio

Austen N. Knapp, MD
Resident Physician
Cole Eye Institute, Cleveland Clinic
Cleveland, Ohio

Thuy K. Le, BA
The Tony and Leona Campane Center for
  Excellence in Image-Guided Surgery and
  Advanced Imaging Research
Cole Eye Institute, Cleveland Clinic
Cleveland, Ohio

Gerardo Ledesma-Gil, MD
Associate Professor
Retina Department
Institute of Ophthmalogy, Conde de Valencianc
Mexico City, Mexico

Henry Li, MS
The Tony and Leona Campane Center for
  Excellence in Image-Guided Surgery and
  Advanced Imaging Research
Cole Eye Institute, Cleveland Clinic
Cleveland, Ohio

Phoebe Lin, MD, PhD
Associate Professor of Ophthalmology
Casey Eye Institute
Oregon Health & Science University
Portland, Oregon

Liang Liu, MD
Research Associate
Casey Eye Institute
Oregon Health & Science University
Portland, Orgeon

Leina M. Lunasco
The Tony and Leona Campane Center for
  Excellence in Image-Guided Surgery and
  Advanced Imaging Research
Cole Eye Institute, Cleveland Clinic
Cleveland, Ohio

Brian Marr, MD
Director of Ophthalmic Oncology, Professor of
  Ophthamalogy
Ophthamalogy
Columbia University
New York, New York
New York Presbyterian
Director of Ophthalmic Oncology
Columbia University Medical Center
New York, New York

Kanwal Singh Matharu, MD
Resident
Cullen Eye Institute
Department of Ophthamalogy
Baylor College of Medicine
Houston, Texas

Nitish Mehta, MD
Clinical Assistant Professor
Ophthalmology
New York University
New York, New York

Thomas A. Mendel, MD, PhD
Vitreoretinal Surgery Fellow
Cole Eye Institute, Cleveland Clinic
Cleveland, Ohio

Ronald Walden Milam Jr, MD
Vitreoretinal Surgery Fellow
Cole Eye Institute, Cleveland Clinic
Cleveland, Ohio

Mihai Mititelu, MD, MPH
Associate Professor
Medical Director, Clinical Eye Research Unit
University of Wisconsin-Madison
Madison, Wisconsin

Yasha Modi, MD
Assistant Professor, Department of
    Ophthalmology
NYU Langone Eye Center
New York, New York

Prithvi Mruthyunjaya, MD
Vitreoretinal and Ocular Oncology Service
Stanford University Byers Eye Institute
Palo Alto, California

Ramsudha Narala, MD
Ocular Oncology Fellow
Ophthamology
Standard University Byers Eye Institute
Palo Alto, California

Archana Nair, MD
Resident Physician
Ophthalmology
New York University
New York, New York

Maura Di Nicola, MD
Clinical Fellow
Ocular Oncology Service
Department of Ophthalmology
University of Cincinnati
Cincinnati, Ohio

Carl Noble, DO, MBA
Surgical Retina Fellow
Ophthalmology
University of Cincinnati
Cincinnati Eye Institute
Cincinnati, Ohio

Yan Nuzbrokh, BS
Clinical Research Fellow
Medical Student
Department of Ophthalmology
Columbia University
New York, New York

Margaret O'Connell, BS
The Tony and Leona Campane Center for
    Excellence in Image-Guided Surgery and
    Advanced Imaging Research
Cole Eye Institute, Cleveland Clinic
Cleveland, Ohio

Sally Shin Yee Ong, MD
Vitreoretinal Fellow
Department of Ophthamology, Wilmer Eye
    Instiute
Johns Horkins University
Baltimore, Maryland

Joseph F. Panarelli, MD
Associate Professor
Ophthalmology
NYU School of Medicine
New York, New York

Dong-wouk Park, MD
Medical Retina Fellow
Cole Eye Institute, Cleveland Clinic
Cleveland, Ohio

Paula Eem Pecen, MD
Assistant Professor
Department of Ophthmology
University of Colorado
Aurora, Colorado

Marco Pellegrini, MD
Consultant – Head of Ocular Oncology Service
Department of Biomedical and Clinical
    Sciences "Luigi
Eye Clinic, Luigi Sacco Hospital
University of Milan
Milan, Italy

Prof. Giuseppe Querques, MD, PhD
Associate Professor
Ophthalmology
University Vita-Salute San Raffaele,
Milan, Italy

Aleksandra V. Rachitskaya, MD
Assistant Professor of Ophthamology
Cole Eye Institute, Cleveland Clinic
Cleveland, Ohio

Joseph James Raevis, MD
Surgical Retina Fellow
Ophthamology
University of Wisconsin
Madison, Wisonsin

Spoorti Krishna Reddy Mandadi, MS
Former fellow in Medical Retina and Uveitis
Department of Retina and Uveitis
L V Prasad Eye Institute, Kallam Anji Reddy
    Campus
Hyderabad, Telangana, India

Riccardo Sacconi, MD, FEBO
PhD Candidate
Ophthalmology
University Vita-Salute San Raffaele
Milan, Italy
Consultant
Ophthalmology
IRCCS San Raffaele Hospital
Milan, Italy

David Sarraf, MD
Clinical Professor of Ophthalmology
Jules Stein Eye Institute
University of California
Los Angeles, California

Jackson Scharf, BS
Medical Student
Vagelos College of Physicians and Surgeons
Columbia University
New York, New York
Research Fellow
Retina Disorders and Ophthalmic Genetics
Jules Stein Eye Institute
University of California
Los Angeles, California

Ioana Scherbakova, BFA
Medical Student and Research Assistant
Columbia University
Irving Medical Center
New York, New York

Adrienne Williams Scott, MD
Associate Professor
The Wilmer Eye Institute
Department of Ophthalmology
Johns Hopkins School of Medicine
Baltimore, Maryland

Duriye Damla Sevgi, MD
The Tony and Leona Campane Center for
    Excellence in Image-Guided Surgery and
    Advanced Imaging Research
Cole Eye Institute, Cleveland Clinic Foundation
Cleveland, Ohio

Sumit Sharma, MD
Assistant Professor of Ophthalmology
Cole Eye Institute, Cleveland Clinic
Cleveland, Ohio

Joseph Michael Simonett, MD
Resident
Department of Ophthalmology
Casey Eye Institute
Oregon Health & Science University
Portland, Orgeon

Arun D. Singh, MD
Professor and Director, Department of
    Ophthalmic Oncology
Cole Eye Insititue, Cleveland Clinic
Cleveland, Ohio

Rishi P. Singh, MD
Associate Professor
Cole Eye Institute, Cleveland Clinic
Cleveland, Ohio

Alsion H. Skalet, MD, PhD
Associate Professor
Casey Eye Institute
Ophthamology, Radiation Medicine &
    Dermatology
Orgeon Health & Science University
Portland, Orgeon
Division Chief, Ocular Oncology
Ophthamology
Casey Eye Institute, OHSU
Portland, Orgeon

Arjun B. Sood, MD
Vitreoretinal Surgery Fellow
Cole Eye Institute, Cleveland Clinic
Cleveland, Ohio

Sunil Srivastava, MD
Staff Physician, Vitreoretinal Service
Cole Eye Institute, Cleveland Clinic
Cleveland, Ohio

Brittney Statler, MD
Medical Retinal Fellow
Cole Eye Institute, Cleveland Clinic
Cleveland, Ohio

Sandip Suresh, MD
Department of Ophthalmology
Jules Stein Eye Institute
University of California
Los Angeles, California

Katherine E. Talcott, MD
Staff Physician
Cole Eye Institute, Cleveland Clinic
Cleveland, Ohio

Elias I. Traboulsi, MD, MEd
Professor of Ophthlamology
Cole Eye Institute, Cleveland Clinic
CCLCM, Case University
Cleveland, Ohio
Director, Center for Genetic Eye Disease
Cole Eye Institute, Cleveland Clinic
Cleveland, Ohio

Stephen H. Tsang, MD, PhD
László Bitó Professor
Ophthalmology, Pathology & Cell Biology
Columbia Stem Cell Initiative
New York, New York
Attending
Department of Ophthalmology
New York-Presbyterian Hospital
New York, New York

Edmund Tsui, MD
Assistant Professor
Jules Stein Eye Institute
University of California
Los Angeles, California

Atsuro Uchida, MD, PhD
Assistant Professor
Department of Ophthalmology
Keio University School of Medicine
Tokyo, Japan

Chukwumamkpam C. Uzoegwu, MS
Tony and Leona Campane Center for
    Excellence in Image-Guided Surgery and
    Advanced Imaging Research
Cole Eye Institute, Cleveland Clinic
Cleveland, Ohio

Derrick Wang, BA
Jules Stein Eye Institute
University of California
Los Angeles, California

Basil K. Williams Jr, MD
Assistant Professor of Ophthamology, Director
    of Ocular Oncology
Department of Ophthamology
University of Cincinnati
Cincinnati, Ohio

Lawrence A. Yannuzzi, MD
Professor of Clinical Ophthamolgy
Coulmbia University School of Medicine,
New York, New York
President & Founder
LuEsther T. Meets Retinal Research Center
Manhattan Eye, Ear &Throat Hospital
New York, New York

CONTENTS

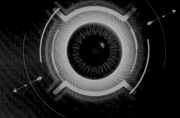

THE VITREORETINAL INTERFACE AND PERIPHERAL RETINAL PATHOLOGY

INFLAMMATION AND INFECTION

INHERITED RETINAL DEGENERATIONS

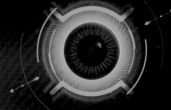

- CNV—choroidal neovascularization
- DCP—deep capillary plexus
- DRIL—disorganization of the retinal inner layers
- EDI-OCT—enhanced depth imaging optical coherence tomography
- ELM—external limiting membrane
- EZ—ellipsoid zone
- FA—fluorescein angiography
- FAF—fundus autofluorescence
- FAZ—foveal avascular zone
- ICG—indocyanine green
- ICG—indocyanine green angiography
- IRF—intraretinal fluid
- IZ—interdigitation zone
- NIR—near infrared reflectance
- OCT—optical coherence tomography
- OCTA—optical coherence tomography angiography
- ONL—outer nuclear layer
- PED—pigment epithelial detachment
- RF—red-free image
- RNFL—retinal nerve fiber layer
- RPE—retinal pigment epithelium
- SCP—superficial capillary plexus
- SD-OCT—spectral domain optical coherence tomography
- SRF—subretinal fluid
- SS-OCT—swept source optical coherence tomography
- SS-OCTA—swept source optical coherence tomography angiography
- VEGF—vascular endothelial growth factor

Part 1
Introduction

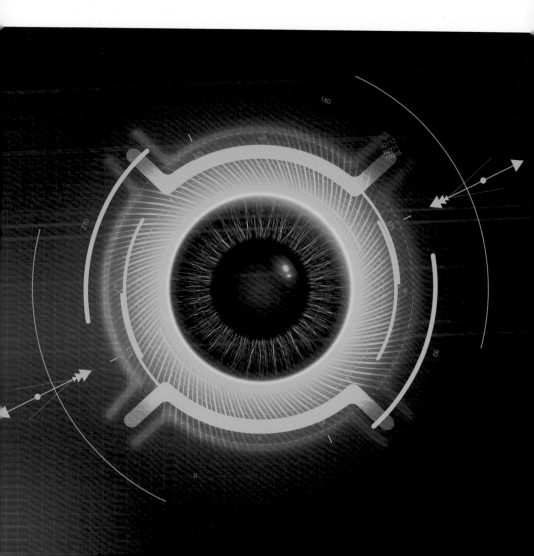

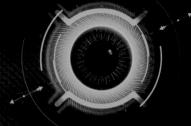

CHAPTER 1

Optical Coherence Tomography Overview

SALIENT FEATURES

- Optical coherence tomography (OCT) allows the visualization of retina and choroid through a noninvasive procedure and plays a pivotal role in modern ophthalmic multimodal imaging. In many ways, OCT has become the most valuable diagnostic imaging tool in the vitreoretinal clinic.
- OCT technology has continuously evolved and expanded from its inception as time-domain OCT. The advent of Fourier domain detection techniques with either spectrometer-based system referred to as spectral-domain OCT (SD-OCT), or frequency swept laser-based system referred to as swept-source OCT (SS-OCT), has enabled OCT imaging with unprecedented scanning speeds and sensitivities leading to widespread clinical utilization of OCT. Faster scanning speeds is crucial for in vivo imaging as it can minimize motion artifacts and also permit the acquisition of volumetric OCT data.
- OCT angiography (OCTA) provides detailed information on the microvascular flow of the individual layers within the retina and choroid. The large volume of OCTA data is amenable to software-based image processing and may provide quantitative biomarkers that reflect vascular pathology.
- Microscope-integrated intraoperative OCT provides real-time feedback on the tissue-instrument interactions during vitreoretinal surgery.

OCT IMAGING

- OCT allows real-time, high-resolution, noninvasive optical biopsy of the tissue, including the retina.[1,2] OCT utilizes a concept known as interferometry. The technology is based on the detection and analysis of interference between two low-coherence (broadband width) light beams (eg, superluminescent diode [SLD] or a pulsed laser); reference signal; and reflected signal from the tissue. The high-reflective areas of the tissue will create greater interference. The distance (depth) of the tissue can be determined when the reference and reflected signal paths length are matched or have only a small difference (ie, within the coherence length of the light source).

- The reflectivity profile of a single scanning line on the tissue is referred to as an A-scan (1D) and contains information of distance (depth) and signal intensity. A cross-sectional tomographic image (B-scan, 2D) of the tissue can be obtained by combining a series of A-scans (Figure 1.1). Similarly, a volumetric image (3D) of the tissue can be obtained by assembling closely spaced and rapidly acquired B-scans. A volume scan can be processed to reconstruct and view OCT images from any perspective, including rotated B-scans, en-face scans at a specific depth, and thickness maps.

- SD-OCT instruments include a spectrometer and line scan camera that analyzes the spectrum of reflected light and capable of generating A-scan by the application of the Fourier transform. This technology detects signals from the full depth of the tissue simultaneously and eliminates a mechanically moving scanning reference arm employed in time-domain OCT. This facilitated the consequent 50 to 100 times

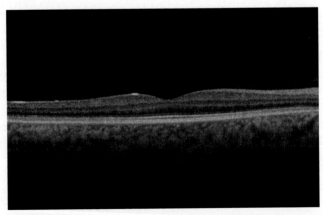

FIGURE 1.1 Swept-source optical coherence tomography macular B-scan of a healthy control.

increase in the scanning speed. Increased scanning speed helps reduce motion artifacts that may degrade image quality and permits the acquisition of a volume scan.

- In SD-OCT, scanning speeds are determined (or limited) by the camera reading rate. Due to the finite spectral resolution of the spectrometer, SD-OCT is susceptible to loss of detection sensitivity at deeper axial ranges, a phenomenon known as sensitivity roll-off.

- SS-OCT equipped with a rapidly tunable laser and a photodetector can achieve faster scanning speeds and higher detection efficiencies than SD-OCT as it does not require a spectrometer and line scan camera. Recent-generation commercial SD-OCT instruments acquire 70,000 to 85,000 A-scans/second, while SS-OCT instruments acquire 100,000 A-scans/second or faster, and the latest research prototype SS-OCT instruments may acquire up to several million A-scans/second. Compared with SD-OCT (scanning wavelength centered around 850 nm), SS-OCT operating at longer scanning wavelength (centered at 1050 nm) offers improved visualization of the choroid and optic nerve with longer imaging range.

- Scanning wavelengths centered around 850 or 1050 nm minimize the signal absorption or attenuation in water (ocular media), and thus are suitable for retinal and choroidal imaging.

- Performance characteristics of OCT, including the scanning speed, axial resolution, and imaging depth, are highly dependent on the design of the instrument. The axial resolution of OCT can be improved by either reducing the coherence length of the light source (broadband light sources have shorter coherence length) or reducing the center wavelength. The lateral resolution is generally limited by the optical properties of the eye. Specific trade-offs between optical parameters exist; (1) a higher A-scan rate results in lower sensitivity, (2) improving axial resolution decreases the maximum imaging depth, and (3) improving lateral scan density leads to a smaller field of view.

- To compensate for eye motion, commercial instruments utilize the fundus image from scanning laser ophthalmoscopy or infrared camera for active eye tracking. Additional utilization of software registration and motion correction has been proposed to further reduce artifacts.

- Averaging multiple scans can reduce (speckle) noise and improve the signal-to-noise ratio (image quality). Utilization of adaptive optics that compensate for ocular aberrations can improve lateral resolution.

- Enhanced depth imaging technique (usually reserved for SD-OCT) utilizes the sensitivity roll-off phenomenon; a vertically inverted structural image can be obtained by placing an objective lens closer to the eye, bringing choroid-sclera interface at the zero-decay line, which thus allows for better visualization of the choroid.

References

1. Fujimoto J, Swanson E. The development, commercialization, and impact of optical coherence tomography. *Invest Ophthalmol Vis Sci.* 2016;57(9):OCT1-OCT13.

2. Aumann S, Donner S, Fischer J, Müller F. Optical coherence tomography (OCT): principle and technical realization. In: Bille JF, ed. *High resolutionImaging in Microscopyand Ophthalmology.* Gewerbestrasse, Switzerland: Springer; 2019:59-85.

3. Spaide RF, Fujimoto JG, Waheed NK, Sadda SR, Staurenghi G. Optical coherence tomography angiography. *Prog Retin Eye Res.* 2018;64(5):1-55.

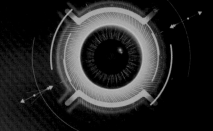

CHAPTER 2

Optical Coherence Tomography Angiography Overview

OPTICAL COHERENCE TOMOGRAPHY ANGIOGRAPHY BASIC PRINCIPLES

- Based on optical coherence tomography (OCT).
- Noninvasive method allowing for visualization of functional blood vessels in the eye producing a three-dimensional reconstruction of vascular networks.
- Achieved by using variation in the OCT signal caused by moving red blood cells (RBCs).
  - To differentiate dynamic particles (predominantly RBCs) from static structural tissues of the eye, repeated scans are taken at the same location.
  - Produces a static map of the vascular network without providing any true information regarding blood flow or vascular leakage.
- Provides ability to view optical coherence tomography angiography (OCTA) images with corresponding en-face images.

OCTA TECHNIQUES[1]

- Phase signal–based OCTA technique
  - Phase variance
    - Measurement of phase variance between adjacent B-scans or the motion-contrast technique.
    - Quantifies axial blood flow parallel to the direction of the imaging acquisition device.

- Intensity-based OCTA technique
  - Amplitude decorrelation
    - Performed through analysis of amplitude changes in the OCT signal.
    - Split-spectrum amplitude decorrelation angiography (SSADA) acts to partition the spectrum into smaller spectra and performs the repeated B-scan decorrelation separately for each subspectrum.
    - Improves the signal-to-noise ratio.
  - Speckle variance
    - An extension of Doppler OCT which is a phase-based technology that was adapted using laser speckle technique.
    - Measurement of the speckle variance within the OCT signal and adjacent region using only amplitude information.
- Complex signal–based OCTA technique
  - OCT microangiography (OMAG) algorithm
    - Uses variations in both the intensity and phase information between sequential B-scans at the same position.
    - Coherent information used to calculate flow signal.

SPECTRAL-DOMAIN OCTA VERSUS SWEPT-SOURCE OCTA

- Spectral-domain OCTA (SD-OCTA)[2]
  - Operates at ~840 nm wavelength.
  - A-scan rate of typically 70,000-100,000 scans per second to obtain SSADA.
  - Resolution is limited by the spectrometers used.
- Swept-source OCTA (SS-OCTA)[3]
  - Operates at ~1050 nm wavelength.
  - A-scan rate of 100,000 scans per second or higher with an intensity- and phase-based algorithm.
  - Does not use spectrometer-based detection.
  - Instantaneous line-width of the swept light system.
  - Axial resolution of 5µm and lateral resolution of 14µm.
  - Less variation in sensitivity with depth.
    - Improved visualization of the choroid.

OCTA VASCULATURE SEGMENTATION

- The segmentation on OCTA systems is usually performed through an automated process and has preset layers of interest. In addition, manual segmentation can be performed.

- The retinal vasculature is depth encoded on OCTA which can be split into various layers: a superficial layer, slab, or plexus and a deep layer, slab, or plexus by machine software which varies slightly between systems.[2]
  - Superficial plexus is located predominantly within the ganglion cell layer (Figure 2.1).
  - Deep plexus is located at the outer boundary of the inner nuclear layer (Figure 2.2).
  - Superficial and deep capillary plexuses may be affected differently by different retinal diseases.
- Most systems provide an avascular or outer retinal slab.
  - Segments between the outer plexiform layer and Bruch membrane.
  - This region is devoid of vascular flow.
  - Useful in detecting choroidal neovascular membranes.
- Choroidal vasculature often is divided into a choriocapillaris and/or choroid slab (Figure 2.3).
- As technology and speed improve, additional slabs and segmentation approaches are being utilized and explored.

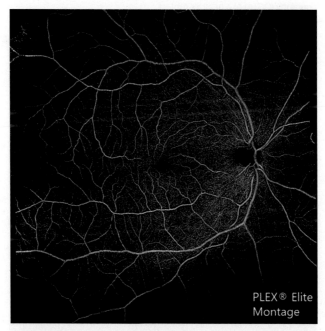

PLEX® Elite
Montage

FIGURE 2.1 En-face superficial retina segmentation slab from a swept-source 12 × 12 mm optical coherence tomography angiography (OCTA) of a healthy subject.

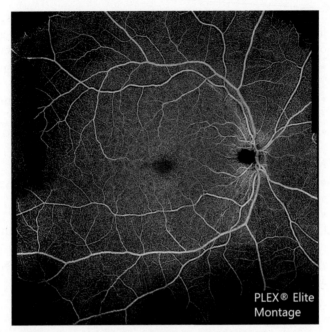

FIGURE 2.2 En-face deep retina segmentation slab from a swept-source 12 × 12 mm optical coherence tomography angiography (OCTA) of a healthy subject.

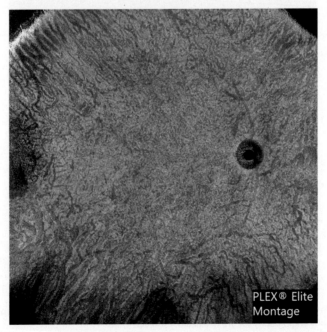

FIGURE 2.3 En-face choroid segmentation slab from a swept-source 12 × 12 mm optical coherence tomography angiography (OCTA) of a healthy subject.

OCTA ARTIFACTS

- Occur due to scanning methodology used to generate the motion-contrast signal, image acquisition, image processing and display, eye motion, and intrinsic properties of the eye and related pathology.[4]
- Because scans are repeated over the same area more than once in OCTA, motion artifacts are more likely to occur from microsaccades, breathing, and cardiac cycle changes.
- Refracted, reflected, absorbed, or passing of the OCT beam through a vessel generating false blood flow signals.
- Fluctuating shadows from RBCs in superficial vessels can cast extra flow signals to deeper vascular networks leading to projection artifact.[5,6]
- Software segmentation errors.

References

1. Kashani AH, Chen CL, Gahm JK, et al. Optical coherence tomography angiography: a comprehensive review of current methods and clinical applications. *Prog Retin Eye Res.* 2017;60:66-100. doi:10.1016/j.preteyeres.2017.07.002.
2. de Carlo TE, Bonini Filho MA, Chin AT, et al. Spectral-domain optical coherence tomography angiography of choroidal neovascularization. *Ophthalmology.* 2015;122(6):1228-1238. doi:10.1016/j.ophtha.2015.01.029.
3. Zhang Q, Wang RK, Chen CL, et al. Swept source optical coherence tomography angiography of neovascular macular telangiectasia Type 2: *Retina.* 2015;35(11):2285-2299. doi:10.1097/IAE.0000000000000840.
4. Spaide RF, Fujimoto JG, Waheed NK. Image artifacts in optical coherence tomography angiography: *Retina.* 2015;35(11):2163-2180. doi:10.1097/IAE.0000000000000765.
5. Zhang A, Zhang Q, Wang RK. Minimizing projection artifacts for accurate presentation of choroidal neovascularization in OCT micro-angiography. *Biomed Opt Express.* 2015;6(10):4130. doi:10.1364/BOE.6.004130.
6. Zhang M, Hwang TS, Campbell JP, et al. Projection-resolved optical coherence tomographic angiography. *Biomed Opt Express.* 2016;7(3):816. doi:10.1364/BOE.7.000816.

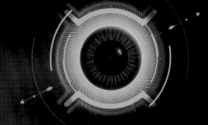

CHAPTER 3

OCT and OCTA Interpretation

OCT SALIENT FEATURES

- Spectral-domain optical coherence tomography (SD-OCT) provides high-resolution cross-sectional images of the retina and is the diagnostic imaging test of choice to assess many vitreoretinal diseases.[1]
- There are several commercially available SD-OCT devices on the market, including Zeiss Cirrus, Heidelberg Spectralis, Topcon 3D OCT, and Optovue Avanti RTVue.
- The international nomenclature for OCT panel reported a consensus paper on the retinal and choroidal landmarks on SD-OCT (Figure 3.1).[2]

OCT INTERPRETATION

- OCT interpretation should be done in a systematic fashion and focus on scan quality, pattern, reflectivity, quantitative analysis, and qualitative analysis.[1]
- OCT scan characteristics:
  - Scan quality:
    - Some devices provide a quantitative output of signal strength that may be used as a surrogate.
    - Artifacts should be identified and can be caused by the patient (poor fixation), operator (decentered or out-of-focus scans), or software issues (failed or incorrect segmentation).
  - Scan pattern—the two most common scan protocols for OCT devices are macular cube and line scans.

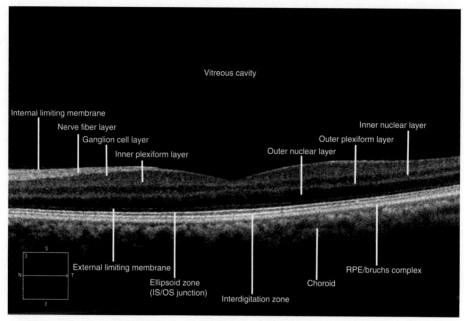

Vitreous cavity

Internal limiting membrane
Nerve fiber layer
Ganglion cell layer
Inner plexiform layer

Inner nuclear layer
Outer plexiform layer
Outer nuclear layer

External limiting membrane
Ellipsoid zone
(IS/OS junction)
Interdigitation zone

Choroid

RPE/bruchs complex

FIGURE 3.1 Normal optical coherence tomography (OCT) horizontal raster scan of the left eye with labels of the retina and choroid. Note the nerve fiber layer (NFL) is thicker on the left side, which corresponds to nasal retina and identifies the image as the left eye. IS/OS, inner and outer segments; RPE, retinal pigment epithelium.

- Macular cube:
  - The composition of the scans varies based on device and user input. These are usually moderately densely sampled with variable B-scan densities.
  - The overall size of the macular cube (eg, 6 × 6 mm) can be varied.
  - These scans are typically utilized for line-by-line review, thickness map construction, change analysis, and three-dimensional (3D) reconstruction.
- Line scans (horizontal, vertical, radial):
  - Raster scans are often higher A-scan density with averaging that produce higher signal-to-noise images.
  - These may provide better visualization of subtle pathology.
- Appearance of the reflectivity profile:
  - Gray scale and false-color visualization is an option and is based on clinician preference.
- Quantitative analysis:
  - Commercial software systems provide automated segmentation of various retinal layers. These values are then compared to normative data (age-matched patients).

- Qualitative analysis:
  - Review strategies include cross-sectional review of individual B-scans and/or en-face review.
  - Systematic approach to evaluation of OCT features is key.
  - One approach is to evaluate OCT structural features by interpreting from inner to outer:
    - Vitreous cell or media opacities (eg, hemorrhage, asteroid hyalosis, gas or silicone oil tamponade).
    - Vitreoretinal interface: vitreomacular traction and epiretinal membrane.
    - Retinal/choroidal layers—(eg, nerve fiber layer infarct or thinning, cystoid macular edema, ellipsoid zone attenuation, subretinal fluid, drusen, pigment epithelial detachment, choroidal thinning, and pachychoroid).

OCTA SALIENT FEATURES

- OCT angiography (OCTA) is an extension of OCT and allows for noninvasive imaging of the retinal and choroidal vasculature.
- Serial OCT B-scans of the same location are acquired. Variation in light backscatter (decorrelation of signal amplitude) can detect static tissue versus erythrocyte flow. This information is used to generate a 3D vascular flow map.[3]
- Software within each OCTA device automatically segments the retina and choroid into various layers. The 3D flow data from each layer are converted into a two-dimensional en-face image report (Figure 3.2).
- There are several OCTA devices available including Zeiss AngioPlex, Optovue AngioVue, and Heidelberg Spectral. Each device has its own segmentation software.[4]

OCTA INTERPRETATION

- Interpretation of OCTA information relies on accurate segmentation and limiting artifacts (eg, motion, projection) (Figure 3.3).
- Automated segmentation software may misidentify anatomic boundaries in a pathologic retina. Manual segmentation can overcome this issue but is labor intensive and not ideal for a busy clinical practice.[5]
- Combined viewing of en-face OCTA images and OCT B-scan with decorrelation overlay has been reported to have higher sensitivity to detecting choroidal neovascular membranes.[6]

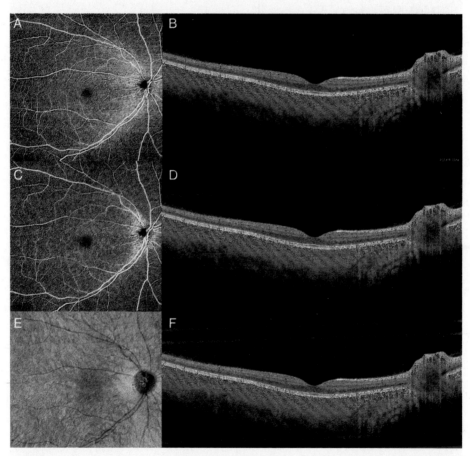

FIGURE 3.2 Normal swept-source optical coherence tomography (OCT) angiography showing a 12 × 12 mm two-dimensional en-face image report and corresponding B-scan of the superficial retina (A and B), deep retina (C and D), and choroid (E and F).

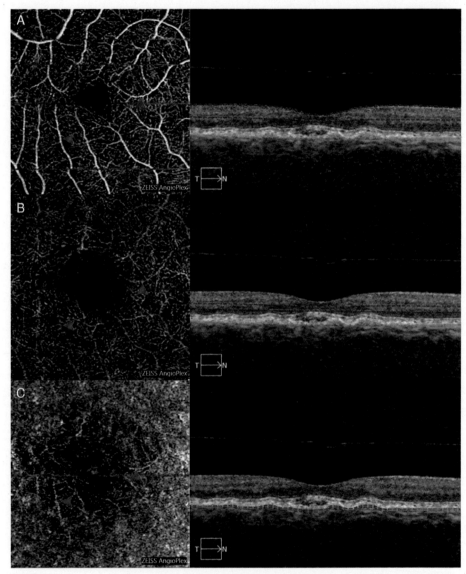

FIGURE 3.3 Optical coherence tomography (OCT) angiography showing a 3 × 3 mm two-dimensional en-face imaging report and corresponding B-scan of the superficial retina (A), deep retina (B), and chorio-capillaris (C). The red arrowheads identify superficial vessels that are projecting into the deep and chorio-capillaris layers.

References

1. Bhende M, Shetty S, Parthasarathy MK, Ramya S. Optical coherence tomography: a guide to interpretation of common macular diseases. *Indian J Ophthalmol*. 2018;66:20-35.

2. Staurenghi G, Sadda S, Chakravarthy U, Spaide RF. Proposed lexicon for anatomic landmarks in normal posterior segment spectral-domain optical coherence tomography: the IN*OCT consensus. *Ophthalmology*. 2014;121:1572-1578.

3. Spaide RF, Fujimoto JG, Waheed NK, Sadda SR, Staurenghi G. Optical coherence tomography angiography. *Prog Retin Eye Res*. 2018;64:1-55.

4. Kashani AH, Chen CL, Gahm JK, et al. Optical coherence tomography angiography: a comprehensive review of current methods and clinical applications. *Prog Retin Eye Res*. 2017;60:66-100.

5. Spaide RF, Fujimoto JG, Waheed NK. Image artifacts in optical coherence tomography angiography. *Retina*. 2015;35:2163-2180.

6. Babiuch AS, Uchida A, Figueiredo N, et al. Impact of optical coherence tomography angiography review strategy on detection of choroidal neovascularization. *Retina*. 2020;40(4):672-678.

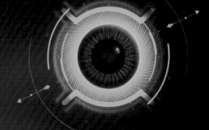

CHAPTER 4

The Normal Retina and Choroid

OCT IMAGING

- **The basic principles for tissue reflectivity:** Retinal layers with cellular components yield low reflectivity. In contrast, retinal layers with synaptic or fiber layers yield high reflectivity. The boundaries also produce high reflectivity. Therefore, nuclear layers generally appear hyporeflective, whereas retinal nerve fiber layer and plexiform layers appear hyperreflective. A structural spectral-domain optical coherence tomography (OCT) image from a healthy subject is shown in Figure 4.1.

- **Vitreous:** The posterior hyaloid face with incomplete posterior vitreous detachment (PVD) may be visible on the OCT scan. A separation of the posterior hyaloid face from the neurosensory retina and optic disc on structural OCT scans can help determine whether a PVD is present or absent. Retrohyaloid space is between the posterior hyaloid face and internal limiting membrane (ILM). Premacular bursa or posterior precortical vitreous pocket is an optically empty liquid space overlying the macula caused by degenerative liquefaction of the vitreous.

- **Cellular layers:** Retinal layers where cellular body exists, such as the ganglion cell layer, inner nuclear layer (INL), and outer nuclear layer (ONL), pose low reflectivity. The ONL may be thinner than what it appears as it may include Henle fiber layer, as discussed below.

- **Retinal nerve fiber layer and plexiform layers:** Retinal nerve fiber layer and inner plexiform layer (IPL) typically pose high reflectivity as they are located parallel to the retinal surface and perpendicular to the beam direction of the OCT light source. The exception is the outer

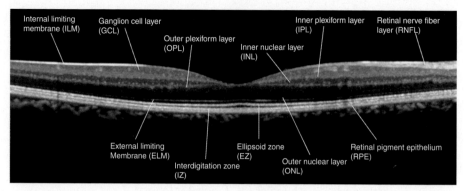

Internal limiting membrane (ILM)   Ganglion cell layer (GCL)   Outer plexiform layer (OPL)   Inner nuclear layer (INL)   Inner plexiform layer (IPL)   Retinal nerve fiber layer (RNFL)

External limiting Membrane (ELM)   Interdigitation zone (IZ)   Ellipsoid zone (EZ)   Outer nuclear layer (ONL)   Retinal pigment epithelium (RPE)

FIGURE 4.1 Foveal cross-sectional optical coherence tomography (OCT) imaging of healthy subject.

plexiform layer (OPL); Henle fiber layer within OPL has variable reflectivity depending on the orientation of the light source relative to the plane of the retina. Henle fiber layer contains obliquely oriented photoreceptor axons and is almost isoreflective with the ONL in untilted B-scans. Henle fiber layer can be recognized when the OCT light source is inserted at the edge of the pupil that will induce the tilting of OCT images.

- **Outer retinal bands:** The integrity of the outer retinal hyperreflective bands on structural OCT, including the external limiting membrane (ELM), ellipsoid zone (EZ), and interdigitation zone (IZ), reflects the health of photoreceptors. The elevation of the ELM and EZ band at the central fovea termed foveal bulge is present in healthy subjects. The foveal bulge represents the crowding and thinning of cone photoreceptors and elongation of cone outer segment. It is considered a biomarker for predicting foveal function.

- **Ellipsoid zone:** Also referred to as the inner segment/outer segment (IS/OS) junction. EZ reflects the mitochondrial-rich band in the inner segment of photoreceptors. Loss or discontinuation of the EZ band represents defects or dysfunction in the photoreceptors, which typically has a profound negative effect on the visual function.

- **Interdigitation zone:** Also referred to as cone outer segment tip (COST). A hyperreflective band below EZ and above retinal pigment epithelium (RPE) on Fourier-domain structural OCT. The IZ band corresponds to the contact cylinders formed by the apices of the RPE cells.

- **Retinal pigment epithelium:** Observed as the outermost and thickest hyperreflective band on structural OCT. This hyperreflectivity is due to the presence of melanin. The high melanin scattering of the RPE can obscure adjacent layers. Under normal conditions, melanin scattering of the RPE thereby limits the visibility of Bruch membrane.

- **Choroid:** Imaging of the choroid using conventional spectral-domain OCT platforms has been challenging, due to the decreased signal transmission beyond the RPE. The attenuation is caused by the presence of melanin deposits in the RPE or hemoglobin within red blood cells in the choroid; both strongly absorb light. The use of enhanced depth imaging technique on spectral-domain OCT allows the visualization of the choroid in reasonable clarity (Figure 4.2). More detail of the choroid can be visualized with the use of high-penetration swept-source OCT platforms. The Sattler layer containing medium-sized vessels is seen as a layer of round or oval hyporeflective spaces, and the outermost Haller layer containing large choroidal vessels can be distinguished with lower OCT signal intensity.

OCTA IMAGING

- OCT angiography (OCTA) allows the depth-resolved en-face visualization of the different retinal capillary plexuses that cannot be distinguished by fluorescein angiography (Figure 4.3). The retinal capillary network at the posterior pole is comprised of four layers: the radial peripapillary capillary plexus (RPCP) around the optic disc, the superficial vascular plexus (SVP), intermediate capillary plexus (ICP), and deep capillary plexus (DCP).
- Most OCTA platforms separate these four capillary plexuses into two major plexuses, namely superficial vascular complex (SVC) and deep vascular complex (DVC).[1] SVC contains RPCP and SVP. DVC includes ICP and DCP and is treated as a single vascular network; until recently, these two plexuses cannot be easily differentiated due to the flow projection artifact caused by superficial vessels and inaccurate segmentation process. Projection resolved SSADA OCTA platform successfully demonstrated the separate visualization of the four capillary plexuses.

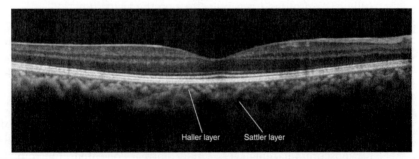

FIGURE 4.2 Foveal cross-sectional optical coherence tomography (OCT) imaging applying the enhanced depth imaging technique of healthy subjects.

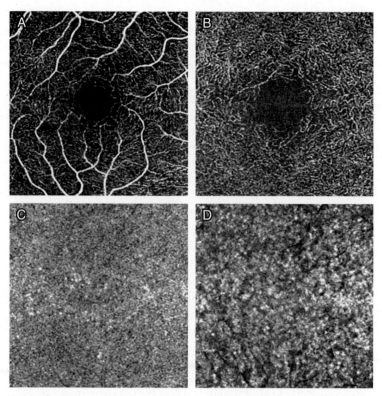

FIGURE 4.3 Normal optical coherence tomography (OCT) angiography showing 3 × 3 mm two-dimensional en-face image report of the superficial capillary plexus (A), deep capillary plexus (B), choriocapillaris (C), and choroid (D).

- During the segmentation process, specific parameters that concern the intraretinal level (eg, ILM, IPL, RPE) are defined, and the offset is used to include all the vessels of the specific capillary plexuses. For example, the assessment of the SVC typically uses a slab from ILM to IPL -10 μm, and DVC uses a slab from IPL -10 μm to OPL +10 μm.
- Most OCTA platforms generate en-face OCTA and B-scan OCT images with vascular flow overlay. The detected flow signals are superimposed onto a gray-scale structural B-scan OCT image in a color-coded overlay.
- Most OCTA platforms allow quantitative analysis of vessel density, flow area, and the area measurements of foveal avascular zone (FAZ). OCTA platforms equipped with panoramic imaging function can deliver widefield montage OCTA.
- **Radial peripapillary capillary plexus:** This layer forms within the retinal nerve fiber layer. Long capillary segments are oriented radially around the optic disc resembling the orientation of the retinal nerve fiber layer.

- **Superficial vascular plexus:** This layer located in the ganglion cell layer consists of arterioles and venules that emanate from the superior and inferior vascular arcades and connected by transverse capillaries. The vascular pattern converges toward the fovea with a centripetal pattern.

- **Intermediate capillary plexus and deep capillary plexus:** The two plexuses ICP and DCP are part of DVC and visualized as a single vascular network in most OCTA platforms. ICP is formed at the IPL/INL interface, whereas DCP is formed at the INL/OPL interface. DVC consists of a close-knit pattern of capillaries with numerous horizontal and radial interconnections. The vascular pattern is orderly distributed around the FAZ. Both ICP and DCP are supplied by vertical interconnecting anastomoses from the SVP.

- **Foveal avascular zone:** A region of absent capillaries at the center of the macula surrounded by interconnected capillary networks. The FAZ can vary considerably in size and shape, even among healthy individuals.

- **Outer retina:** In a healthy subject, the outer retina appears avascular as there should be no vascular components.

- **Choriocapillaris:** Accounts for the inner portion of the choroid, containing small vessels with fenestrated endothelial cells. En-face OCTA of the choriocapillaris can be generated by projecting a thin slab below the Bruch membrane, visualized as confluent, lobular flow in the central macula. More lobular and less dense structures can be observed toward the periphery. The image quality of the choriocapillaris slab can be enhanced by multiple en-face OCTA averaging.

- **Choroid:** The visualization of the choroidal vessels is challenging because the light is scattered or attenuated by the pigmented RPE and choriocapillaris with dense vascular structure. In healthy subjects without high myopia, even using swept-source OCT, vascular flow in the larger vessels cannot be visualized due to signal loss with depth, projection artifact from overlying retinal vessels and choriocapillaris.

Reference

1. Campbell JP, Zhang M, Hwang TS, et al. Detailed vascular anatomy of the human retina by projection-resolved optical coherence tomography angiography. *Sci Rep.* 2017;7:42201.

Part 2
Retinal Vascular Disease

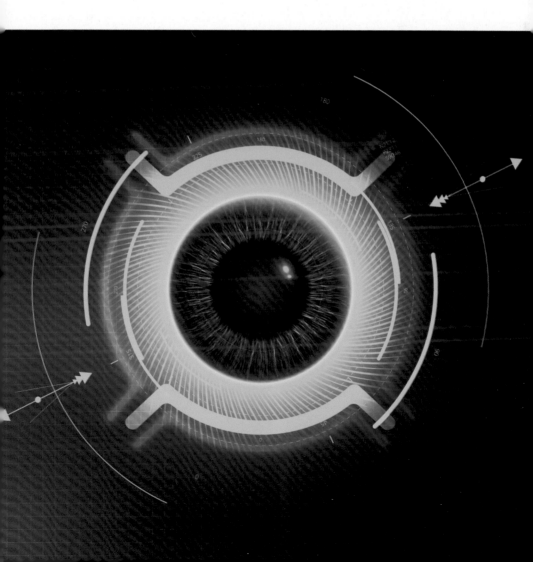

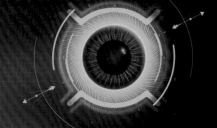

CHAPTER 5

Nonproliferative Diabetic Retinopathy

SALIENT FEATURES

- Nonproliferative diabetic retinopathy (NPDR) is a constellation of retinal changes due to a chronic hyperglycemia-induced microangiography that is staged as mild, moderate, or severe.
- Mild NPDR is defined as the presence of at least one microaneurysm.
- Eyes that have hard exudates, cotton wool spots, microaneurysms, and intraretinal hemorrhages, but that do not qualify for severe NDPR, are considered moderate NDPR.
- Severe NPDR is defined by the "4:2:1: rule," which is the presence of intraretinal hemorrhage in all four quadrants, venous beading in at least two quadrants, or intraretinal microvascular abnormality (IRMA) in at least one quadrant.
- Optical coherence tomography (OCT) and optical coherence tomography angiography (OCTA) are not required for the diagnosis of any stage of diabetic retinopathy (DR), but the above findings can be seen readily with OCT.

OCT IMAGING

- One key role for OCT is the identification of diabetic macular edema (DME). This may include intraretinal fluid and/or subretinal fluid. On OCT, intraretinal fluid consists of hyporeflective cystic spaces within the retina for intraretinal fluid (Figure 5.1, white asterisks). Subretinal fluid consists of hyporeflective fluid beneath the retina and above the retinal pigment epithelium (see Chapter 13).

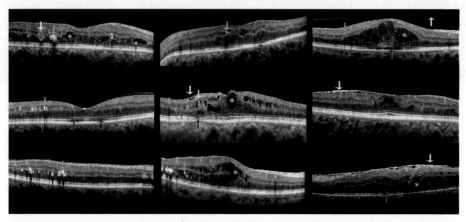

FIGURE 5.1 Foveal optical coherence tomography (OCT) images from several patients with nonproliferative diabetic retinopathy (NPDR) with and without diabetic macular edema (DME). Microaneuryms are highlighted with yellow arrows. Green arrows indicate hyperreflective dots. Ellipsoid disruption is commonly present and is highlighted by red arrows. White arrows are vitreoretinal abnormalities such as epiretinal membrane, vitreomacular traction/adhesion, and thickened posterior hyaloid. Cystoid macular edema when present is identified with a white asterisk, and focal retinal atrophy is shown in one image with a green asterisk.

- Microaneurysms on OCT may be seen as round hyperreflective structures with hyporeflective lumens (Figure 5.1, yellow arrows).
- Hard exudates are seen on OCT as small hyperreflective spots 20 to 40 µm in diameter often seen in clusters (Figure 5.1, green arrows). Smaller hyperreflective dots may indicate inflammatory aggregates.[1]
- Cotton wool spots and intraretinal hemorrhages manifest as patches of hyperreflectivity within the nerve fiber layer with posterior shadowing (Figure 5.1, red asterisk).
- Epiretinal membrane (ERM), vitreomacular traction (VMT), vitreomacular adhesion (VMA), and thickened, taut posterior hyaloid membranes on OCT may be comorbid in DR (Figure 5.1, white arrows).
- More subtle findings such as ellipsoid zone (EZ) loss (Figure 5.1, red arrows), focal retinal atrophy (Figure 5.1, green asterisk), disorganization of the retinal inner layers (DRILs), and generalized retinal atrophy may also be seen and often reflect greater severity of diabetic manifestations (eg, ischemia).
- Integrity of the outer retinal structural lines including the ellipsoid zone, interdigitation zone (IZ), and external limiting membrane (ELM) on OCT is associated with visual outcomes in patients with DR and DME (Figure 5.1).[2]

OCTA IMAGING

- Retinal vascular abnormalities in DR such as capillary dilation, clustering, tortuosity, microaneurysm formation, and nonperfusion can be seen with OCTA (Figure 5.2).
- OCTA can be used to help stage DR by distinguishing IRMAs from neovascularization (NV) which extends above the retinal surface (Figures 5.3 and 6.5).
- OCTA may also help to identify enlargement/irregularity to the foveal avascular zone which correlates with visual acuity and DR severity (Figure 5.2B and C).[3]

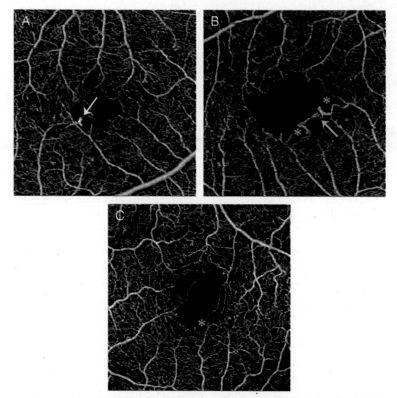

FIGURE 5.2 En-face superficial retina segmentation slabs from 3 × 3 spectral-domain en-face optical coherence tomography angiography (OCTA) imaging of patients of moderate to severe diabetic retinopathy severity. A microaneurysm is identified as a fusiform enlargement of a capillary in (A) (yellow arrow). A cluster of abnormally dilated and tortuous parafoveal capillaries (teal arrow) is present in (B). Enlargement and irregularity of the foveal avascular zone (green asterisks) are present in (B and C). A varying degree of capillary nonperfusion (red asterisks) is present in all images.

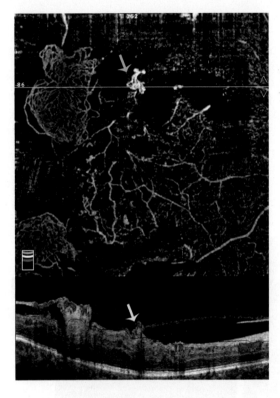

FIGURE 5.3 Optical coherence tomography angiography (OCTA) of a patient with proliferative diabetic retinopathy and advanced preretinal neovascularization (green arrow). Segmentation at the level of the vitreoretinal interface identifies tortuous preretinal vasculature. Confirmation of preretinal location is performed by identification of a positive flow signal within the preretinal hyperreflective membranes on the corresponding structural OCT (yellow arrow).

- OCTA-measured decreases in vascular density and branching morphology as well as increases in average vascular caliber have been associated with worse DR severity.[4]
- Significant disruption of tissue architecture, such as intraretinal fluid or vitreomacular traction, can make interpretation of the OCTA difficult.
- Widefield OCTA may provide critical information regarding the retinal periphery including identification of neovascularization and underlying ischemia.

References

1. Vujosevic S, Torresin T, Bini S, et al. Imaging retinal inflammatory biomarkers after intravitreal steroid and anti-VEGF treatment in diabetic macular oedema. *Acta Ophthalmol.* 2017;95:464-471.
2. Otani T, Yamaguchi Y, Kishi S. Correlation between visual acuity and foveal microstructural changes in diabetic macular edema. *Retina.* 2010;30:774-780.
3. Lee H, Lee M, Chung H, Kim HC. Quantification of retinal vessel tortuosity in diabetic retinopathy using optical coherence tomography angiography. *Retina.* 2018;38:976-985.
4. Kim AY, Chu Z, Shahidzadeh A, Wang RK, Puliafito CA, Kashani AH. Quantifying microvascular density and morphology in diabetic retinopathy using spectral-domain optical coherence tomography angiography. *Invest Ophthalmol Vis Sci.* 2016;57:OCT362-OCT370.

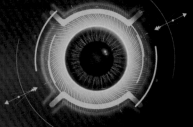

CHAPTER 6

Proliferative Diabetic Retinopathy

SALIENT FEATURES

- Any appearance of neovascularization (NV) in an eye with underlying diabetic retinopathy qualifies as proliferative diabetic retinopathy (PDR).
- Neovascularization can present as neovascularization of the disc (NVD), neovascularization of the iris (NVI), or neovascularization elsewhere (NVE).
- Fibrosis from the scaffold of neovascular vessels growing at the vitreoretinal interface can coalesce into tractional membranes with resultant tractional retinal detachment, combined rhegmatogenous/traction retinal detachment, vitreous hemorrhage, and potentially severe vision loss.
- Color and red-free fundus photography and red-free imaging can identify the irregular fine vascular networks extending from the optic disc or retina.
- Fluorescein angiography is a useful adjunct imaging modality that can readily identify NV as leakage from irregular vascular networks.
- Preretinal hemorrhages and/or vitreous hemorrhage can be seen on fundus photography and is considered a PDR equivalent.

OCT IMAGING

- The typical findings of microaneurysms, dot blot hemorrhages, exudates, and cotton wools spots that are seen in NDPR (see Chapter 5) are also seen in PDR. The differentiating feature is the presence of NVD, NVE, or NVI or hemorrhagic equivalent. This is often accompanied by more severe underlying ischemia.

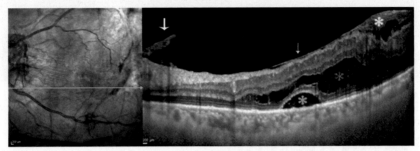

FIGURE 6.1 Optical coherence tomography (OCT) image of a patient with a proliferative diabetic retinopathy with neovascularization of the disc and preretinal tractional membranes. Neovascularization of the disc is evident as a hyperreflective loop extending from the optic disc into the vitreous cavity (white arrow). A broad neovascular tractional membrane is visible temporally as a preretinal hyperreflective sheet (yellow asterisk). Note the continuity of the temporal neovascular membrane with the central epiretinal membrane (yellow arrow). There is traction-induced subretinal (green asterisk) and intraretinal (pink asterisk) fluid present.

- Neovascular vessels are seen on optical coherence tomography (OCT) as hyperreflective loops extending from the optic disc or retinal surface that project into the vitreous space and may be adherent to the posterior hyaloid (Figures 6.1 and 6.4).
- These may be small foci of hyperreflective protrusions (Figure 6.4, yellow arrow) or larger hyperreflective sheets (Figure 6.1, yellow asterisk).

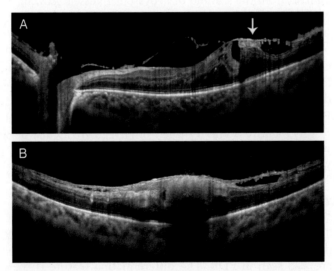

FIGURE 6.2 (A) Optical coherence tomographies (OCTs) from a patient with preretinal neovascular complexes with adhesion to the posterior hyaloid (yellow arrow). (B) Subhyaloid hemorrhage elsewhere is visible as a homogenous hyperreflective preretinal mass (red asterisk).

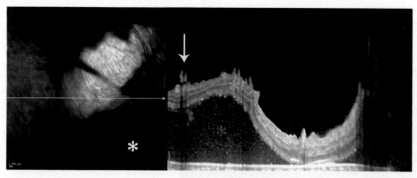

FIGURE 6.3 Optical coherence tomography (OCT) of a patient with proliferative diabetic retinopathy and a tractional retinal detachment. Complete neurosensory detachment is noted with overlying traction-inducing preretinal membranes (yellow arrow). There are intraretinal (green asterisk) and subretinal (red asterisk) hyperreflective dots consistent with hard exudates in the former and possible mild subretinal hemorrhage in the latter. There is media opacity from vitreous hemorrhage (white asterisk).

- A broad spectrum of vitreoretinal interface abnormalities from the epiretinal membrane to vitreomacular traction/adhesion is commonly present in patient with PDR (Figures 6.1 and 6.2).
- Tractionally detached retina is defined by the presence of subretinal fluid on OCT frequently due to overlying hyperreflective tractional bands. The retina itself is often thickened with cystoid degeneration (Figure 6.3).
- Disorganization of the retinal inner layers (DRILs) as seen by OCT is more commonly identified in patients with PDR (Figure 7.3).
- Regression of hyperreflective vascular loops on OCT may be seen after treatment of PDR with anti–vascular endothelial growth factor (VEGF) (fast regression) or panretinal photocoagulation (PRP) (slower regression) (Figure 6.4).

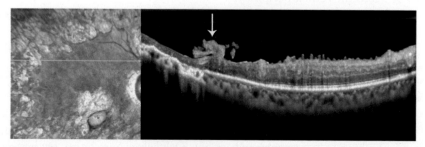

FIGURE 6.4 Optical coherence tomography (OCT) of a patient that received panretinal photocoagulation for proliferative diabetic retinopathy. Partially regressed preretinal neovascularization visualized as a collapsed hyperreflective loop temporally (yellow arrow).

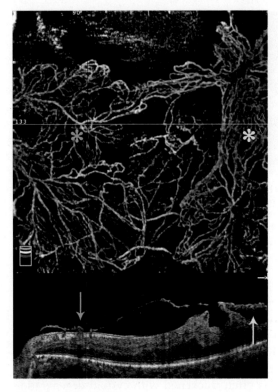

FIGURE 6.5 Optical coherence tomography angiography (OCTA) of a patient with proliferative diabetic retinopathy and advanced neovascularization of the disc (yellow asterisk) and temporal retina (green asterisk). Segmentation at the level of the vitreoretinal interface identifies tortuous preretinal vasculature. Confirmation of preretinal location is performed by identification of a positive flow signal within the preretinal hyperreflective membranes on the corresponding structural OCT (yellow and green arrows).

OCTA IMAGING

- Neovascularization is readily seen on optical coherence tomography angiography (OCTA) as irregular proliferation of small-caliber new vessels with saccular and dilated terminal loops and anastomotic connections of the outer borders. This is best seen by segmenting the OCTA image at the level of the vitreoretinal interface (Figure 6.5).[1]
- Extensive capillary nonperfusion is often present both in the macula and the retinal periphery.
- Widefield OCTA may provide visualization of the peripheral nonperfusion and NVE.
- Following anti-VEGF therapy and/or laser therapy, reduction in flow through neovascular loops may be visualized with OCTA.

Reference

1. de Carlo TE, Bonini Filho MA, Baumal CR, et al. Evaluation of preretinal neovascularization in proliferative diabetic retinopathy using optical coherence tomography angiography. *Ophthalmic Surg Lasers Imaging Retin.* 2016;47:115-119.

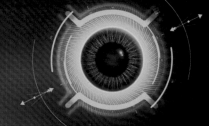

CHAPTER 7

Diabetic Macular Edema

SALIENT FEATURES

- Diabetic macular edema (DME), the most common cause of visual loss in patients with diabetic retinopathy (DR), is prevalent in 4.2% to 12.8% of patients with diabetes.[1]
- DME may appear in patients with nonproliferative diabetic retinopathy (NPDR) or proliferative diabetic retinopathy (PDR).
- The pathogenesis of DME is multifactorial and incompletely understood; however, both vascular permeability and inflammation have been implicated in its development.[2]

OCT IMAGING

- Optical coherence tomography (OCT) is considered the gold standard for the diagnosis and monitoring of DME.
- The basic morphologic features of DME include intraretinal fluid, which presents on OCT as focal hyporeflective circular structures within the retinal tissue, and subretinal fluid, which presents as a hyporeflective space between the retina the retinal pigment epithelium (RPE) (Figure 7.1).
- There are some data to suggest that patients that present with primarily subretinal fluid experience greater visual acuity gain after treatment than those with cystoid macular edema.[3]
- Central foveal thickness (CFT) and mean central subfield thickness (CST) are standardized OCT-derived measurements thickening that may help to identify abnormal thickening and can track changes over time (Figure 7.2C and D).

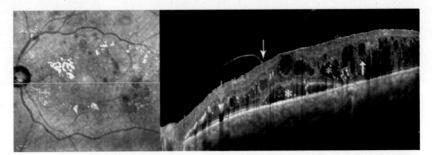

FIGURE 7.1 Optical coherence tomography (OCT) of a patient with diabetic macular edema highlighting many common features of diabetic retinopathy and diabetic macular edema including hyperreflective dots (green arrow), subretinal fluid (yellow asterisk), intraretinal fluid (green asterisk), vitreomacular adhesion (white arrow), epiretinal membrane (pink asterisk), and microaneurysm (yellow arrow).

- CFT and CST are not accurate predictors of visit to visit best corrected visual acuity (BCVA).[4]
- A visually prognostic spectral-domain OCT (SD-OCT) imaging biomarker is disorganization of retinal inner layers (DRILs), defined as the inability to identify boundaries between the ganglion cell/inner plexiform layer complex, inner nuclear layer, and outer plexiform layer (Figure 7.3). Patients with DRIL have worse VA at baseline and poorer responses to treatment.[5]
- DRIL, however, is difficult to quantitate with high interobserver variability.

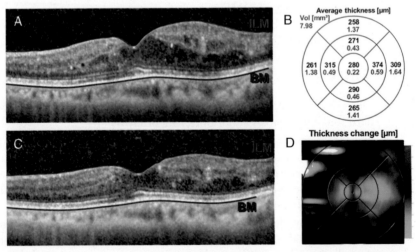

FIGURE 7.2 Optical coherence tomography (OCT) derived central retinal thickness (CRT) as a clinical marker in the treatment of diabetic macular edema (DME). A, Foveal OCT of a patient with DME demonstrates cystoid macular edema, hyperreflective dots (HRDs), and mild attenuation of the ellipsoid zone. B, Automatic measurements show moderate thickening. C, After antivascular endothelial growth factor therapy, OCT demonstrates reduction of cystoid spaces and improved integrity of the ellipsoid zone. There was an accompanying one-line improvement in visual acuity. D, Automatic thickness change maps provide a rapid assessment of macular thickness change.

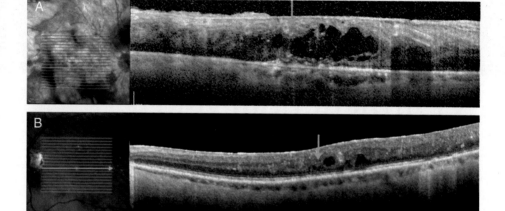

FIGURE 7.3 Foveal optical coherence tomography (OCT) images from patients with chronic diabetic macular edema significant for loss of inner retinal layer laminations characteristic of disorganization of retinal inner layers (DRILs) (green arrows) more prominent in (A) than (B).

OCTA IMAGING

- Optical coherence tomography angiography (OCTA) in the setting of macular edema can be difficult to interpret due to the retinal architectural disruptions of the cystic changes. In addition, the areas of fluid have no vascular flow and may masquerade as more severe retinal ischemia than is actually present.

References

1. Lee R, Wong TY, Sabanayagam C. Epidemiology of diabetic retinopathy, diabetic macular edema and related vision loss. *Eye Vis (Lond)*. 2015;2:17.
2. Antcliff RJ, Marshall J. The pathogenesis of edema in diabetic maculopathy. *Semin Ophthalmol*. 1999;14:223-232.
3. Sophie R, Lu N, Campochiaro PA. Predictors of functional and anatomic outcomes in patients with diabetic macular edema treated with ranibizumab. *Ophthalmology*. 2015;122:1395-1401.
4. Browning DJ, Glassman AR, Aiello LP, et al; Diabetic Retinopathy Clinical Research Network. Relationship between optical coherence tomography-measured central retinal thickness and visual acuity in diabetic macular edema. *Ophthalmology*. 2007;114:525-536.
5. Fickweiler W, Schauwvlieghe ASME, Schlingemann RO, et al. Predictive value of optical coherence tomographic features in the bevacizumab and ranibizumab in patients with diabetic macular edema (BRDME) study. *Retina*. 2018;38:812-819.

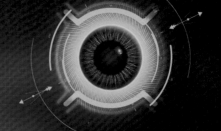

CHAPTER 8

Central Retinal Vein Occlusion

SALIENT FEATURES

- Retinal vein occlusion is the second most common retinal vascular disease after diabetic retinopathy.[1]
- In central retinal vein occlusion (CRVO), the occlusion is at or proximal to the lamina cribosa of the optic nerve. CRVO is divided into two categories which affect treatment and prognosis: nonischemic and ischemic.[2]
- CRVOs are most commonly associated with advanced age and hypertension, but other risk factors include glaucoma, diabetes, hyperlipidemia, and various hypercoagulable conditions.[2]
- Acute CRVO is a clinical diagnosis manifesting intraretinal hemorrhages in all quadrants, dilated tortuous retinal vasculature, cotton wool spots, optic disc edema, and macular edema.[2]
- In nonischemic CRVOs, visual acuity (VA) is typically better than 20/200 with no relative afferent pupillary defect (RAPD) and an overall good prognosis for visual recovery. In ischemic CRVOs, VA is typically worse than 20/200 with an RAPD, a high chance of anterior segment neovascularization, and an overall poor prognosis for visual recovery.[3]
- In chronic CRVO, small vessels that normally connect the retinal and choroidal circulation near the optic nerve head expand and develop into optociliary shunt vessels which redirect venous drainage from the occluded central retinal vein to the choroid, vortex veins, and ophthalmic veins.[3]

OCT IMAGING

- One key role for optical coherence tomography (OCT) in this diagnosis is identification of macular edema. This may include intraretinal and/or subretinal edema, characterized on OCT as hyporeflective cystoid spaces within the retina (Figure 8.1, white asterisks) or subretinal (Figure 8.1, yellow asterisks), respectively.[4]
- There may be hyperreflective foci (HF; Figure 8.1, green arrows) in any layer of the retina and even within the vitreous. HF are thought to be extravasated lipoproteins, and they may serve as a negative prognostic biomarker for final visual acuity.[5]
- In acute disease, there may be inner retinal hyperreflectivity, which may represent ischemic damage or retinal disruption.[6]
- There may be microaneurysms, hard exudates, cotton wool spots, or neovascularization.
- There may be disorganization of the retinal inner layers (DRILs), ellipsoid zone (EZ) and external limiting membrane (ELM) disruption, reduced cone outer segment tip (COST) visibility, and epiretinal membrane.[4]
- En-face structural OCT may reveal cystoid spaces, characterized by dark spaces without vessel signal (Figure 8.2).
- Treatment with intravitreal anti–vascular endothelial growth factor (VEGF) therapy and/or intravitreal corticosteroids may improve macular edema. This can be serially followed via change analysis software (Figure 8.3) which may guide retreatment decisions.

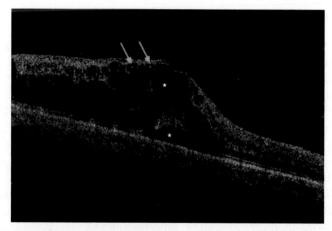

FIGURE 8.1 Foveal optical coherence tomography (OCT) images from a patient with central retinal vein occlusion (CRVO)–related macular edema. Green arrows indicate hyperreflective foci (HF). There is both intraretinal and subretinal edema, characterized on OCT as hyporeflective cystoid spaces within the retina (white asterisks) and beneath the retina and above the retinal pigment epithelium (yellow asterisks).

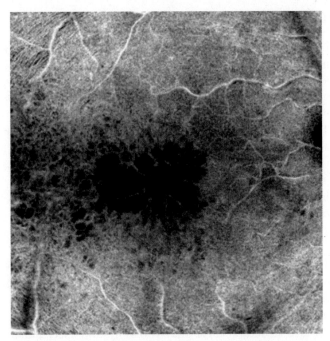

FIGURE 8.2 En-face optical coherence tomography (OCT) at the level of the superficial capillary plexus showing the presence of cystoid edema, which corresponds to dark hyporeflective areas.

OCTA IMAGING

- While ultra-widefield fluorescein angiography may be used to evaluate for peripheral retinal ischemia and neovascularization, optical coherence tomography angiography (OCTA) can provide useful information about macular nonperfusion and/or neovascularization. Additionally, OCTA allows for better visualization through intraretinal hemorrhage due to a longer wavelength light.[1,7]
- OCTA clearly delineates areas of nonperfusion (Figure 8.4). This is typically more extensive in the deep capillary plexus than in the superficial capillary plexus.[1,7]
- There may be vascular tortuosity or fusiform dilation of vessels (Figure 8.5), collateral vessel formation (Figure 8.6), microaneurysms, intraretinal hemorrhages, and nonperfused ghost vessels.[1,7]
- OCTA may reveal optic disc collaterals at the level of the superficial peripapillary plexus, neovascularization of the disc (NVD) above the retina at the level of the vitreous, or neovascularization elsewhere.[1]

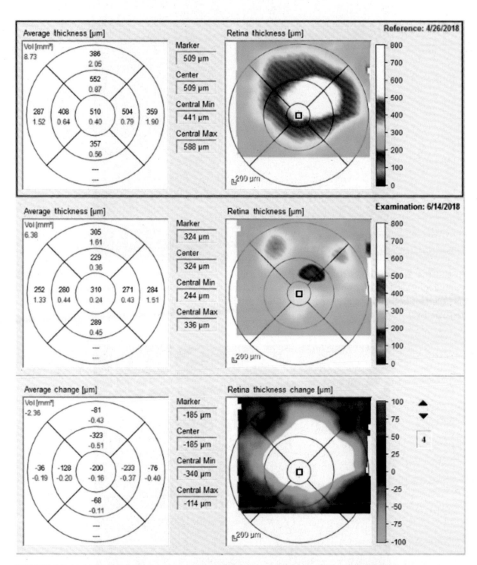

FIGURE 8.3 Heidelberg optical coherence tomography (OCT) Spectralis change analysis image demonstrating improved macular edema after administration of an anti–vascular endothelial growth factor (anti-VEGF) agent in a patient with central retinal vein occlusion (CRVO)-related macular edema.

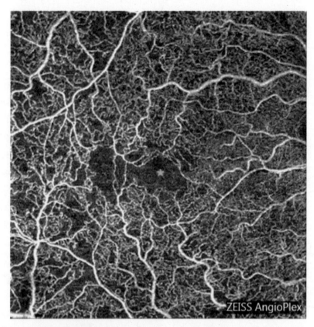

FIGURE 8.4 En-face superficial segmentation of a 6 × 6 spectral-domain optical coherence tomography angiography (OCTA) slab from a patient with central retinal vein occlusion (CRVO) reveals irregularity and enlargement of the foveal avascular zone (green asterisk) and multifocal areas of capillary nonperfusion (red asterisks).

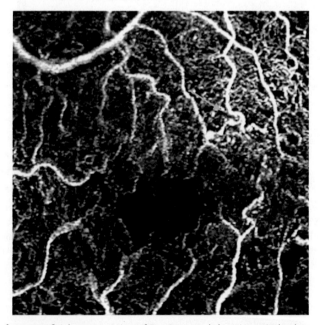

FIGURE 8.5 En-face superficial segmentation of 3 × 3 spectral-domain optical coherence tomography angiography (OCTA) showing fusiform dilation and tortuosity of vessels (green arrow).

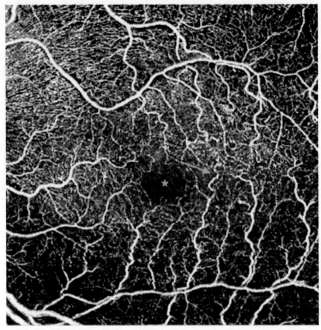

FIGURE 8.6 En-face superficial retina segmentation of 6 × 6 spectral-domain optical coherence tomography angiography (OCTA) showing collateral vessel formation (green arrow) and irregularity of the foveal avascular zone (green asterisk).

References

1. Mastropasqua R, Toto L, Di Antonio L, et al. Optical coherence tomography angiography microvascular findings in macular edema due to central and branch retinal vein occlusions. *Sci Rep.* 2017;7(1):40763. doi:10.1038/srep40763.

2. Chatziralli I, Theodossiadis G, Chatzirallis A, Parikakis E, Mitropoulos P, Theodossiadis P. Ranibizumab for retinal vein occlusion: predictive factors and long-term outcomes in real-life data. *Retina.* 2018;38(3):559-568. doi:10.1097/IAE.0000000000001579.

3. Blair K, Czyz C. In: *Central Retinal Vein Occlusion.* Treasure Island, FL: Ohio University, StatPearls [Internet]; 2019.

4. Chan EW, Eldeeb M, Sun V, et al. Disorganization of retinal inner layers and ellipsoid zone disruption predict visual outcomes in central retinal vein occlusion. *Ophthalmol Retina.* 2019;3(1):83-92. doi:10.1016/j.oret.2018.07.008.

5. Bo B, Zhao H-Y, Jiao X, Zhang F. Evaluation of hyperreflective foci as a prognostic factor of visual outcome in retinal vein occlusion. *Int J Ophthalmol.* 2017;10(4). doi:10.18240/ijo.2017.04.17.

6. Mehta N, Lavinsky F, Gattoussi S, et al. Increased inner retinal layer reflectivity in eyes with acute CRVO correlates with worse visual outcomes at 12 months. *Invest Ophthalmol Vis Sci.* 2018;59(8):3503. doi:10.1167/iovs.18-24153.

7. Tsai G, Banaee T, Conti F, Singh R. Optical coherence tomography angiography in eyes with retinal vein occlusion. *J Ophthalmic Vis Res.* 2018;13(3):315. doi:10.4103/jovr.jovr_264_17.

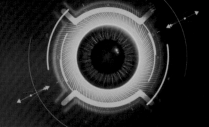

CHAPTER 9

Branch Retinal Vein Occlusion

SALIENT FEATURES

- Branch retinal vein occlusion (BRVO) is a venous occlusion at any branch of the central retinal vein. It is thought to be secondary to venous compression or narrowing.
- Other possible causes include vascular degenerative changes and hypercoagulable states. Risk factors include hypertension and hyperlipidemia.[2]
- Occurring more commonly than central retinal vein occlusion (CRVO), the prevalence of BRVO is 4.42 per 1000 people, with an estimated 13.9 million persons affected worldwide.[1]
- The diagnosis of BRVO is clinical, relying on fundoscopic evaluation for hemorrhages, cotton wool spots, exudates, edema, and tortuous veins along the distribution of the occluded vein.[3] Chronic changes include vessel sclerosis and collateral formation.
- Complications include macular edema, ischemic maculopathy, retinal neovascularization, and vitreous hemorrhage. Macular edema is the most common of these complications leading to reduced visual acuity.[2]

OCT IMAGING

- OCT is helpful in diagnosis and monitoring therapeutic responses of macular-involving BRVO-associated edema. The classic morphologic features of edema include intraretinal fluid which appears as hyporeflective cystic spaces within the retina (Figure 9.1). Subretinal fluid

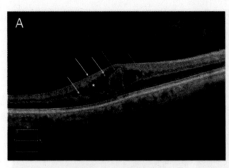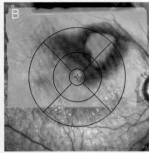

FIGURE 9.1 A, Optical coherence tomography (OCT) of a patient with branch retinal vein occlusion (BRVO)–associated macular edema highlighting hyporeflective cystoid spaces (white asterisk), hyperreflective foci (green arrows) within the retina, as well as hyperreflective material within the cystic spaces (red arrows). Close examination demonstrates disorganization of the retinal inner layer (DRIL) (yellow arrow). B, OCT volumetric data displayed on a near-infrared imaging of the macula in a patient with superior BRVO demonstrate superonasal retinal thickening respecting the median raphe.

may also be present as a hyporeflective space between the retina and RPE. Volumetric analysis demonstrates edema respecting the horizontal raphe.

- Intraretinal hemorrhages and cotton wool spots appear as areas of hyperreflectivity within the nerve fiber layer with associated posterior shadowing.
- Disruption of the ellipsoid zone (EZ) and disorganization of the retinal inner layers (DRILs) is believed to be associated with ischemia and corresponds to poorer visual outcomes (Figure 9.1).[4]
- Hyperreflective foci may also be present in all retinal layers (Figure 9.1) and are associated with worse visual prognosis.[5] They are thought to represent extravasated lipids and proteins.[6]

OCTA FINDINGS

- Vascular abnormalities such as decreased capillary density, capillary nonperfusion, enlargement of the foveal avascular zone (FAZ), and venous dilation can be seen in both superficial and deep vascular plexuses on optical coherence tomography angiography (OCTA) (Figure 9.2A and B).[7-9]
- Decreased vascular density and enlargement of the FAZ on OCTA have been shown to correlate with visual acuity (Figure 9.2A).
- Collateral formation around the parafovea and crossing the raphe can be visualized on OCTA in cases of chronic BRVO (Figure 9.2A).

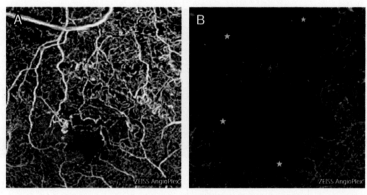

FIGURE 9.2 A, En-face superficial retina segmentation slab from 3 × 3mm spectral-domain optical coherence tomography angiography (OCTA) image from a patient with a superior branch retinal vein occlusion shows a large fusiform dilated capillary (yellow arrow). There is also a cluster of abnormally dilated and tortuous parafoveal collateral vessels (teal arrow). The foveal avascular zone is irregular in shape (green asterisk), and there are areas of nonperfusion and decreased vascular density (red asterisks). B, An en-face deep retina segmentation slab OCTA images shows extensive vascular drop out in the deep capillary plexus (green asterisks).

References

1. Rogers S, McIntosh RL, Cheung N, et al. The prevalence of retinal vein occlusion: pooled data from population studies from the United States, Europe, Asia, and Australia. *Ophthalmology.* 2010;117(2):313-319.e1. doi:10.1016/j.ophtha.2009.07.017.

2. Jaulim A, Ahmed B, Khanam T, Chatziralli IP. Branch retinal vein occlusion: epidemiology, pathogenesis, risk factors, clinical features, diagnosis, and complications. An update of the literature. *Retina.* 2013;33(5):901-910. doi:10.1097/IAE.0b013e3182870c15.

3. Spaide RF, Fujimoto JG, Waheed NK, Sadda SR, Staurenghi G. Optical coherence tomography angiography. *Prog Retin Eye Res.* 2018;64:1-55. doi:10.1016/j.preteyeres.2017.11.003.

4. Babiuch AS, Han M, Conti FF, Wai K, Silva FQ, Singh RP. Association of disorganization of retinal inner layers with visual acuity response to anti–vascular endothelial growth factor therapy for macular edema secondary to retinal vein occlusion. *JAMA Ophthalmol.* 2019;137(1):38-46. doi:10.1001/jamaophthalmol.2018.4484.

5. Mo B, Zhou H-Y, Jiao X, Zhang F. Evaluation of hyperreflective foci as a prognostic factor of visual outcome in retinal vein occlusion. *Int J Ophthalmol.* 2017;10(4):605-612. doi:10.18240/ijo.2017.04.17.

6. Ogino K, Murakami T, Tsujikawa A, et al. Characteristics of optical coherence tomographic hyperreflective foci in retinal vein occlusion. *Retina.* 2012;32(1):77-85. doi:10.1097/IAE.0b013e318217ffc7.

7. Rispoli M, Savastano MC, Lumbroso B. Capillary network anomalies IN branch retinal vein occlusion ON optical coherence tomography angiography. *Retina.* 2015;35(11):2332-2338. doi:10.1097/IAE.0000000000000845.

8. Samara WA, Shahlaee A, Sridhar J, Khan MA, Ho AC, Hsu J. Quantitative optical coherence tomography angiography features and visual function in eyes with branch retinal vein occlusion. *Am J Ophthalmol.* 2016;166:76-83. doi:10.1016/j.ajo.2016.03.033.

9. Mastropasqua R, Toto L, Di Antonio L, et al. Optical coherence tomography angiography microvascular findings in macular edema due to central and branch retinal vein occlusions. *Sci Rep.* 2017;7(1):40763. doi:10.1038/srep40763.

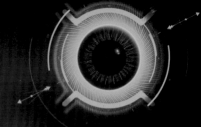

CHAPTER 10

Central Retinal Artery Occlusion

SALIENT FEATURES

- Central retinal artery occlusion (CRAO) results most commonly due to embolism or intravascular thrombosis causing sudden, painless, monocular visual loss as a result of loss of blood supply to the inner retinal layers.
- Acute CRAO is one of the major causes of acute visual loss with incidence estimated to be 1 to 10 in 100,000.[1]
- About 15% to 30% of the population have a cilioretinal artery that may provide additional blood supply to the fovea which may preserve central vision.[2]
- Classic ischemic fundus findings include cotton wool spots (CWSs), retinal whitening, "cherry-red spot," foveola, and "box-carring" appearance (ie, segmentation of blood in retinal vessels).
- Fluorescein angiography (FA) shows clear retinal vascular delay and capillary nonperfusion.
- Optical coherence tomography (OCT) and optical coherence tomography angiography (OCTA) are useful to evaluate the presence and extent of retinal nonperfusion, increased inner retinal reflectivity, and areas of atrophy and to visualize changes in the capillary network.
- Reperfused CRAO may occur with transient symptoms and minimal signs on examination. Residual findings may be noted on OCT and/or OCTA during both the acute and chronic phase.

OCT IMAGING

- Acute CRAO is characterized on OCT by increased reflectivity and thickness of the inner retina due to ischemia, corresponding with retinal whitening and cotton wool spots on biomicroscopy. Increased reflectivity results in shadowing for outer structures. This hyperreflectivity crosses retinal layers often resulting in loss of the retinal laminar appearance (Figure 10.1).[3]
- A hyperreflective band at the level of the inner nuclear layer (INL) may be present, also termed paracentral acute middle maculopathy (PAMM), which represents ischemia of the intermediate and deep retinal capillary plexuses. This may also be present in eyes with reperfused CRAO (Figure 10.2).[4]
- Thickness of the inner retina layer decreases in the middle period of the retinal artery occlusion, but the hyperreflective band remains and helps for the diagnosis.

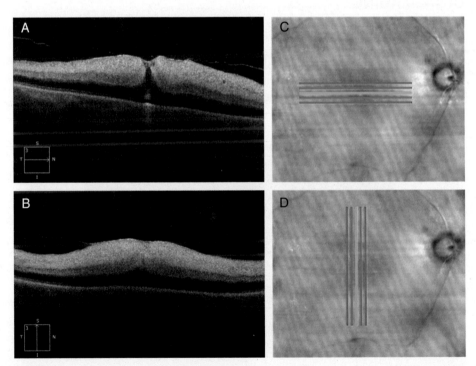

FIGURE 10.1 Horizontal (A) and vertical (B) B-scans of spectral domain optical coherence tomography (SD OCT) in the acute phase of central retinal artery occlusion (CRAO) showing thickening and hyperreflectivity of the inner and middle retinal layers owing to the presence of significant retinal ischemia. C and D, *En-face* images showing the direction of the OCT B-scans.

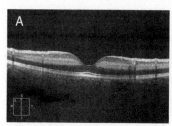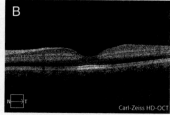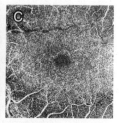

FIGURE 10.2 Foveal optical coherence tomography (OCT) of the eye from a patient with paracentral acute middle maculopathy (PAMM)–like findings secondary to reperfused central retinal artery occlusion (CRAO) shows a hyperreflective band in the inner nuclear layer (A) with OCTA of the deep plexus (B) showing decreased perfusion (C). OCTA, optical coherence tomography angiography.

- In the chronic stage, OCT reveals moderate-severe inner retinal atrophy (thinning) with often relative preservation of outer retinal lines including outer nuclear layer and ellipsoid zone (EZ) (Figure 10.3).[5]
- OCT imaging can be utilized to determine the severity of retinal atrophy during the chronic phase.

OCTA IMAGING

- OCTA *en-face* images are useful to evaluate nonperfusion at different levels including the superficial capillary plexus (SCP), the radial peripapillary capillary plexus (RPCP), and the deep capillary plexus (DCP), revealing varying degrees of vascular nonperfusion in the superficial versus the deep capillary network in CRAO eyes, and these areas do not necessarily overlap (Figure 10.4).[3,6]

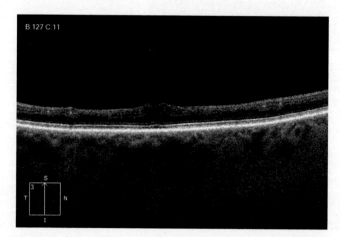

FIGURE 10.3 Foveal OCT of the right eye from a patient with chronic CRAO. Note the severe retinal atrophy and absence of foveal depression and stratification of inner retinal layers. The inner retina is reduced into a single thick hyperreflective band with marked EZ and RPE lines. CRAO, central retinal artery occlusion; EZ, ellipsoid zone; OCT, optical coherence tomography; RPE, retinal pigment epithelium.

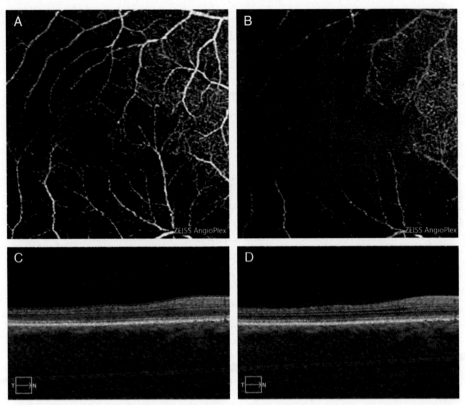

FIGURE 10.4 OCTA of chronic CRAO shows decreased capillary perfusion in both superficial and deep capillary network slabs. The deep capillary plexus reveals more areas of nonperfusion compared to the superficial. Nevertheless, larger vessels remained perfused as well as capillaries in the nasal part of the macula. Color-coded perfusion maps show the extent of nonperfusion observed most significantly temporal to the fovea (C and D). CRAO, central retinal artery occlusion; OCTA, optical coherence tomography angiography.

- Decorrelation overlays typically demonstrate absence of flow signal corresponding to areas of hyperreflectivity.
- OCTA may show partial reperfusion of DCP in areas where SCP is still abnormal after reorganization of vascular interconnections. However, caution should be taken when interpreting abnormal deep plexus perfusion because there might be signal attenuation artifact from inner retinal layer reflectivity masking as hypoperfusion.[6]
- In eyes with PAMM associated with CRAO, the DCP may demonstrate reduction in perfusion. Hyperreflective bandlike lesions of INL are typically seeing in the acute phase on B-scan images followed by corresponding thinning of INL over weeks (Figure 10.4).[4,7]
- Preservation or diffuse attenuation of the RPCP system has been observed on OCTA imaging in CRAO.[6] In chronic stages, RPCP attenuation may be correlated with a decrease in nerve fiber layer (NFL) thickness.[6]

References

1. Leavitt JA, Larson TA, Hodge DO, Gullerud RE. The incidence of central retinal artery occlusion in Olmsted County, Minnesota. *Am J Ophthalmol.* 2011;152(5):820-823.e2. doi:10.1016/j.ajo.2011.05.005.

2. Lorentzen SE. Incidence of cilioretinal arteries. *Acta Ophthalmol.* 1970;48(3):518-524. doi:10.1111/j.1755-3768.1970.tb03753.x.

3. Spaide RF, Klancnik JM, Cooney MJ. Retinal vascular layers imaged by fluorescein angiography and optical coherence tomography angiography. *JAMA Ophthalmol.* 2015;133(1):45-50. doi:10.1001/jamaophthalmol.2014.3616.

4. Chen X, Rahimy E, Sergott RC, et al. Spectrum of retinal vascular diseases associated with paracentral acute middle maculopathy. *Am J Ophthalmol.* 2015;160(1):26-34.e1. doi:10.1016/j.ajo.2015.04.004.

5. Falkenberry SM, Ip MS, Blodi BA, Gunther JB. Optical coherence tomography findings in central retinal artery occlusion. *Ophthalmic Surg Lasers Imaging.* 2006;37(6):502-505. doi:10.3928/15428877-20061101-12.

6. Bonini Filho MA, Adhi M, de Carlo TE, et al. Optical coherence tomography angiography in retinal artery occlusion. *Retina.* 2015;35(11):2339-2346. doi:10.1097/IAE.0000000000000850.

7. Nemiroff J, Kuehlewein L, Rahimy E, et al. Assessing deep retinal capillary ischemia in paracentral acute middle maculopathy by optical coherence tomography angiography. *Am J Ophthalmol.* 2016;162:121-132.e1. doi:10.1016/j.ajo.2015.10.026.

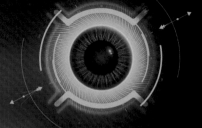

CHAPTER 11

Branch Retinal Artery Occlusion

SALIENT FEATURES

- Branch retinal artery occlusion (BRAO) usually results from occlusion of a division of the retinal artery due to embolism leading to sudden segmental visual loss.
- Retinal opacification in the distribution of the affected vessel caused by infarction of the inner retina along with retinal whitening cotton wool spots (CWSs) can be seen on fundus examination in the acute phase. A Hollenhurst plaque may be visualized at the site of occlusion.
- Fluorescein angiography (FA) usually demonstrates a capillary non-perfusion in the distribution of the occluded artery.

OCT IMAGING

- Acute BRAO is characterized by significant increased hyperreflectivity inner retina including inner nuclear, inner plexiform, and ganglion cell layers, as a hyperreflective band with possible mild increased thickness, which is contrasted by the normal corresponding layers of the unaffected macula[1] (Figure 11.1).
- Paracentral acute middle maculopathy (PAMM) that is seen in central retinal artery occlusion (CRAO) may also be seen in BRAO indicating deep capillary ischemia[2] (Figure 11.2).
- In chronic BRAO, optical coherence tomography (OCT) can be a great toll in diagnosing inner retinal atrophy corresponding to thinning and loss of the inner retinal layer architecture (Figures 11.3 and 11.4).

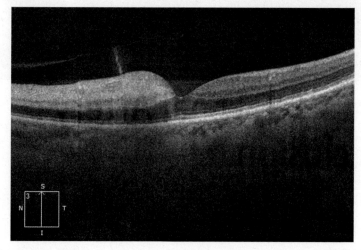

FIGURE 11.1 Optical coherence tomography (OCT) image of the left eye with hyperreflective inner retinal layers and increased thickness consistent with an acute branch retinal artery occlusion (BRAO).

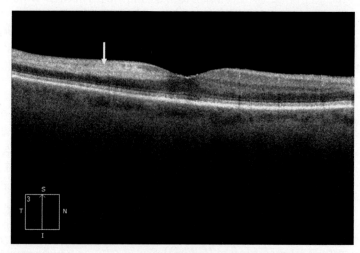

FIGURE 11.2 Optical coherence tomography (OCT) image of the right eye with inner retinal hyperreflectivity and paracentral acute middle maculopathy (PAMM)–like (white arrow) lesions suggestive of deep capillary ischemia and branch retinal artery occlusion (BRAO).

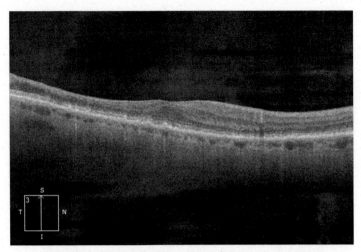

FIGURE 11.3 Optical coherence tomography (OCT) image of the right eye with chronic branch retinal artery occlusion (BRAO) and inner retinal atrophy.

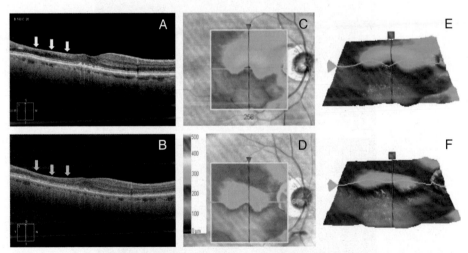

FIGURE 11.4 Optical coherence tomography (OCT) images of the right eye with sequelae of inferior branch retinal artery occlusion (BRAO) demonstrating transition from subacute to chronic stage (A and B). A, Subacute BRAO: Inner retina shows resolving hyperreflective band and retinal atrophy on B-scan inferiorly (white arrows) which is contrasted by the superior unaffected region. B, Progression to chronic BRAO: profound inner retina atrophy and loss of retinal layer architecture inferiorly to the fovea (gray arrows). C and F, En-face mapping of macular thickness (C) and three-dimensional (3D) thickness map (E) depict area of retinal thinning inferiorly which is more prominent in the chronic phase (D and F).

OCTA IMAGING

- Retinal nonperfusion areas and localization of the foci of retinal ischemia can be seen with optical coherence tomography angiography (OCTA).[3]
- OCTA may enable quantification of alterations in vascular density in the superficial capillary plexus (SCP) and deep capillary plexus (DCP), which correlates with the area of hypofluorescence in FA.[4]

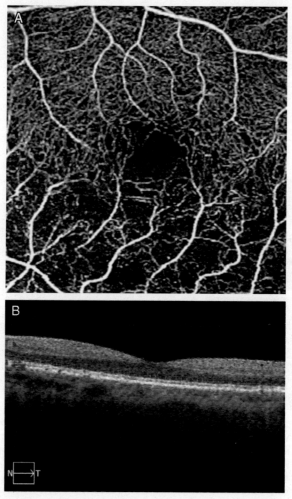

FIGURE 11.5 A, A 3 × 3 mm macular cube optical coherence tomography angiography (OCTA) with *enface* projection capturing the retinal layer of the left eye from a patient with acute branch retinal artery occlusion (BRAO). Slab shows perfusion superior to the fovea while prominent decreased capillary perfusion inferiorly. B, B-scan centered on the fovea shows the segmentation of the retinal layers.

- Areas of PAMM lesions associated with BRAO demonstrate variable defects of the DCP.[6]
- Radial peripapillary capillary (RPC) may be focally attenuated in the arterial occlusion quadrant accompanied by retinal nerve fiber layer thinning.[3]
- *En-face* image can demonstrate the presence of ischemia-induced area of flow voids (Figures 11.5-11.7).

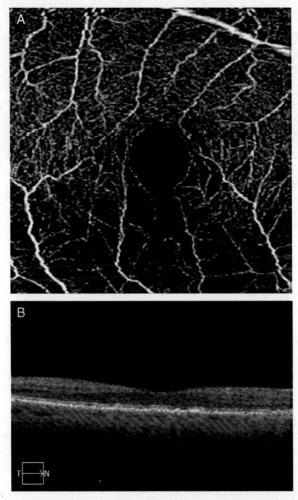

FIGURE 11.6 A, A 3 × 3 mm macular cube optical coherence tomography angiography (OCTA) with *en-face* projection capturing the retinal layer of the right eye from a patient with chronic branch retinal artery occlusion (BRAO) and atrophy. Slab shows perfusion superior to the fovea while prominent decreased capillary perfusion inferiorly. B, B-scan centered on the fovea shows the segmentation of the retinal layers.

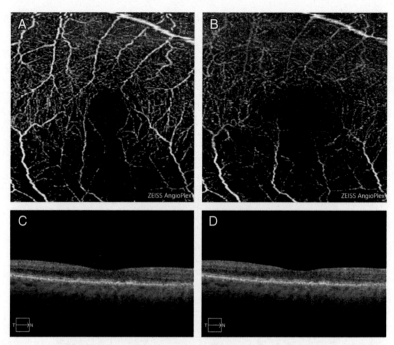

FIGURE 11.7 A and B, A 3 × 3 mm macular cube optical coherence tomography angiography (OCTA) with *en-face* projection capturing the superficial and deep capillary plexuses of the right from a patient with chronic branch retinal artery occlusion (BRAO). Both segmentation slabs show patent perfusion superior to the fovea while prominent decreased capillary perfusion inferiorly. C and D, B-scans centered on the fovea show the segmentation of the superficial and deep capillary layers. Projection artifact is demonstrated in the figure.

References

1. Chen X, Rahimy E, Sergott RC, et al. Spectrum of retinal vascular diseases associated with paracentral acute middle maculopathy. *Am J Ophthalmol.* 2015;160(1):26-34.e1. doi:10.1016/j.ajo.2015.04.004.

2. Yu S, Pang CE, Gong Y, et al. The spectrum of superficial and deep capillary ischemia in retinal artery occlusion. *Am J Ophthalmol.* 2015;159(1):53-63.e2. doi:10.1016/j.ajo.2014.09.027.

3. Çelik T, Bilen F, Yalçındağ FN, Atilla H. Optical coherence tomography angiography in branch retinal artery occlusion. *Turkish J Ophthalmol.* 2018;48(3):150-154. doi:10.4274/tjo.34270.

4. Yang S, Liu X, Li H, Xu J, Wang F. Optical coherence tomography angiography characteristics of acute retinal arterial occlusion. *BMC Ophthalmol.* 2019;19(1):1-9. doi:10.1186/s12886-019-1152-8.

5. Bonini Filho MA, Adhi M, de Carlo TE, et al. Optical coherence tomography angiography in retinal artery occlusion. *Retina.* 2015;35(11):2339-2346. doi:10.1097/IAE.0000000000000850.

6. Nemiroff J, Kuehlewein L, Rahimy E, et al. Assessing deep retinal capillary ischemia in paracentral acute middle maculopathy by optical coherence tomography angiography. *Am J Ophthalmol.* 2016;162:121-132.e1. doi:10.1016/j.ajo.2015.10.026.

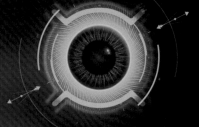
Paracentral Acute Middle Maculopathy

SALIENT FEATURES

- Paracentral acute middle maculopathy (PAMM) is an optical coherence tomography (OCT) finding defined by the presence of a hyperreflective band at the level of the inner nuclear layer (INL) that indicates INL infarction caused by impaired perfusion of the deep vascular complex (ie, intermediate and deep retinal capillary plexus or ICP and DCP) (Figure 12.1).
- Patients present with an acute-onset paracentral negative scotoma and typically experience a permanent visual defect.
- PAMM can complicate a large number of retinal disorders. It is most often secondary to local retinal vascular disease and/or systemic disorders but can be idiopathic.
- Local retinal vascular diseases that can cause PAMM include central retinal vein occlusion, central or branch retinal artery occlusion, diabetic retinopathy, hypertensive retinopathy, sickle cell retinopathy, Purtscher retinopathy, and retinal vasculitis.
- Systemic disorders include migraines, medications (amphetamines, caffeine, vasopressors oral contraceptives), hypovolemia, orbital compression injury, and viral prodromes.
- As such, detection of PAMM should prompt a search for local vascular or systemic risk factors.
- On fundoscopy, PAMM lesions appear gray, smooth in consistency, and deeper within the retina compared to cotton wool spots (Figure 12.1).

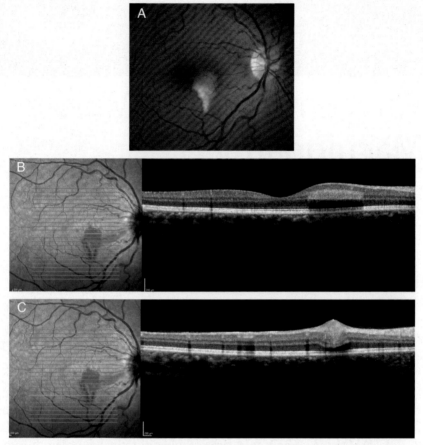

FIGURE 12.1 **Color fundus photography and** spectral-domain optical coherence tomography (OCT) (SD-OCT) of a patient with combined cotton wool spot and paracentral acute middle maculopathy (PAMM) secondary to a branch retinal artery occlusion. A, Color fundus photograph shows a white ischemic lesion with evidence of inner and middle retinal infarction. The latter appears deeper, greyer, and smoother in consistency. B, OCT through the superior region of the lesion shows bandlike inner nuclear layer (INL) hyperreflectivity consistent with a middle retinal infarct or PAMM. C, OCT through the inferior region of the lesion shows evidence of inner retinal infarction. (Courtesy K. Bailey Freund MD).

- As lesions are secondary to an ischemic insult, they are often unilateral but may be bilateral.
- Management is targeted toward the identification and treatment of related vasculopathic and systemic risk factors.

OCT IMAGING

- OCT serves as the mainstay of diagnosis.
- Acute PAMM lesions appear as bandlike, hyperreflective lesions at the level of the INL in the parafovea. The acute lesions leave a legacy of

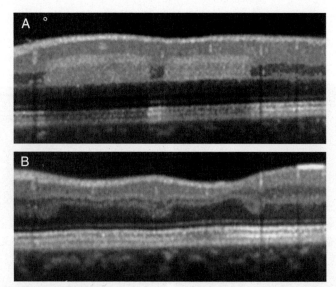

FIGURE 12.2 Spectral-domain optical coherence tomography (OCT) of a patient with paracentral acute middle maculopathy or PAMM. A, OCT at baseline shows two bands of inner nuclear layer (INL) hyper-reflectivity consistent with an INL infarct or PAMM. B, At follow-up, a legacy of middle retinal atrophy corresponding to the baseline PAMM lesions is noted.[1] These lesions may be referred to as old or chronic PAMM. (Reprinted with permission from Yu S, Pang CE, Gong Y, et al. The spectrum of superficial and deep capillary ischemia in retinal artery occlusion. *Am J Ophthalmol.* 2015;159(1):53-63.e2. doi:10.1016/j.ajo.2014.09.027.)

INL thinning or atrophy typical of tissue infarction, ie, old or chronic PAMM (Figure 12.2).

- PAMM lesions can have a diffuse or skip pattern with cross-sectional OCT. With en-face OCT, the skip PAMM lesions typically display a precise perivenular colocalization (Figure 12.3).
- PAMM is a manifestation of the retinal ischemic cascade due to the predominantly physiological vertical flow of blood from the superficial to the deep retinal capillary plexus (Figures 12.3 and 12.4).
- The venular pole of the deep retinal capillary plexus (DCP) is most prone to oxygen desaturation and is the first to exhibit signs of ischemia during periods of impaired vascular flow which manifests as perivenular PAMM with en-face OCT (Figures 12.3 and 12.4).
- With more progressive vascular impairment, PAMM lesions extend diffusely through the INL, and this manifests as globular PAMM with en-face OCT (Figures 12.3 and 12.4).
- With severe blood flow disruption, inner retinal infarction ensues (Figure 12.4).

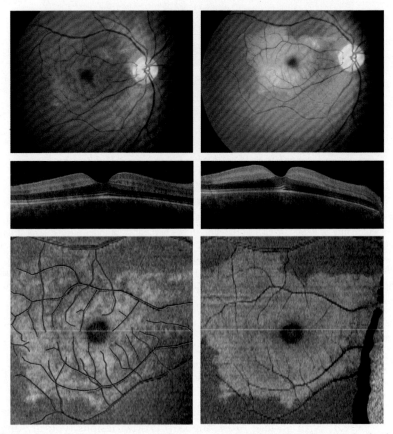

FIGURE 12.3 Spectral-domain optical coherence tomography (OCT) (SD-OCT) and color fundus photography of a patient with cilioretinal artery insufficiency and paracentral acute middle maculopathy (PAMM). **The progressive PAMM lesions are indicative of the ischemic cascade.** At baseline presentation (LEFT), color fundus photograph shows macular whitening. OCT illustrates PAMM or inner nuclear layer (INL) hyperreflectivity in a multifocal skip pattern. Corresponding en-face OCT with vascular overlay of the arteries (red) and veins (blue) illustrates that the fernlike PAMM lesions have a precise perivenular colocalization. 12 hours later (RIGHT), the color fundus photograph shows more diffuse macular whitening and a cherry red spot. OCT shows evolution to diffuse hyperreflectivity of the INL, and corresponding en-face OCT illustrates globular PAMM consistent with the ischemic cascade. (Reprinted with permission from Bakhoum MF, Freund KB, Dolz-Marco R, et al. Paracentral acute middle maculopathy and the ischemic cascade associated with retinal vascular occlusion. *Am J Ophthalmol.* 2018;195:143-153. doi:10.1016/j.ajo.2018.07.031.)

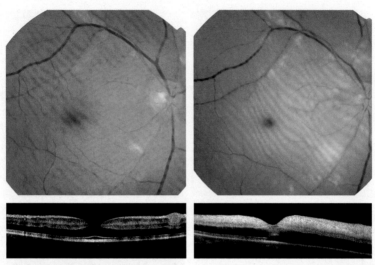

FIGURE 12.4 Spectral-domain optical coherence tomography (OCT) (SD-OCT) and color fundus photography of a patient with progressive central retinal artery occlusion and evidence of the ischemic cascade. At baseline presentation (LEFT), the color fundus photograph illustrates patchy areas of ischemic whitening in the macula consistent with a partial central retinal artery occlusion (CRAO). Corresponding cross-sectional OCT shows inner nuclear layer (INL) hyperreflectivity and PAMM (paracentral acute middle maculopathy) in a multifocal, skip pattern. At the 5-day follow-up interval (RIGHT), the color fundus photograph shows a cherry red spot and progression to a complete CRAO. Corresponding OCT illustrates progression to diffuse middle and inner retinal infarction indicative of the ischemic cascade. (Reprinted with permission from Bakhoum MF, Freund KB, Dolz-Marco R, et al. Paracentral acute middle maculopathy and the ischemic cascade associated with retinal vascular occlusion. *Am J Ophthalmol.* 2018;195:143-153. doi:10.1016/j.ajo.2018.07.031.)

OCTA IMAGING

- Optical coherence tomography angiography (OCTA) of focal PAMM lesions, in the early stages, may or may not show flow deficits within the deep vascular complex (ie, ICP and DCP).
- More severe cases with diffuse PAMM lesions may exhibit attenuation of the deep vascular complex. This is often associated with central retinal artery occlusion. Typically, projection of the superficial retinal capillary plexus will be a sign of impaired perfusion within the deep retinal capillary plexus.
- Chronic PAMM associated with either focal and diffuse lesions often exhibits marked reduction in perfusion of the DCP (Figure 12.5).
- The superficial capillary plexus may in some cases show mild attenuation, particularly in the chronic setting.

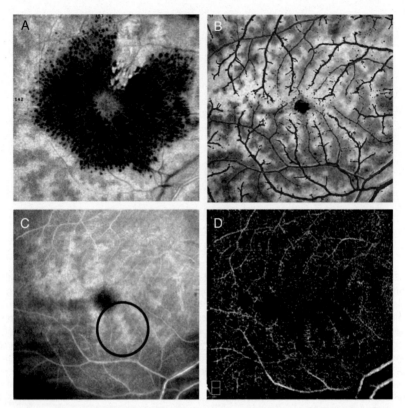

FIGURE 12.5 En-face optical coherence tomography (OCT) and optical coherence tomography angiography (OCTA) images of perivenular fernlike PAMM (paracentral acute middle maculopathy) associated with central retinal vein occlusion. A, En-face OCT segmented at the level of the outer plexiform layer shows cystoid macular edema. B, En-face OCT segmented at the level of the middle retina (ie, inner nuclear layer or INL) with overlay of the arteries (red) and veins (blue) illustrates a precise perivenular colocalization of the hyperreflective fernlike PAMM lesions. On follow-up 6 weeks later, en-face OCT (C) shows persistence of hyperreflective fernlike PAMM lesion (see circle) and OCTA segmented at the level of the deep retinal capillary plexus (DCP) (D) illustrates flow deficit of the DCP (see circle) corresponding with the PAMM lesion on en-face OCT. (Reprinted with permission from Garrity ST, Tseng VL, Sarraf D. Paracentral acute middle maculopathy in a perivenular fern-like distribution with en face optical coherence tomography. *Retin Cases Brief Rep.* 2018;12(suppl 1):S25-S28. doi:10.1097/ICB.0000000000000657.)

References

1. Yu S, Pang CE, Gong Y, et al. The spectrum of superficial and deep capillary ischemia in retinal artery occlusion. *Am J Ophthalmol.* 2015;159(1):53-63. e2. doi:10.1016/j.ajo.2014.09.027.
2. Bakhoum MF, Freund KB, Dolz-Marco R, et al. Paracentral acute middle maculopathy and the ischemic cascade associated with retinal vascular occlusion. *Am J Ophthalmol.* 2018;195:143-153. doi:10.1016/j.ajo.2018.07.031.
3. Garrity ST, Tseng VL, Sarraf D. Paracentral acute middle maculopathy in a perivenular fern-like distribution with en face optical coherence tomography. *Retin Cases Brief Rep.* 2018;12(suppl 1):S25-S28. doi:10.1097/ICB.0000000000000657.

4. Iafe NA, Onclinx T, Tsui I, Sarraf D. Paracentral acute middle maculopathy and deep retinal capillary plexus infarction secondary to reperfused central retinal artery occlusion. *Retin Cases Br Rep.* 2017;11(1):S90-S93. doi:10.1097/ICB.0000000000000424.

5. Sarraf D, Rahimy E, Fawzi AA, et al. Paracentral acute middle maculopathy: A new variant of acute macular neuroretinopathy associated with retinal capillary ischemia. *JAMA Ophthalmol.* 2013;131(10):1275-1287. doi:10.1001/jamaophthalmol.2013.4056.

6. Rahimy E, Kuehlewein L, Sadda SR, Sarraf D. Paracentral acute middle maculopathy: What we knew then and what we know now. *Retina.* 2015;35(10):1921-1930. doi:10.1097/IAE.0000000000000785.

7. Nemiroff J, Kuehlewein L, Rahimy E, et al. Assessing deep retinal capillary ischemia in paracentral acute middle maculopathy by optical coherence tomography angiography. *Am J Ophthalmol.* 2016;162:121-132.e1. doi:10.1016/j.ajo.2015.10.026.

8. Rahimy E, Sarraf D, Dollin ML, Pitcher JD, Ho AC. Paracentral acute middle maculopathy in nonischemic central retinal vein occlusion. *Am J Ophthalmol.* 2014;158(2):372-380.e1. doi:10.1016/j.ajo.2014.04.024.

9. Chen X, Rahimy E, Sergott RC, et al. Spectrum of retinal vascular diseases associated with paracentral acute middle maculopathy. *Am J Ophthalmol.* 2015;160(1):26-34.e1. doi:10.1016/j.ajo.2015.04.004.

10. Ghasemi Falavarjani K, Phasukkijwatana N, Freund KB, et al. En face optical coherence tomography analysis to assess the spectrum of perivenular ischemia and paracentral acute middle maculopathy in retinal vein occlusion. *Am J Ophthalmol.* 2017;177:131-138. doi:10.1016/j.ajo.2017.02.015.

11. Phasukkijwatana N, Rahimi M, Iafe N, Sarraf D. Central retinal vein occlusion and paracentral acute middle maculopathy diagnosed with en face optical coherence tomography. *Ophthalmic Surg Lasers Imaging Retin.* 2016;47(9):862-864. doi:10.3928/23258160-20160901-10.

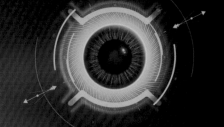

CHAPTER 13

Acute Macular Neuroretinopathy

SALIENT FEATURES

- Acute macular neuroretinopathy (AMN) is a rare condition classically defined by a wedge-shaped or petaloid lesion directed toward the fovea (Figure 13.1).[1,2]
- Patients most commonly complain of a paracentral scotoma with mild vision loss.[1,2]
- This condition is typically found in Caucasian females in the third decade of life.[2]
- The pathogenesis has not been completely elucidated; however, recent studies suggest a microvascular etiology.[3,4] An inflammatory cause is less likely.
- AMN has been shown to be associated with mainly nonspecific illnesses, use of oral contraceptives and vasoconstrictors, and potentially vasoactive events.[2]
- Color fundus photography may illustrate a reddish wedge-shaped parafoveal lesion but can otherwise be normal, and diagnosis usually relies on spectral-domain optical coherence tomography (OCT) and near-infrared reflectance (NIR).[2]

OCT IMAGING

- OCT imaging is critical to make the diagnosis of AMN. NIR is also valuable and displays a tear drop or wedge-shaped hyporeflective lesion in the parafoveal region (Figure 13.2A).[2]
- Acutely, OCT most commonly displays hyperreflectivity of the outer nuclear layer (ONL) with radial extension into the Henle fiber (HFL)

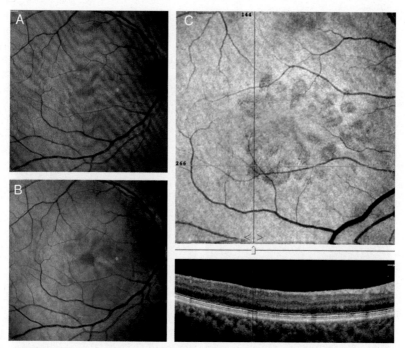

FIGURE 13.1 Multicolor (A), near-infrared reflectance (NIR) (B) and en-face optical coherence tomography (OCT) (C) images of the characteristic petaloid pattern of acute macular neuroretinopathy (AMN). Note that the petaloid lesion identified with NIR and en-face OCT colocalizes with ellipsoid zone attenuation with the corresponding cross-sectional OCT B-scan.

and outer plexiform layers (OPLs), suggesting photoreceptor cell body and axon disruption (Figure 13.2B).[2,5]

- Disruption of the ellipsoid zone (EZ) is an additional feature and, in select cases, may develop after the OPL lesion (Figure 13.2B).[2,5]

- Over time, ONL thinning develops with persistent scotoma, although there is usually recovery of the EZ band.[2,5]

- AMN should not be confused with paracentral acute middle maculopathy (PAMM). While both lesions can be associated with parafoveal hyporeflective features with NIR, PAMM is a middle-level retinal abnormality of the inner nuclear layer (ie, an INL infarct) due to flow impairment of the intermediate or deep retinal capillary plexus. AMN, on the other hand, occurs at the level of the outer retina and may or may not be due to flow impairment in the DCP (Figure 13.3).[3]

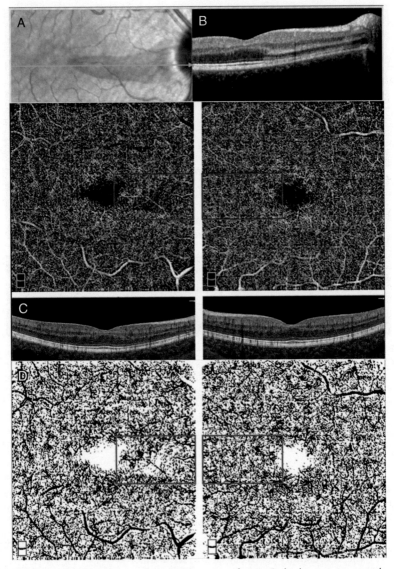

FIGURE 13.2 Near-infrared reflectance (NIR), OCT B-scan, en-face optical coherence tomography angiography (OCTA), and binarized OCTA from a patient with acute macular neuroretinopathy of the right eye. NIR (A) illustrates a wedge-shaped area of hyporeflectivity in the nasal macula corresponding to the acute macular neuroretinopathy (AMN) lesion. The OCT B-scan (B) illustrates a corresponding region of hyperreflectivity within the outer plexiform and the outer nuclear layers with associated disruption of the outer retinal bands including the inner segment ellipsoid zone. En-face OCTA and corresponding OCT B-scan segmentation (C) with red rectangles representing areas of interest illustrates an associated flow deficit of the deep retinal capillary plexus of the right eye (left image) that colocalizes with the AMN lesion OD and normal capillary density in the equivalent area of the left eye (right image). Binarized OCTA (D) with corresponding red rectangles denoting areas of interest reveals reduced capillary density associated with the AMN lesion in the affected right eye (left image) compared to the corresponding area of the normal left eye (right image). (Reprinted with permission from Nemiroff J, Sarraf D, Davila JP, Rodger D. Optical coherence tomography angiography of acute macular neuroretinopathy reveals deep capillary ischemia. *Retin Cases Brief Rep*. 2018;12(suppl 1):S12-S15.)

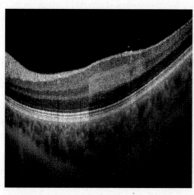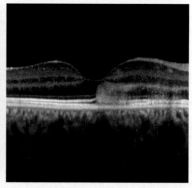

FIGURE 13.3 Side-by-side optical coherence tomography (OCT) B-scan comparisons of paracentral acute middle maculopathy (PAMM, left image) versus acute macular neuroretinopathy (AMN, right image). Note the band of hyperreflectivity at the level of the middle retina or inner nuclear layer for PAMM and at the level of the outer retina for AMN. (Reprinted with permission from Rahimy E, Kuehlewein L, Sadda SR, Sarraf D. Paracentral acute middle maculopathy: what we knew then and what we know now. *Retina*. 2015;35(10):1921-1930.)

OCT ANGIOGRAPHY IMAGING

- Optical coherence tomography angiography (OCTA) flow deficits in both the DCP[6-8] (Figure 13.2C and D) and choriocapillaris[9-11] have been found to colocalize to AMN lesions on OCT.
- Although the definitive site of nonperfusion in the pathogenesis of AMN is unclear, it is suggested that the deficits in either the DCP or choriocapillaris may play a role in the development of AMN given that both contribute to the blood supply of the photoreceptors, the main target of AMN.[11]

References

1. Bos PJ, Deutman AF. Acute macular neuroretinopathy. *Am J Ophthalmol.* 1975;80(4):573-584.
2. Bhavsar KV, Lin S, Rahimy E, et al. Acute macular neuroretinopathy: a comprehensive review of the literature. *Surv Ophthalmol.* 2016;61(5):538-565.
3. Sarraf D, Rahimy E, Fawzi AA, et al. Paracentral acute middle maculopathy: a new variant of acute macular neuroretinopathy associated with retinal capillary ischemia. *JAMA Ophthalmol.* 2013;131(10):1275-1287.
4. Rahimy E, Sarraf D. Paracentral acute middle maculopathy spectral-domain optical coherence tomography feature of deep capillary ischemia. *Curr Opin Ophthalmol.* 2014;25(3):207-212.
5. Fawzi AA, Pappuru RR, Sarraf D, et al. Acute macular neuroretinopathy: long-term insights revealed by multimodal imaging. *Retina.* 2012;32(8):1500-1513.
6. Pecen PE, Smith AG, Ehlers JP. Optical coherence tomography angiography of acute macular neuroretinopathy and paracentral acute middle maculopathy. *JAMA Ophthalmol.* 2015;133(12):1478-1480.

7. Ashraf M, Goldstein D, Fawzi A. Optical coherence tomography angiography: potential artifacts in acute macular neuroretinopathy. *JAMA Ophthalmol.* 2017;135(6):675-676.

8. Nemiroff J, Sarraf D, Davila JP, Rodger D. Optical coherence tomography angiography of acute macular neuroretinopathy reveals deep capillary ischemia. *Retin Cases Brief Rep.* 2018;12(suppl 1):S12-S15.

9. Thanos A, Faia LJ, Yonekawa Y, Randhawa S. Optical coherence tomographic angiography in acute macular neuroretinopathy. *JAMA Ophthalmol.* 2016;134(11):1310-1314.

10. Lee SY, Cheng JL, Gehrs KM, et al. Choroidal features of acute macular neuroretinopathy via optical coherence tomography angiography and correlation with serial multimodal imaging. *JAMA Ophthalmol.* 2017;135(11):1177-1183.

11. Casalino G, Arrigo A, Romano F, Munk MR, Bandello F, Parodi MB. Acute macular neuroretinopathy: pathogenetic insights from optical coherence tomography angiography. *Br J Ophthalmol.* 2019;103(3):410-414.

12. Rahimy E, Kuehlewein L, Sadda SR, Sarraf D. Paracentral acute middle maculopathy: what we knew then and what we know now. *Retina.* 2015;35(10):1921-1930.

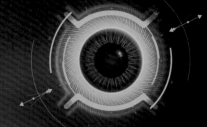

CHAPTER 14

Retinal Macroaneurysm

SALIENT FEATURES

- Retinal artery macroaneurysm (RAM) is a rare, acquired, round or fusiform dilation of the retinal arteriole, most commonly found along the temporal arcades.[1-4]
- RAM is most commonly associated with hypertension and arteriosclerotic disease,[1,2] and in one-third of cases, it is associated with retinal vein occlusion.[3]
- It is more prevalent among females and occurs unilaterally in 90% of cases.[1]
- Diagnosis is made based on clinical examination and fluorescein angiography. Associated signs of aneurysmal rupture include edema, hemorrhage, and exudation, often in a circinate pattern surrounding the aneurysm (Figure 14.1A).[1]
- On fluorescein angiography (FA), RAM is characterized by early uniform filling of the dilated arteriole.[1] Incomplete or absent filling can be seen in thrombosed or involuted macroaneurysms.[1,3]
- Patients are usually asymptomatic unless complicated by macular edema or macroaneurysm rupture, with hemorrhage that can occur in all retinal layers: subretinal, intraretinal, and/or preretinal.[4]

OCT IMAGING

- On optical coherence tomography (OCT), RAM appears as a dilated vessel with a thick hyperreflective wall with a hyporeflective lumen.
- Manifestations of chronic or acute macular edema may be present on OCT including intraretinal edema (hyporeflective cystic spaces),

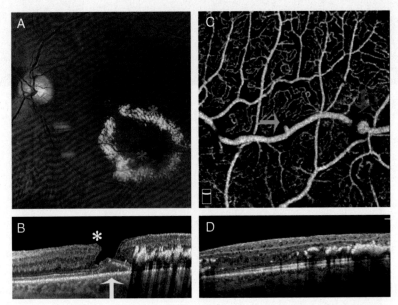

FIGURE 14.1 A, Color fundus photo demonstrating retinal artery macroaneurysm (RAM) with surrounding intraretinal hemorrhage (red asterisk) and circinate pattern of exudation (pink asterisk). B, Optical coherence tomography (OCT) demonstrating lamellar hole with epiretinal proliferation (white asterisk), intraretinal lipid exudation (pink asterisk), and subretinal hyperreflective material (yellow arrow). C, Optical coherence tomography angiography (OCTA) demonstrating fusiform dilation of a retinal arteriole (red arrow) and adjacent smaller aneurysmal dilation (green arrow) on superficial en-face imaging. D, Corresponding B-scan demonstrating intraretinal lipid exudates.

> subretinal fluid (hyporeflective space between the retina and retinal pigment epithelium), and lipid exudation (hyperreflective spots 20-40 um in size clustered in the outer retina) (Figure 14.1B).
>
> - Acute retinal hemorrhage, if present, will appear as an area of homogeneous hyperreflectivity between the internal limiting membrane (ILM) and the inner retina, within the retina, or in the subretinal space.
> - If the hemorrhage is subacute, it can present with both hyporeflective and hyperreflective components as the blood organizes.

OCTA IMAGING

- RAMs are well-delineated on optical coherence tomography angiography (OCTA) as saccular or fusiform outpouching of a retinal arteriole on both en-face and cross-sectional imaging (Figures 14.1C and 14.2).
- OCTA may be useful to identify culprit lesions in patients presenting with acute preretinal hemorrhage where blocking would obscure identification of the RAM on FA.
- Flow signal may decrease if the lesion undergoes thrombosis either spontaneously or after treatment with laser photocoagulation.[5]

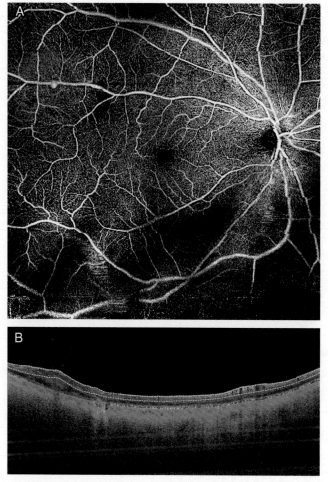

FIGURE 14.2 A, Zeiss PLEX Elite optical coherence tomography angiography (OCTA) demonstrating fusiform dilation of a retinal arteriole (red arrow) on superficial en-face imaging. B, Corresponding B-scan demonstrating flow within the lesion.

References

1. Rabb MF, Gagliano DA, Teske MP. Retinal arterial macroaneurysms. *Surv Ophthalmol.* 1988;33(2):73-96.
2. Panton RW, Goldberg MF, Farber MD. Retinal arterial macroaneurysms: risk factors and natural history. *Br J Ophthalmol.* 1990;74(10):595-600.
3. Hughes EL, Dooley IJ, Kennelly KP, Doyle F, Siah WF, Connell P. Angiographic features and disease outcomes of symptomatic retinal arterial macroaneurysms. *Graefes Arch Clin Exp Ophthalmol Heidelb.* 2016;254(11): 2203-2207.

4. Goldenberg D, Soiberman U, Loewenstein A, Goldstein M. Heidelberg spectral-domain optical coherence tomographic findings in retinal artery macroaneurysm. *Retina*. 2012;32(5):990-995.
5. Astroz P, Miere A, Cohen SY, Querques G, Souied EH. Optical coherence tomography angiography in the Diagnosis and follow-up of retinal arterial macroaneurysms. *Retin Cases Brief Rep*. 2018:1-4.

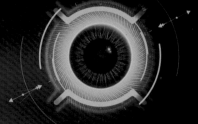

CHAPTER 15

Macular Telangiectasia Type II

SALIENT FEATURES

- Bilateral, slowly progressive condition usually affecting patients between the ages of 40 and 60 years characterized by macular capillary changes, variable foveal cavitations, and loss of outer retinal structure with eventual macular atrophy.[1]
- Muller cell dysfunction and the corresponding photoreceptor loss may be attributable to systemically low serine levels; abnormal serine metabolism results in elevated deoxysphingolipids, which may be associated with macular toxicity as a result of the neurotoxic effects of the metabolite deoxydihydroceramide produced from the hydrolyzation of deoxysphingolipids.[2]
- Hallmarks of the disease include unique zone of "light gray discoloration" in the temporal juxtafoveal macula due to the loss of retinal transparency,[3] presence of telangiectatic macular vessels, retinal pigment epithelial (RPE) hypertrophy, blunted "right-angle" venules, crystalline deposits, and pigmentary migration into the retina.[1]
- Potential complications of the disease include proliferation of pigment plaques, photoreceptor loss, foveal atrophy, and subretinal neovascularization temporal to the fovea that may result in visual loss from hemorrhage or exudation.[4]
- Fluorescein angiography is the historical gold standard to confirm the diagnosis of the disease showing telangiectatic capillaries, most commonly temporal to the foveola, in the early phase and a diffuse hyperfluorescence in the late phase (late hyperfluorescence may even be noted in the absence of telangiectatic alterations, Figure 15.1).[4]

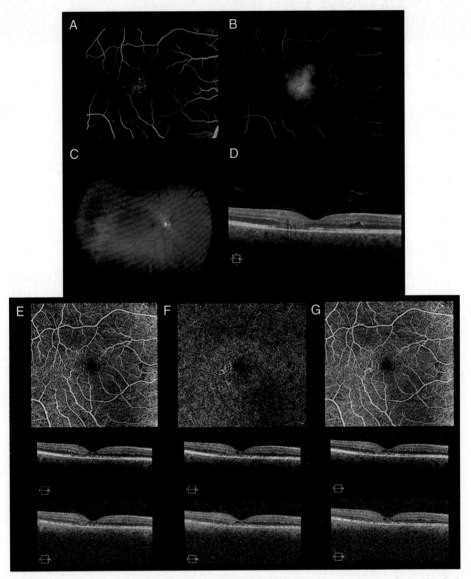

FIGURE 15.1 Early (A) and late (B) fluorescein angiography showing telangieactatic capillaries that leak late in the temporal portions of the macula. Corresponding fundus photo (C). Optical coherence tomography (OCT) (D) shows focal outer retinal loss and ellipsoid zone attenuation. Optical coherence tomography angiography (OCTA) of the superficial (E), deep (F), and whole retina (G) highlights the temporal telangiectatic vessels. Corresponding OCTs demonstrate degenerative cystic changes.

- Lipid exudates, intra- or subretinal hemorrhage, and macular edema are not typical features of this disease and warrant reconsideration for diagnosis and staging.[1]
- Due to the outstanding visualization of the unique anatomic features of macular telangiectasia type II, OCT and optical coherence tomography angiography (OCTA) have become key diagnostic tests that are supplanting fluorescein angiography (FA) as the gold-standard diagnostic test in this condition.

OCT IMAGING

- Characteristic features on spectral-domain OCT (SD-OCT) include macular thinning, plaques and breaks in the ellipsoid zone with progressive outer retinal atrophy, temporal foveal pit enlargement that may progress into large hyporeflective cavitations in the inner and outer retina, and the development of full-thickness macular hole in the absence of vitreoretinal traction.[5]
- In the early stages of disease, subtle splaying of the foveal depression and focal areas of hyporeflectivity in the normally hyperreflective ellipsoid zone can be observed (Figure 15.1).[1]
- Foveal hyporeflective spaces may present in the early or late course of the disease and must be distinguished from cystoid cavities (seen in macular edema) and pseudohole formation (as seen with the epiretinal membrane).[1]
- The degenerative cystic spaces are often within the fovea and begin in the sub–internal limiting membrane (ILM) space. These cystic changes tend to not have an "exudative" appearance without an increase in retinal thickness and do not have a convex appearance.
- Progression of the disease is indicated by shrinkage of the outer layers and reduction in the central foveal thickness.[4]
- In more advanced disease, clusters of intraretinal RPE migration and hyperplasia may present as hyperreflective intraretinal lesions.[1]

OCTA IMAGING

- Microvascular changes on OCTA are shown to arise first from the deep capillary plexus of the retina, then to the superficial plexus, and finally extend circumferentially around the fovea with concomitant formation of telangiectatic, microaneurysmal-like changes (Figures 15.2-15.4).[6]
- Loss of capillaries may be present in both the inner and outer plexus in the macular region (often presenting more so in the outer plexus).[7]

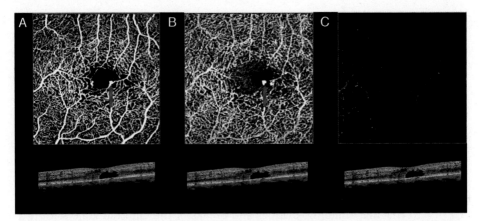

FIGURE 15.2 Optical coherence tomography angiography (OCTA) of the superficial plexus (A), deep plexus (B), and avascular zone (C) showing a nasal telangiectatic vessel (arrow) with flow in the corresponding OCT images with flow overlay (red and green). Note the lack of flow and lack of vessels in the avascular zone as well as the cavitary hyporeflective spaces on the OCT B-scans.

- In advanced diseases, the vessels in the outer plexus may appear thinner and less densely packed and may present with an abnormal arrangement.[7]
- Imaging findings of advanced disease may also demonstrate increased loss of the perifoveal capillaries of the inner plexus and invasion of deeper layers and the subretinal space with new vessels.[5,7]
- Retinal-choroidal anastomosis (RCA) may also be present before the development of subretinal neovascularization; right-angle veins, focal

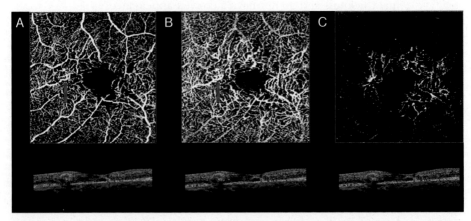

FIGURE 15.3 Optical coherence tomography angiography (OCTA) of the superficial plexus (A), deep plexus (B), and avascular zone (C) showing a telangiectatic vessels (arrow) that actually course around nearly the entire fovea with flow in the corresponding OCT images with flow overlay (red and green) and also extend into the avascular area.

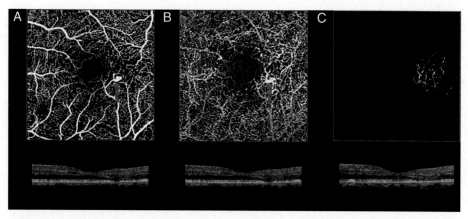

FIGURE 15.4 Optical coherence tomography angiography (OCTA) of the superficial plexus (A), deep plexus (B), and avascular zone (C) showing a nasal telangiectatic vessel (arrow) with flow in the corresponding OCT images with flow overlay (red and green). There is also flow extending into the avascular zone.

hyperpigmentation, ellipsoid zone defects, and hyperreflective outer retinal lesions are all intercorrelated findings with RCA.[4,6,7]

- OCTA provides clinical utility over FA in detecting subretinal neovascularization in patients presenting with no macular hemorrhage and prominent temporal leakage on FA.[8]
- One-year follow-up OCTA results of patients with proliferative and nonproliferative disease have shown marked reduction in the vascular density of the superficial and deep capillary plexuses with changes most prominent in the latter, suggesting a role for ischemia in the pathogenesis and progression of the disease.[9]

References

1. Christakis PG, Fine HF, Wiley HE. The diagnosis and management of macular telangiectasia. *Ophthalmic Surg Lasers Imaging*. 2019;50(3):139-144.
2. Gantner ML, Eade K, Wallace M, et al. Serine and Lipid metabolism in macular disease and peripheral neuropathy. *N Engl J Med*. 2019;381:1422-1433.
3. Breazzano MP, Yannuzzi LA, Spaide RF. Characterizing retinal-choroidal anastomosis in macular telangiectasia type 2 with optical coherence tomography angiography. *Retina*. 2020;40(1):92-98.
4. Chidambara L, Gadde SG, Yadav NK. Characteristics and quantification of vascular changes in macular telangiectasia type 2 on optical coherence tomography angiography. *Br J Ophthalmol*. 2016;100(11):1482-1488.
5. Nalci H, Sermet F, Demirel S, Ozmert E. Optic coherence angiography findings in type-2 macular telangiectasia. *Turk J Ophthalmol*. 2017;47(5):279-284.
6. Zhang Q, Wang RK, Chen CL, et al. Swept source OCT angiography of neovascular macular telangiectasia type 2. *Retina*. 2015;35(11):2285-2299.

7. Spaide RF, Klancnik JM Jr, Cooney MJ. Retinal vascular layers in macular telangiectasia type 2 imaged by optical coherence tomographic angiography. *JAMA Ophthalmol.* 2015;133(1):66-73.

8. Villegas V, Kovach JL. Optical coherence tomography angiography of macular telangiectasia type 2 with associated subretinal neovascular membrane. *Case Rep Ophthalmol Med.* 2017;2017:8186134.

9. Demir ST, Guven D, Karatas ME, Dirim AB, Sendul SY, Ustaoglu M. Evaluation of 1-year follow-up results of macular telangiectasia type 2 cases by optical coherence tomography angiography. *GMS Ophthalmol Cases.* 2019;9:Doc29.

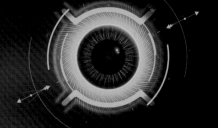

CHAPTER 16

Coats Disease

SALIENT FEATURES

- Coats disease is a predominantly unilateral, idiopathic, nonhereditary, congenital retinal vascular abnormality.
- A variant of type 1 macular telangiectasia; it involves telangiectasias of small- and medium-sized retinal blood vessels without vitreoretinal traction.[1]
- Males in their first or second decade of life are typically affected, with an earlier onset portending a worse visual prognosis.
- Vascular leakage typically leads to a peripheral exudative retinal detachment, most commonly in the inferior and temporal quadrants.
- Coats disease is staged according to the funduscopic presence of telangiectasias, exudates, foveal involvement, and exudative retinal detachment. Progression to end stage is characterized by total retinal detachment, glaucoma, and phthisis.
- Other characteristic findings include light bulb aneurysms, vascular sheathing, and vascular beading.
- Fluorescein angiography can demonstrate leakage from peripheral and macular telangiectatic vasculature. Capillary rarefaction and nonperfusion may be seen. Fellow eyes may demonstrate mild, asymptomatic peripheral vascular abnormalities.[2]
- A vision-threatening exudative maculopathy occurs in about a quarter to 40% of patients. Later in the disease course, macular fibrosis appears as a dull-gray sheet or nodule and is associated with visual loss.

- Treatment options for the exudative maculopathy include cryo-therapy and laser photocoagulation to areas of telangiectatic, leaking vessels, and intravitreal anti–vascular endothelial growth factor therapy.
- Various permutations of vitreoretinal surgery including pars plana vitrectomy, cryotherapy, laser photocoagulation, intraocular tamponade, and external drainage of subretinal fluid may be employed in cases with exudative retinal detachment.
- Despite therapy, poorer visual prognosis is correlated to increased disease stage. Advanced-stage eyes may require enucleation.[3,4]

OCT IMAGING

- Even in eyes without obvious macular involvement on fundus examination, optical coherence tomography (OCT) imaging can reveal intraretinal fluid, intraretinal exudates, subretinal fluid, subretinal exudates, and disruption of the external limiting membrane and ellipsoid zone.[5]
- Outer retinal layer disruption and subfoveal hyperreflective nodules (sharply demarcated hyperreflective subfoveal lesions with posterior shadowing) are associated with poorer visual prognosis.[6]
- Macular atrophy and fibrosis may develop in up to 50% of cases despite therapy. The presence of subretinal fluid or subretinal exudates at baseline has been associated with higher likelihood of macular fibrosis development in retrospective study (Figures 16.1-16.5).[7]

OCTA IMAGING

- Qualitative changes on optical coherence tomography angiography (OCTA) include capillary telangiectasias, aneurysms, nonperfusion, and dilatation in both the superficial and deep vascular plexuses (SCP and DCP).
- Positive flow signal within hyperreflective fibrotic nodules may be seen.[8]
- Increased foveal avascular zone (FAZ) area and decreased vascular density in both the SCP and DCP can be seen in eyes affected with early-stage Coats disease.[9]
- Increased FAZ area in the SCP has noted in the fellow eyes when compared to healthy controls (Figures 16.6 and 16.7).[10]

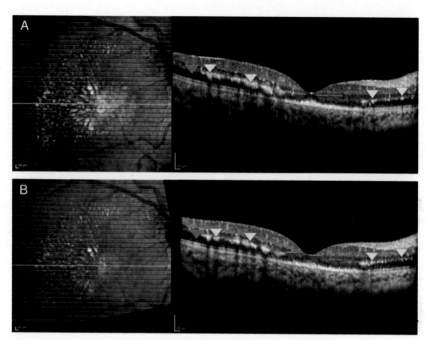

FIGURE 16.1 Optical coherence tomography (OCT) of a patient with Coats disease, showing features before (A) and after (B) treatment with multiple intravitreal anti–vascular endothelial growth factor (VEGF) and photocoagulation therapies. Intraretinal exudates at the level of the outer plexiform layer (yellow arrows), as well as hyporeflectivity in the outer retinal layers (blue arrow), are diminished after treatment. Thickening at the level of the retinal pigment epithelium (RPE) with ellipsoid disruption (EZ) persists (red arrows).

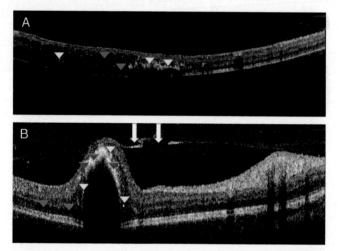

FIGURE 16.2 Optical coherence tomographies (OCTs) from a patient with Coats disease showing classic OCT features. The patient received multiple treatments with laser photocoagulation and intravitreal bevacizumab over their disease course. A, Intraretinal edema (blue arrows) and intraretinal hyperreflective foci/hard exudates (yellow arrows) are present. B, A hyperreflective nodule with posterior shadowing (red arrows) and vitreous traction along the margin of the nodule (white arrows) is noted in this particular patient.

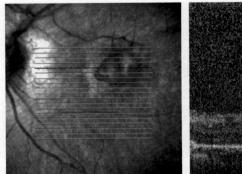
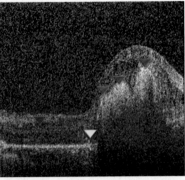

FIGURE 16.3 Optical coherence tomography (OCT) of a patient with Coats disease who underwent treatment with multiple intravitreal bevacizumab and laser photocoagulation applications over a 38-month period. The near-infrared image demonstrates a focal hyper- and hyporeflective lesion. There is a characteristic subfoveal hyperreflective nodule (red arrows) on spectral-domain optical coherence tomography (SD-OCT). Trace intraretinal fluid (blue arrow) and hard exudates (yellow arrow) are also present.

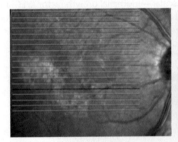
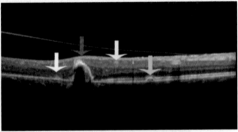

FIGURE 16.4 Optical coherence tomography (OCT) of a patient with Coats disease who underwent treatment with multiple intravitreal bevacizumab and laser photocoagulation applications. An extrafoveal small fibrotic nodule is present temporally (red arrow). Intraretinal hard exudates are present (yellow arrow). A small retinal pigment epithelium abnormality is highlighted with a white arrow, and a small retinal pigment epithelial detachment is shown with a green arrow. The pretreatment images are unavailable.

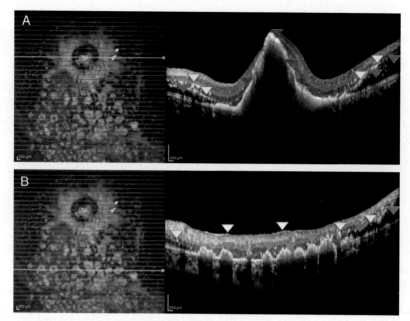

FIGURE 16.5 Optical coherence tomography (OCT) of a patient with Coats disease who underwent treatment with multiple intravitreal bevacizumab and laser photocoagulation applications. Highlighted are extensive hard exudates (yellow arrows), a thickened outer nuclear layer (blue arrows), a mild epiretinal membrane (white arrow), and a large subfoveal fibrotic nodule (red arrows) in the central (A) and inferior (B) scans, corresponding with the infrared images to the left. The green arrows highlight excrescences in the retinal pigment epithelium in the setting of chorioretinal atrophy.

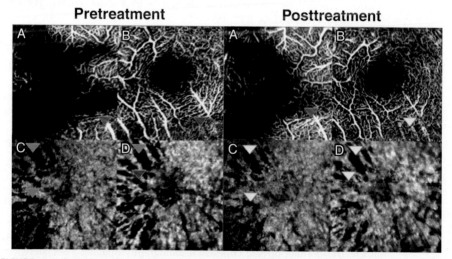

FIGURE 16.6 Optical coherence tomography angiography (OCTA) of a patient with Coats disease, showing features before (left) and after (right) treatment in the superficial vascular plexus (A), deep vascular plexus (B), choriocapillaris (C), and choroid (D). The presence of microaneurysms (red arrows) and capillary nonperfusion (blue arrows) is shown. Vascular reperfusion of the deep vascular plexus, choriocapillaris, and choroid following treatment with anti–vascular endothelial growth factor (VEGF) and laser photoablation was noted in this patient (yellow arrows).

Pretreatment   **Posttreatment**

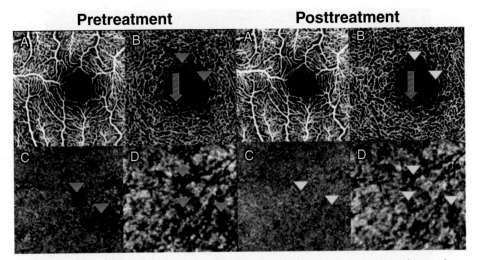

FIGURE 16.7 Optical coherence tomography angiography (OCTA) of a patient with Coats disease, showing features in the superficial vascular plexus (A), deep vascular plexus (B), choriocapillaris (C), and choroid (D). The presence of abnormal vessels within the foveal avascular zone (red arrows) and capillary nonperfusion (blue arrows) are shown before and after treatment with intravitreal bevacizumab and laser photocoagulation. Vascular reperfusion of the deep vascular plexus, choriocapillaris, and choroid following treatment was seen in this case (yellow arrows).

References

1. Sen M, Shields CL, Honavar S, Shields J. Coats disease: an overview of classification, management and outcomes. *Indian J Ophthalmol*. 2019;67(6):763-771. doi:10.4103/ijo.IJO_841_19.

2. Jeng-Miller KW, Soomro T, Scott NL, et al. Longitudinal examination of fellow-eye vascular anomalies in coats' disease with widefield fluorescein angiography: a multicenter study. *Ophthalmic Surg Lasers Imaging Retina*. 2019;50(4):221-227. doi:10.3928/23258160-20190401-04.

3. Dalvin LA, Udyaver S, Lim LAS, et al. Coats disease: clinical features and outcomes by age category in 351 cases. *J Pediatr Ophthalmol Strabismus*. 2019;56(5):288-296. doi:10.3928/01913913-20190716-01.

4. Shields CL, Udyaver S, Dalvin LA, et al. Visual acuity outcomes in Coats disease by classification stage in 160 patients. *Br J Ophthalmol*. 2020;104(3):422-431. doi:10.1136/bjophthalmol-2019-314363.

5. Gupta MP, Dow E, Jeng-Miller KW, et al. Spectral domain optical coherence tomography findings in coats disease. *Retina*. 2019;39(6):1177-1185. doi:10.1097/IAE.0000000000002120.

6. Ong SS, Mruthyunjaya P, Stinnett S, Vajzovic L, Toth CA. Macular features on spectral-domain optical coherence tomography imaging associated with visual acuity in coats' disease. *Invest Ophthalmol Vis Sci*. 2018;59(7):3161-3174. doi:10.1167/iovs.18-24109.

7. Ong SS, Cummings TJ, Vajzovic L, Mruthyunjaya P, Toth CA. Comparison of optical coherence tomography with fundus photographs, fluorescein angiography, and histopathologic analysis in assessing coats disease. *JAMA Ophthalmol.* 2019;137(2):176-183. doi:10.1001/jamaophthalmol.2018.5654.

8. Rabiolo A, Marchese A, Sacconi R, et al. Refining coats' disease by ultra-widefield imaging and optical coherence tomography angiography. *Graefes Arch Clin Exp Ophthalmol.* 2017;255(10):1881-1890. doi:10.1007/s00417-017-3794-7.

9. Schwartz R, Sivaprasad S, Macphee R, et al. Subclinical macular changes and disease laterality in pediatric coats disease determined BY quantitative optical coherence tomography angiography. *Retina.* 2019;39(12):2392-2398.

10. Stanga PE, Romano F, Chwiejczak K, et al. Swept-source optical coherence tomography angiography assessment of fellow eyes in coats disease. *Retina.* 2019;39(3):608-613. doi:10.1097/IAE.0000000000001995.

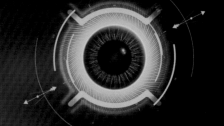

CHAPTER 17

Sickle Cell Retinopathy and Carrier States

SALIENT FEATURES

- Sickle cell retinopathy is an ocular complication of sickle cell carrier states or sickle cell disease, a common and life-threatening hemoglobinopathy affecting 1 in every 365 children born in the United States of African origin.[1]
- In sickle cell disease, abnormal sickle-shaped erythrocytes cause repeated cycles of vaso-occlusion and inflammation in small blood vessels. In the eye, these microvascular insults can lead to nonproliferative and proliferative sickle cell retinopathy.[2]
- Findings consistent with nonproliferative retinopathy include salmon patches (intraretinal hemorrhages), iridescent spots (deposition of hemosiderin and macrophages under the internal limiting membrane after hemorrhage resorption), and black sunbursts (retinal pigment epithelium migration and proliferation as a result of hemorrhage).
- In proliferative sickle cell retinopathy, localized retinal ischemia may lead to upregulation of vascular growth factors, and this in turn can cause retinal neovascularization, vitreous hemorrhage, and tractional retinal detachment.
- In 1971, Goldberg described five stages of proliferative sickle cell retinopathy[3]:
  - Stage I: peripheral arteriolar occlusions
  - Stage II: peripheral arteriovenular anastomoses
  - Stage III: neovascular and fibrous proliferations
  - Stage IV: vitreous hemorrhage
  - Stage V: retinal detachment

- The homozygous HbSS is the most common sickle cell disease genotype. HbSS patients also have the most severe systemic complications when compared to patients with compound heterozygous conditions, such as HbSC and HbS with β-thalassemia. Interestingly, however, proliferative sickle cell retinopathy is more commonly observed in HbSC and HbS with β-thalassemia patients when compared to HbSS patients.[3]
- Sickle cell trait (HbAS) occurs when both HbA and HbS are inherited and strictly is not a form of sickle cell disease. However, reports of sickle cell retinopathy have been published in patients with sickle cell trait who have a concomitant-associated systemic disease such as diabetes, hypertension, syphilis, tuberculosis, or sarcoidosis.[4]

OCT IMAGING

- Optical coherence tomography (OCT) has shown characteristic temporal macular thinning in seemingly visually asymptomatic patients with sickle cell disease (Figure 17.1).
- Macular thinning has been reported to be more common in HbSS patients as compared to HbSC and HbS with β-thalassemia patients.[5]
- Macular thinning has also been shown to correlate with paracentral scotomas on automated perimetry in patients with sickle cell disease.[6]
- Local ischemic events including paracentral acute middle maculopathy and acute macular neuroretinopathy in sickle cell disease can present as hyperreflectivity of the middle and outer retinal layers on OCT (Figure 17.2). Ellipsoid zone disruption can also be demonstrated on OCT with acute choroidal infarction in sickle cell disease (Figure 17.3).
- OCT can also demonstrate retinal thickening in the acute phase and thinning in the chronic phase when central retinal arterial/vein occlusion occurs in sickle cell disease (Figures 17.4 and 17.5).[7] Furthermore, cystoid macular edema in central retinal vein occlusion can be monitored using OCT.[7]

OCTA IMAGING

- Studies have shown that flow loss is more common in the temporal macula, a known watershed zone in the macular vasculature, and can localize to the superficial and deep capillary plexus in patients with sickle cell disease (Figure 17.1).[8,9]

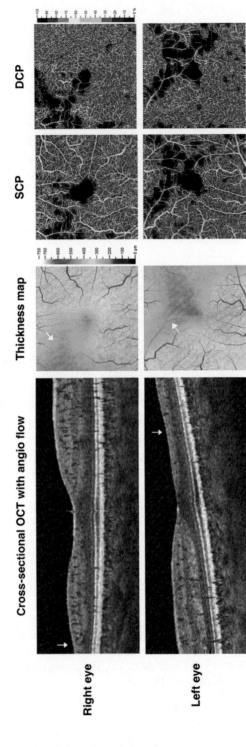

FIGURE 17.1 A 33-year-old man with HbSS disease had mild nonproliferative changes and maintained 20/16 distance visual acuity in both eyes. The cross-sectional optical coherence tomography (OCT) with angiographic flow and retinal thickness map (internal limiting membrane to retinal pigment epithelium) demonstrated superotemporal and temporal thinning (white arrows) in both eyes. The OCT angiography vascular density maps demonstrated corresponding superficial capillary plexus (SCP) and deep capillary plexus (DCP) flow loss in the superotemporal and temporal quadrants (red arrows) in both eyes. The extent of flow loss was more extensive in the deep than superficial capillary plexus.

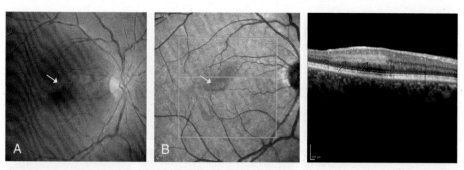

FIGURE 17.2 A 29-year-old man with HbSS disease presented with acute decrease in vision in the right eye. Visual acuity was 20/30. A, Fundus photography revealed a placoid-shaped area of retinal whitening in the superior juxtafoveal region (white arrow). B, This corresponded to an area of hyporeflectivity on the en-face infrared image (yellow arrow), and hyperreflectivity predominantly in the inner nuclear layer (red arrows). These findings were consistent with paracentral acute middle maculopathy.

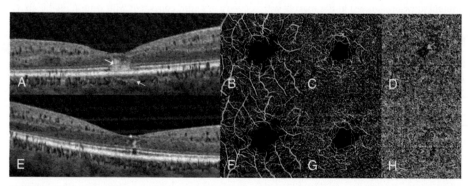

FIGURE 17.3 A 41-year-old man with HbSS disease reported sudden onset of a central scotoma in the right eye. Visual acuity was decreased to 20/63. A, The cross-sectional optical coherence tomography (OCT) with angiographic flow demonstrated foveal hyperreflectivity at the outer nuclear layer with disruption of the external limiting membrane and ellipsoid zone (white arrow) and loss of flow in the choriocapillaris (yellow arrow). OCT angiography of the (B) superficial capillary plexus, (C) deep capillary plexus, and (D) choriocapillaris demonstrates flow loss in the choriocapillaris (green arrow). One year after initial presentation, the patient's scotoma had improved, and his visual acuity was slightly improved to 20/40. E, The cross-sectional OCT with angiographic flow revealed improvement of the outer retinal hyperreflectivity, recovery of the external limiting membrane and ellipsoid zone, and recovery of flow in the choriocapillaris. OCT angiography of the (F) superficial capillary plexus, (G) deep capillary plexus, and (H) choriocapillaris demonstrates improvement of flow in the choriocapillaris. These findings suggest that choriocapillaris flow loss may be involved in the pathogenesis of acute macular neuroretinopathy.

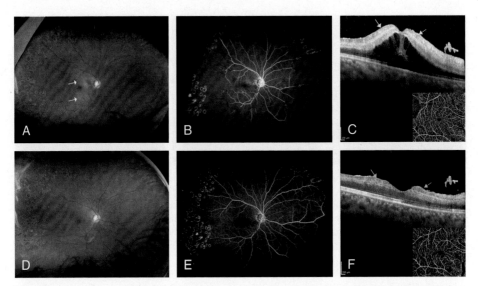

FIGURE 17.4 A 35-year-old man with HbSC disease and a history of stage IV sickle cell retinopathy status post scatter laser photocoagulation in both eyes presented for acute painless visual loss in the right eye. Visual acuity was 20/400. A, Examination and ultra-wide-field fundus photography showed retinal whitening (white arrows) in the macula with a cherry red spot consistent with central retinal artery occlusion. B, Fluorescein angiography at 5 minutes also revealed loss of arterial (red arrows) and venous (blue arrows) flow in the superotemporal macula, and the nasal, inferior and temporal midperiphery. C, Optical coherence tomography (OCT) demonstrated inner retinal thickening and hyperreflectivity (yellow arrows) as well as cystoid macular edema. (Inset) A 6 × 6mm OCT angiography scan of the entire retina also showed loss of superficial and deep capillary plexus flow in the superotemporal macula (purple arrow). The patient received emergent red blood cell exchange transfusion. Two weeks later, he reported subjective visual improvement although acuity had only improved to 20/250. D, Ultra-wide-field photography showed resolution of retinal whitening in the macula. E, Fluorescein angiography at 5 minutes demonstrated reperfusion of the arteries and veins that previously had no flow. F, OCT showed resolution of macular edema and residual inner retinal thinning (green arrows). (Inset) A 6 × 6mm OCT angiography scan of the entire retina showed recovery of superficial and deep capillary plexus flow in the superotemporal macula.

- Flow loss has also been shown to correlate to macula thinning on OCT, worse visual acuity, HbSC genotype, and presence of proliferative sickle cell retinopathy.[9]
- Optical coherence tomography angiography (OCTA) has also been used to show hypoperfusion of the choriocapillaris in sickle cell patients (Figure 17.3).[10]
- Other OCTA findings reported in sickle cell disease patients include foveal avascular zone enlargement, foveal avascular zone contour irregularity, and decreased parafoveal capillary density (Figures 17.4 and 17.5).[7,11]

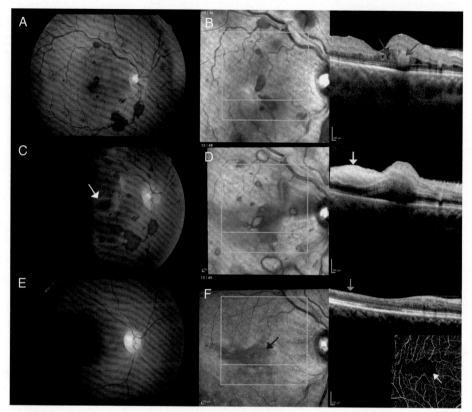

FIGURE 17.5 A 43-year-old woman with HbSS disease presented with acute decrease in vision in the right eye. Visual acuity was hand motions. A, Color photography revealed optic nerve hyperemia, dilated and tortuous vessels, and diffuse intraretinal and subinternal limiting membrane hemorrhages, consistent with a central retinal vein occlusion. B, Optical coherence tomography (OCT) showed intraretinal hyperreflectivity in areas of intraretinal hemorrhage (red arrow) and intraretinal fluid (blue arrow). The patient received emergent exchange transfusion. Five days after initial presentation, her visual acuity improved to 4/200. C, Color photography showed improvement of optic nerve hyperemia, persistent diffuse hemorrhages, and worsening retinal whitening in the macula (white arrow). D, On OCT, there was severe inner retinal hyperreflectivity and thickening (yellow arrow). These findings suggest the interval development of a combined central retinal artery and vein occlusion. Three months after presentation, her visual acuity had improved to 20/160. E, Color photography showed resolution of hemorrhages and retinal whitening and attenuated vasculature. F, OCT illustrated generalized thinning of both the inner and outer retina involving the fovea and temporal macula (orange arrow). (Inset) The en-face 6 × 6mm OCT angiography scan of the entire retina showed an enlarged and irregular foveal avascular zone (white arrow) that matched the shape of an area of hyporeflectivity on the en-face infrared scan (purple arrow).[7] Cai S, Bressler NM. Outcome after exchange transfusion for central retinal vein occlusion associated with extensive capillary and arteriolar nonperfusion in a patient With hemoglobin SS disease. *JAMA Ophthalmology.* 2019; 137 (6).

References

1. Li J, Bender L, Shaffer J, Cohen D, Ying G, Binenbaum G. Prevalence and onset of pediatric sickle cell retinopathy. *Ophthalmology.* 2019;126(7):1000-1006.

2. Ware RE, de Montalemberg M, Tshilolol L, Abboud MR. Sickle cell disease. *Lancet.* 2017;390(10091):311-323.

3. Goldberg M. Classification and pathogenesis of proliferative sickle retinopathy. *Am J Ophthalmol.* 1971;71(3):649-665.

4. Nagpal K, Asdourian GK, Patrianakos D, et al. Proliferative retinopathy in sickle cell trait: report of seven cases. *Arch Intern Med.* 1977;137(3):325-328.

5. Lim JI, Cao D. Analysis of retinal thinning using spectral-domain optical coherence tomography imaging of sickle cell retinopathy eyes compared to age- and race-matched control eyes. *Am J Ophthalmol.* 2018;192:229-238.

6. Martin GC, Denier C, Zambrowski O, et al. Visual function in asymptomatic patients with homozygous sickle cell disease and temporal macular atrophy. *JAMA Ophthalmol.* 2017;135(10):1100-1105.

7. Cai S, Bressler NM, Linz MO, Scott AW. Outcome after exchange transfusion for central retinal vein occlusion associated with extensive capillary and arteriolar nonperfusion in a patient with hemoglobin SS disease. *JAMA Ophthalmol.* 2019;137(6):718-720.

8. Ong S, Linz MO, Liu X, Liu TYA, Han IC, Scott AW. Retinal thickness and microvascular changes in children with sickle cell disease evaluated by optical coherence tomography (OCT) and OCT angiography. *Am J Ophthalmol.* 2019;209:88-98.

9. Han IC, Linz MO, Liu TYA, Zhang AY, Tian J, Scott AW. Correlation of ultra-widefield fluorescein angiography and OCT angiography in sickle cell retinopathy. *Ophthalmol Retina.* 2018;2(6):599-605.

10. Lee SY, Cheng JL, Gehrs KM, et al. Choroidal features of acute macular neuroretinopathy via optical coherence tomography angiography and correlation with serial multimodal imaging. *JAMA Ophthalmol.* 2017;135(11):1177-1183.

11. Lynch G, Scott AW, Linz MO, et al. Foveal avascular zone morphology and parafoveal capillary perfusion in sickle cell retinopathy. *Br J Ophthalmol.* 2019;104(4):473-479.

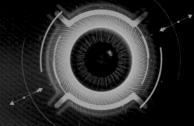

CHAPTER 18

Radiation Retinopathy

SALIENT FEATURES

- Radiation retinopathy (RR), characterized as nonproliferative or proliferative, is a slowly progressive retinal vasculopathy that develops following exposure to ocular irradiation from plaque brachytherapy, external beam radiation, proton beam radiotherapy, helium ion radiotherapy, or gamma knife radiotherapy.[1]
- Clinical features of RR are similar to diabetic retinopathy (DR) and develop typically within 18 months to 3 years after radiation exposure.[1,2]
- Nonproliferative RR features include microaneurysms, cotton wool spots, hemorrhages, vascular occlusion, telangiectasias, exudates, and macular edema (Figure 18.1A).[2]
- In contrast to early pericyte loss in DR, the primary insult in RR is early endothelial cell damage with relative preservation of pericytes.[1,2]
- Endothelial cell loss in capillaries leads to microaneurysm formation, capillary occlusion with ischemia, and telangiectatic vessels or collateral vasculature at the edges of capillary occlusions.[1,2]
- Proliferative RR can develop secondary to retinal ischemia. This is characterized by retinal neovascularization with possible neovascular glaucoma, vitreous hemorrhage, and/or tractional retinal detachment.[3]

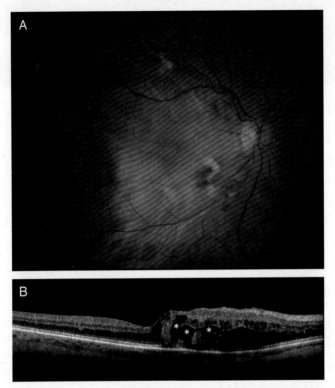

FIGURE 18.1 A, Fundus photograph of the right eye with nonproliferative radiation retinopathy (RR) 18 months after plaque brachytherapy for choroidal melanoma–displaying hemorrhages, cotton wool spots, and microaneurysms. B, Corresponding foveal optical coherence tomography (OCT) image showing cystoid macular edema with intraretinal fluid (white asterisks).

OCT IMAGING

- Optical coherence tomography (OCT) allows for the identification of macular edema, one of the earliest signs of RR.[4]
- Macular edema can comprise of intraretinal fluid, visualized as hyporeflective cystoid spaces within the retina on OCT (Figure 18.1B), and/or subretinal fluid, visualized as hyporeflective spaces between the retina and retinal pigment epithelium on OCT. When macular edema is severe, there may be loss of the foveal contour.[4]
- Cotton wool spots, ischemic infarcts of the nerve fiber layer, manifest as inner retinal hyperreflective areas within the nerve fiber layer (see NPDR chapter).[5]

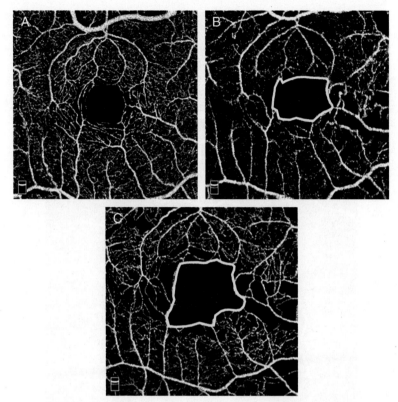

FIGURE 18.2 A. 3 × 3mm macular optical coherence tomography angiogram (OCTA) of the right eye prior to plaque brachytherapy surgery with normal foveal avascular zone (FAZ). B, Eighteen months following plaque brachytherapy, there is an increase in the FAZ (yellow outline). C, Further increase in the FAZ is seen at postoperative month 24 (yellow outline).

- Hard exudates or lipid deposits that accumulate in the neural retina due to loss of retina vessel integrity can be seen as bright, hyperreflective lesions with sharp borders on OCT (see NPDR chapter).[6]
- RR with severe ischemia and/or prolonged macular edema can lead to retinal atrophy and photoreceptor loss on OCT (see NPDR chapter).[6]

OCTA

- Optical coherence tomography angiography (OCTA) can demonstrate subclinical early microvascular changes in the capillary network that are not yet visible clinically or on OCT.[7]
- A decrease in the capillary density in the superficial and/or deep capillary plexuses with an increase in the foveal avascular zone (FAZ) can

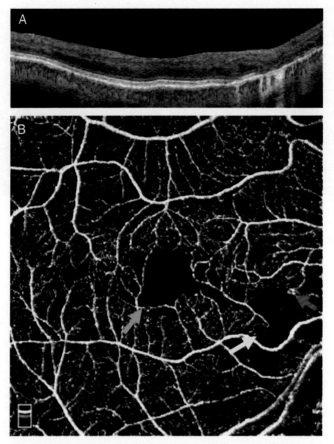

FIGURE 18.3 En-face superficial retina segmentation slabs from 6 × 6 macular optical coherence tomography angiogram (OCTA) image demonstrating fusiform dilatation of a capillary consistent with a microaneurysm (A and B, red arrow). In addition, there is an increase in the foveal avascular zone (FAZ) (green arrow) and loss of capillary density (yellow arrow).

be demonstrated on OCTA in patients with RR (Figure 18.2A-C). The area and diameter of the FAZ have been shown to be enlarged compared to fellow nonirradiated eyes.[7]

- OCTA may show the presence of microaneurysms (Figure 18.3A and B) and telangiectatic vessels (Figure 18.4).[7]
- When the peripapillary retina is exposed to high doses of radiation, a decrease in peripapillary capillary density can be seen on OCTA (Figure 18.5).[8] The decrease in peripapillary capillary density is greater in the hemiretina of radiation treatment (Figure 18.5).[8]

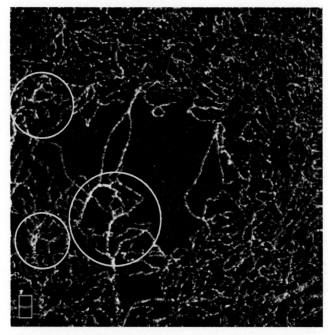

FIGURE 18.4 En-face deep retina segmentation slabs from 3 × 3 macular optical coherence tomography angiogram (OCTA) image showing irregular vasculature consistent with telangiectasias (yellow circles) and areas of decrease in capillary density.

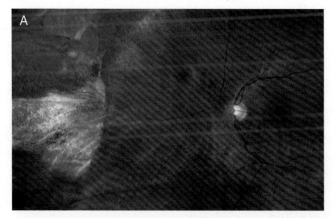

FIGURE 18.5 A, Wide-field fundus photograph of the left eye showing a regressed-appearing superonasal choroidal melanoma after plaque brachytherapy treatment. There is chorioretinal atrophy inferior to the lesion and significant secondary and tertiary vessel dropout in the nasal hemiretina. B, En-face superficial retina slab from a 3 × 3 optic nerve head optical coherence tomography angiogram (OCTA) image demonstrates a decrease in peripapillary capillary density that is more significant in the irradiated nasal hemiretina compared to the temporal hemiretina.

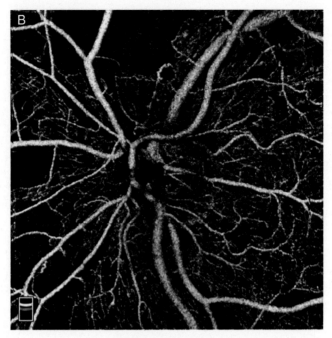

FIGURE 18.5 Cont'd

References

1. Krema H, Xu W, Payne D, Vasquez LM, Pavlin CJ, Simpson R. Factors predictive of radiation retinopathy post 125 Iodine brachytherapy for uveal melanoma. *Can J Ophthalmol.* 2011;46(2):158-163.

2. Spielberg L, De Potter P, Leys A. Radiation retinopathy. In: Ryan SJ, ed. *Retina.* 2nd ed. St Louis: Mosby; 1994:1083-1090.

3. Biancitto C, Shields CL, Pirondini C, Mashayekhi A, Furuta M, Shields JA. Proliferative radiation retinopathy after plaque radiotherapy for uveal melanoma. *Ophthalmology.* 2010;117:1005-1012.

4. Horgan N, Shields CL, Mashayekhi A, Teixeira LF, Materin MA, Shields JA. Early macular morphological changes following plaque radiotherapy for uveal melanoma. *Retina.* 2008;28:263-273.

5. Kozak I, Bartsch DU, Cheng L, Freeman WR. In vivo histology of cotton wool spots using high resolution optical coherence tomography. *Am J Ophthalmol.* 2006;141:748-750.

6. Srinivas S, Nittala MG, Hariri A, et al. Quantification of intraretinal hard exudates in eyes with diabetic retinopathy by optical coherence tomography. *Retina.* 2018;38(2):231-236.

7. Shields CL, Say EAT, Samara WA, Khoo CTL, Mashayekhi A, Shields JA. Optical coherence tomography angiography of the macula after plaque radiotherapy of choroidal melanoma. *Retina.* 2016;36:1493-1505.

8. Skalet AH, Liu L, Binder C, et al. Quantitative OCT angiography evaluation of peripapillary retinal circulation after plaque brachytherapy. *Ophthalmol Retina.* 2018;2(3):244-250.

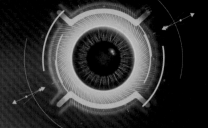

CHAPTER 19

Hypertensive Retinopathy

SALIENT FEATURES

- Hypertensive retinopathy develops when retinal vascular damage occurs secondary to either hypertensive emergency acutely or chronically elevated blood pressure.
- Hypertensive retinopathy may be asymptomatic or, in acute crisis, can present with new-onset symptoms, including blurred vision and visual field defects.[1]
- Slit-lamp examination may reveal cotton wool spots, flame-shaped hemorrhage, exudates, arteriolar narrowing, Elschnig spots, subretinal fluid, pigment epithelial detachments, and papilledema. Less commonly with severe ischemia, retinal neovascularization may develop.[1]
- Microvascular retinal changes during chronic hypertension occur prior to most reporting of visual symptoms.[1]

OCT FEATURES

- Hypertension is associated with inner retinal atrophy/thinning.[2]
  - Thinning of the ganglion cell inner plexiform layer in hypertensive eyes correlates with decrease in retinal blood flow per optical coherence tomography angiography (OCTA).
  - Peripapillary retinal nerve fiber layer (RNFL) and central macular thickness in eyes manifesting significant ischemia are significantly reduced.

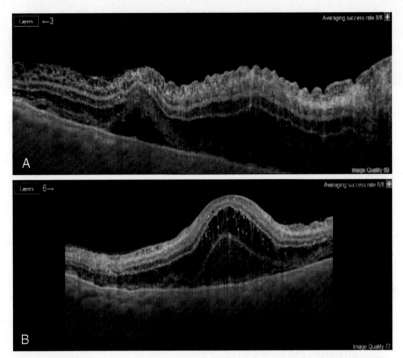

FIGURE 19.1 (A and B) Swept-source optical coherence tomography (SS-OCT) with macular subretinal fluid, solid hyperreflective deposits overlying the retinal pigment epitheium (RPE) and splitting of the ganglion cell and nerve fiber layer with retinal irregularity. (Reprinted with permission from Rotsos T, Andreanos K, Blounas S, Brouzas D, Ladas DS, Ladas ID. Multimodal imaging of hypertensive chorioretinopathy by swept-source optical coherence tomography and optical coherence tomography angiography: case report. *Medicine (Baltimore)*. 2017;96(39):e8110.)

- Cotton wool spots are hyperreflective on optical coherence tomography (OCT), a finding which may persist on imaging even after they become unobservable on examination. Focal thinning in the RNFL and inner retina may be noted following cotton wool spot resolution.
- In hypertensive emergency, OCT can show well-described features such as subretinal fluid and hyperreflective fibrin deposits overlying the RPE (Figure 19.1).[4]
- Severe acute hypertension may result in subretinal fluid accumulation, retinal layer splitting (ie, retinoschisis), and eventual exudative retinal detachment (Figures 19.1 and 19.2).[6]
- Outer retinal atrophy with ellipsoid zone loss and outer nuclear layer thinning may develop following resolution of subretinal fluid, particularly in areas of choroidal atrophy (Figure 19.3).

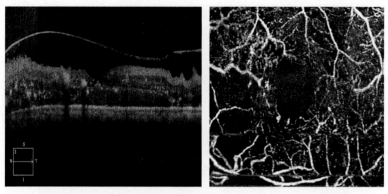

FIGURE 19.2 Spectral-domain optical coherence tomography (SD-OCT) B-scan showing macular subretinal fluid with hyperreflective deposits with corresponding 3 × 3 retinal slab optical coherence tomography angiography (OCTA) demonstrating diffuse ischemia secondary to malignant hypertensive retinopathy.

OCTA IMAGING

- OCTA allows for observation of such pathological retina distortions in addition to quantifying hypertension-induced retinal ischemia and arteriolar narrowing (Figure 19.2).[2]
- Flow void areas can be visualized in the choriocapillaris in acute HTNR (Figure 19.4).
- Patients with HTNR and chronic hypertension without observable retinopathy both show decreased macular vessel and perfusion densities and increased foveal avascular zones compared to healthy controls.

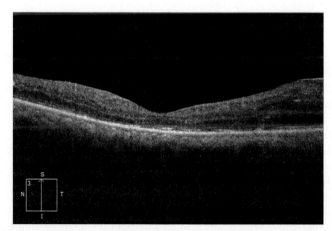

FIGURE 19.3 Macular optical coherence tomography (OCT) B-scan of same eye from Figure 19.2 demonstrating retinal thinning and outer retinal loss after resolution of subretinal fluid with improved blood pressure control.

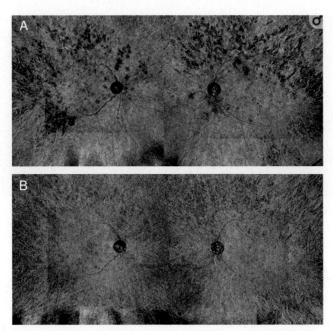

FIGURE 19.4 Swept-source optical coherence tomography angiography (SS-OCTA) showing flow voids in the choriocapillaris slab on initial presentation during acute hypertensive episode (A) showing significant improvement of vascular flow at 1 month (B). (Reprinted with permission from Rezkallah A, Kodjikian L, Abukhashabah A, Denis P, Mathis T. Hypertensive choroidopathy: multimodal imaging and the contribution of wide-field swept-source oct-angiography. *Am J Ophthalmol Case Rep.* 2019;13:131-135.)

References

1. Lee WH, Park J-H, Won Y, et al. Retinal microvascular change in hypertension as measured by optical coherence tomography angiography. *Sci Rep.* 2019;9:156. doi:10.1038/s41598-018-36474-1.

2. Donati S, Maresca AM, Cattaneo J, et al. Optical coherence tomography angiography and arterial hypertension: a role in identifying subclinical microvascular damage? *Eur J Ophthalmol.* 2019:1120672119880390. doi:10.1177/1120672119880390.

3. Lim HB, Lee MW, Park JH, Kim K, Jo YJ, Kim JY. Changes in ganglion cell–inner plexiform layer thickness and retinal microvasculature in hypertension: an optical coherence tomography angiography study. *Am J Ophthalmol.* 2019;199:167-176.

4. Suzuki M, Minamoto A, Yamane K, Uka J, Aoki S, Mishima HK. Malignant hypertensive retinopathy studied with optical coherence tomography. *Retina.* 2005;25(3):383-384.

5. Kozak I, Bartsch DU, Cheng L, Freeman WR. In vivo histology of cotton-wool spots using high-resolution optical coherence tomography. *Am J Ophthalmol.* 2006;141(4):748-750.

6. Rotsos T, Andreanos K, Blounas S, Brouzas D, Ladas DS, Ladas ID. Multimodal imaging of hypertensive chorioretinopathy by swept-source optical coherence tomography and optical coherence tomography angiography: case report. *Medicine (Baltimore)*. 2017;96(39):e8110.

7. Lee HM, Lee WH, Kim KN, Jo YJ, Kim JY. Changes in thickness of central macula and retinal nerve fibre layer in severe hypertensive retinopathy: a 1-year longitudinal study. *Acta Ophthalmol*. 2018;96(3):e386-e392.

8. Shukla D, Ramchandani B, Vignesh TP, Rajendran A, Neelakantan N. Localized serous retinal detachment of macula as a marker of malignant hypertension. *Ophthalmic Surg Lasers Imaging*. 2010;1-7.

9. Rezkallah A, Kodjikian L, Abukhashabah A, Denis P, Mathis T. Hypertensive choroidopathy: multimodal imaging and the contribution of wide-field swept-source oct-angiography. *Am J Ophthalmol Case Rep*. 2019;13:131-135.

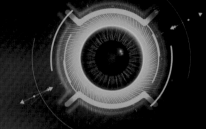

CHAPTER 20

Preeclampsia

SALIENT FEATURES

- Preeclampsia is a multisystemic syndrome specific to pregnancy, a leading cause of maternal and neonatal morbidity and mortality with complex relations to various organs and systems of the body.
- Ocular findings include retinopathy, optic neuropathy, retinal edema, subretinal fluid, retinal hemorrhages, Elschnig spots, cotton wool spots, segmental or generalized constriction of the retinal arterioles, and exudative retinal detachment.
- Preeclampsia usually presents in the third trimester of the pregnancy. Visual symptoms are considered a manifestation of severe preeclampsia.
- Pathological retinal characteristics and proximity of the lesions to the fovea predict visual symptoms.
- Fundus photographs can show decreased retinal arterial-to-vein ratio.
- Fluorescien angiography (FA) has been used to evaluate the vascular findings of preeclampsia in the retina, but due to the dye-based injection requirement, noninvasive imaging is often preferred during pregnancy.

OCT IMAGING

- Optical coherence tomography (OCT) provides a noninvasive means to image the retina in pregnant patients without risk to the fetus.
- OCT findings are variable and may include foveal contour flattening, diffuse intraretinal edema that slowly resolves postpartum, subretinal fluid, serous retinal detachments, photoreceptor layer disruption, highly reflective retinal pigment epithelium (RPE) with thickened choriocapillaris, and V-shaped adhesions disrupting the outer retina reflecting Elschnig spots (Figures 20.1 and 20.2)

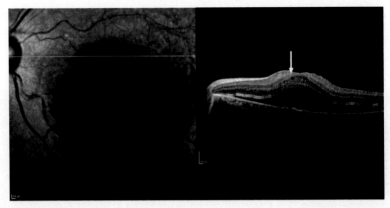

FIGURE 20.1 Preeclampsia-induced serous retinal detachment with intraretinal cysts (white arrow) and macular thickening.

- Choroidal and retinal nerve fiber layer (RNFL) thickness changes from normal pregnancy may also be observed in preeclampsia.
  - Pregnancy is associated with increased choroidal thickness compared to nonpregnant women, but preeclamptic women have a less increase in choroidal thickening. This difference has been attributed to preeclampsia-related systemic vascular vasospasm.
  - RNFL thickening has also been described in preeclampsia and may reflect subclinical involvement of the central nervous system in their disease.

OCTA IMAGING

- Even without visible abnormal findings on slit-lamp examination, optical coherence tomography angiography (OCTA) has demonstrated microvascular changes.
- Preeclampsia is associated with decreased superficial and deep foveal vascular density compared to healthy women who were not pregnant.

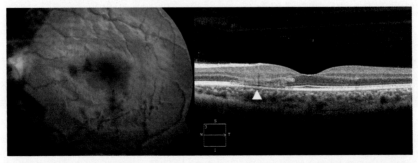

FIGURE 20.2 Fundus photograph in preeclampsia demonstrating optic disc and retinal hemorrhages, as well as possible alterations in appearance of the choroid/outer retina (left). Optical coherence tomography (OCT) demonstrating outer retinal disruption with increased reflectivity of the outer nuclear layer (ONL) and ellipsoid zone (EZ) loss (arrowhead, right). This may be consistent with focal choroidal ischemia.

- Other reports have identified decreased choriocapillaris and optic disc flow in preeclamptic women compared to healthy pregnant women but no abnormalities in other layers (Figure 20.3).

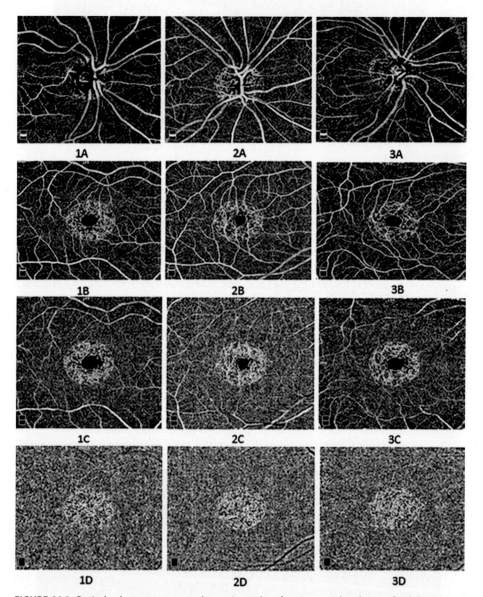

FIGURE 20.3 Optical coherence tomography angiography of optic nerve head, superficial-deep blood flow area, and choriocapillaris blood flow area of patients in three different groups. (1) Preeclamptic pregnant women. (2) Healthy pregnant women. (3) Control nonpregnant women. (Reprinted with permission from Urfalıoglu S, Bakacak M, Özdemir G, Güler M, Beyoglu A, Arslan G. Posterior ocular blood flow in preeclamptic patients evaluated with optical coherence tomography angiography. *Pregnancy Hypertens*. 2019;17:203-208.)

References

1. Ataş M, Açmaz G, Aksoy H, et al. Evaluation of the macula, retinal nerve fiber layer and choroid in preeclampsia, healthy pregnant and healthy non-pregnant women using spectral-domain optical coherence tomography. *Hypertens Pregnancy*. 2014;33(3):299-310. doi:10.3109/10641955.2013.877924.
2. Neudorfer M, Spierer O, Goder M, et al. The prevalence of retinal and optical coherence tomography findings in preeclamptic women. *Retina*. 2014;34(7):1376-1383. doi:10.1097/IAE.0000000000000085.
3. AlTalbishi AA, Khateb S, Amer R. Elschnig's spots in the acute and remission stages in preeclampsia: spectral-domain optical coherence tomographic features. *Eur J Ophthalmol*. 2015;25(5):e84-e87.
4. Theodossiadis PG, Kollia AK, Gogas P, Panagiotidis D, Moschos M, Theodossiadis GP. Retinal disorders in preeclampsia studied with optical coherence tomography. *Am J Ophthalmol*. 2002;133(5):707-709.
5. Sayin N, Kara N, Pirhan D, et al. Subfoveal choroidal thickness in preeclampsia: comparison with normal pregnant and nonpregnant women. *Semin Ophthalmol*. 2014;29(1):11-17.
6. Ciloglu E, Okcu NT, Dogan NÇ. Optical coherence tomography angiography findings in preeclampsia. *Eye*. 2019;33(12):1946-1951.
7. Urfalıoglu S, Bakacak M, Özdemir G, Güler M, Beyoglu A, Arslan G. Posterior ocular blood flow in preeclamptic patients evaluated with optical coherence tomography angiography. *Pregnancy Hypertens*. 2019;17:203-208.

Part 3
Outer Retinal and Choroidal Disease

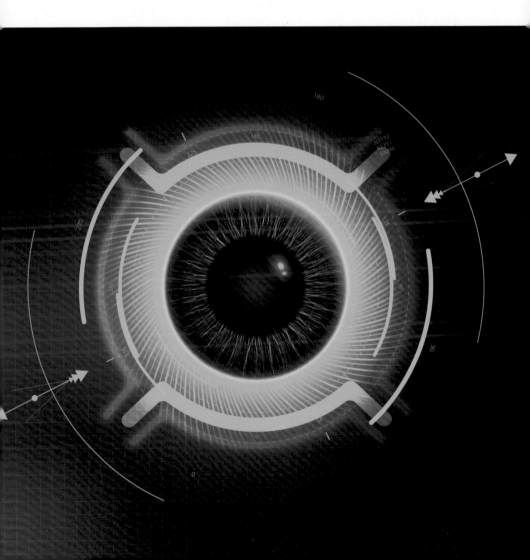

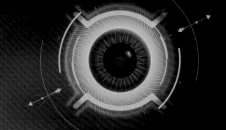

CHAPTER 21

Nonexudative Age-Related Macular Degeneration

SALIENT FEATURES

- Nonexudative age-related macular degeneration (AMD), otherwise known as "dry AMD," is associated with the presence of small deposits (ie, drusen), under the macula, and areas of retinal pigment epithelium (RPE) loss and outer retinal atrophy in the more advanced stages.[1,4]
- AMD is a leading cause of central vision loss worldwide.[4]
- Currently, there is no therapeutic for reversing dry AMD, but results from the AREDS and AREDS 2 clinical trials indicated that increased antioxidant and zinc intake were associated with reduced risk of progression to late-stage AMD.[3]
- Late-stage AMD may progress to neovascular AMD (see Chapter 21) and/or atrophy of photoreceptive layers (ie, geographic atrophy [GA]).
- GA is the concurrent atrophy/loss of the RPE, photoreceptors, and choriocapillaris and can cause significant irreversible vision loss.[5]
- Decreased choriocapillaris flow has been associated with progression of dry AMD.[4]
- With the advent of optical coherence tomography angiography (OCTA), a new entity has been described: neovascular nonexudative AMD. In these eyes, a choroidal neovascular complex is present on OCTA but is quiescent without any evidence of exudation (eg, intraretinal fluid, subretinal fluid).

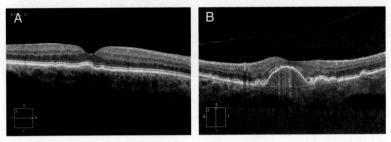

FIGURE 21.1 Optical coherence tomography (OCT) for dry age-related macular degeneration (AMD). Drusen results in retinal pigment epithelium (RPE) deflections that may be mild (A) or signficant (B) with associated pigment epithelial detachment and overlying ellipsoid zone (EZ) loss.

OCT IMAGING

- A hallmark diagnostic feature includes the RPE deflections related to drusen deposits (Figure 21.1). Overall, drusen burden may be a risk factor for progression and may be best documented on optical coherence tomography (OCT).
- Early outer retinal attenuation and loss of ellipsoid zone may be identified in eyes overlying drusen or in areas of early atrophy.
- Complete GA can be identified by attenuation of the ellipsoid zone (EZ) and loss of the RPE (Figures 21.2 and 21.3). This is associated with increased transmission and "illumination" of the underlying choroid due to the decreased attenuation from the loss of the retinal layers and RPE.
- Multiple potential imaging biomarkers have been identified that may result in increased risk of progression to advanced disease,

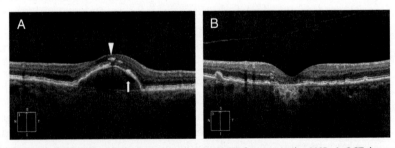

FIGURE 21.2 Predictive optical coherence tomography (OCT) features in dry AMD. A, OCT demonstrates inwardly migrating hyperreflective foci (arrowhead), heterogeneity within the pigment epithelial detachment (arrow), and large drusen volume and area. No choroidal neovascularization (CNV) was identified on optical coherence tomography angiography (OCTA) or fluorescein angiogram (FA). B, These features have all been identified as risk factors for progression to atrophy. As demonstrated in this case, subfoveal atrophy develops of both the retinal pigment epithelium (RPE) and ellipsoid zone (EZ) with collapse of the large pigment epithelial detachment.

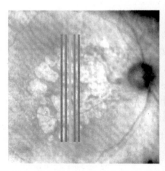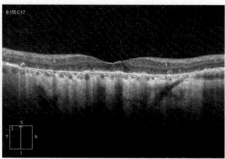

FIGURE 21.3 Late-stage age-related macular degeneration (AMD) can manifest as geographic atrophy corresponding to the near-infrared image (left). On optical coherence tomography (OCT), geographic atrophy consists of the loss of the choriocapillaris, retinal pigment epithelium (RPE), ellipsoid zone (EZ), and outer nuclear layer (ONL) (right). Bruch membrane remains. Increased transmission of the OCT signal to the choroid results in greater visualization of the choroid details (ie, brighter signal) as noted in this signal diffusely across the macula. A small island of subfoveal RPE preservation appears to be present.

including hyperreflective foci (thought to represent pigment migration), increased heterogeneity of reflectivity signal within a drusen, and larger drusen volume/area (Figure 21.2).

- In areas of GA, Bruch membrane maybe be hyperreflective due to loss of overlying RPE.
- OCT has been the gold standard for detecting intraretinal or subretinal fluid that may be indicative of conversion to neovascular AMD. The "double-layer" sign is also strongly associated with underlying inactive choroidal neovascularization (Figures 21.4 and 21.7).

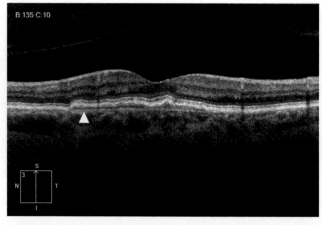

FIGURE 21.4 Double-layer sign on optical coherence tomography (OCT) showing retinal pigment epithelium (RPE) and Bruch membrane (BM) (arrowhead) represents inactive (ie, nonexudative neovascular AMD) choroidal neovascularization.

OCTA IMAGING

- Reduced flow of choriocapillaris, known as flow voids, can be identified as darkened spots on the en-face image (Figure 21.5).[5]
- *En-face* images of eyes with GA demonstrate loss of choriocapillaris with associated prominent large choroidal vessels that may be mistaken for choroidal neovascularization (Figure 21.6).[4,5]
- OCTA is frequently used to evaluate for possible underlying inactive choroidal neovascularization that may suggest neovascular nonexudative AMD (Figure 21.7).

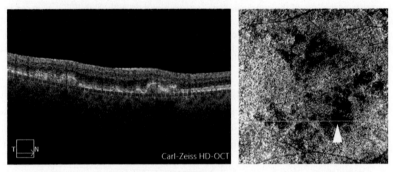

FIGURE 21.5 Flow voids in the choriocapillaris caused by drusen (arrowhead).

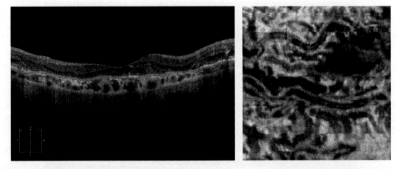

FIGURE 21.6 Optical coherence tomography (OCT) and optical coherence tomography angiography (OCTA) of a patient with geographic atrophy. OCT demonstrates diffuse outer retinal loss. OCTA demonstrates robust visualization of the large choroidal vessels on the en-face choroid slab due to increased transmission of signal and loss of the overlying choriocapillaris.

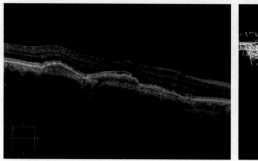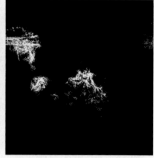

FIGURE 21.7 Optical coherence tomography (OCT) and optical coherence tomography angiography (OCTA) of a patient with inactive choroidal neovascularization indicative of neovascular nonexudative age-related macular degeneration (AMD). OCTA (right) provides excellent visualization of the underlying choroidal neovascularization (CNV).

References

1. Christenbury JG, Folgar FA, O'Connell RV, Chiu SJ, Farsiu S, Toth CA. Age-related eye disease study 2 ancillary spectral domain optical coherence tomography study group. Progression of intermediate age-related macular degeneration with proliferation and inner retinal migration of hyperreflective foci. *Ophthalmology*. 2013;120(5):1038-1045.

2. Veerappan M, El-Hage-Sleiman AK, Tai V, et al. Optical coherence tomography reflective drusen substructures predict progression to geographic atrophy in age-related macular degeneration. *Ophthalmology*. 2016;123(12):2554-2570.

3. Sleiman K, Veerappan M, Winter KP, et al. Optical coherence tomography predictors of risk for progression to non-neovascular atrophic age-related macular degeneration. *Ophthalmology*. 2017;124(12):1764-1777.

4. Sadda SR, Guymer R, Holz FG, et al. Consensus definition for atrophy associated with age-related macular degeneration on OCT: classification of atrophy report 3. *Ophthalmology*. 2018;125(4):537-548.

5. Arya M, Sabrosa AS, Duker JS, Waheed NK. Choriocapillaris changes in dry age-related macular degeneration and geographic atrophy: a review. *Eye Vis*. 2018;5(1):22.

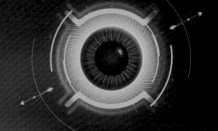

CHAPTER 22

Subretinal Drusenoid Deposits

SALIENT FEATURES

- Subretinal drusenoid deposits (SDDs), also known as reticular pseudodrusen, are aggregations of material that exist inside the retinal pigment epithelium (RPE). These deposits may penetrate internally through the ellipsoid zone (EZ).
- SDDs are associated with type 3 neovascularization, outer retinal atrophy, and progression to geographic atrophy.
- Often regression of SDDs may result in the development of outer retinal atrophy.
- Occurs most commonly in advanced age groups. These SDDs are frequently associated with age-related macular degeneration (AMD) and age-related choroidal atrophy.

OCT IMAGING

- SDDs appear on optical coherence tomography (OCT) imaging as small elevations of material resting on top of the RPE. These accumulations are often isoreflective with the RPE and can be fairly subtle on imaging. This is in contrast to drusen which are under the RPE but above the Bruch membrane (see Chapter 21).
- On OCT imaging, SDDs may be accompanied with EZ loss around the peak of the material deposit and also may be associated with outer retinal thinning.
- Other concurrent associated signs may also be noted including peripapillary atrophy and choroidal thinning.
- Choroidal neovascularization and geographic atrophy may also be associated with the presence of SDDs.

OCTA IMAGING

- Compared to conventional drusen, SDDs of the same size demonstrate increased flow voids/nonperfusion within the choriocapillaris, providing a possible mechanistic explanation for worse visual deficits in AMD patients with SDDs compared to those without.
- In areas of choriocapillaris density defects, ghostlike vessels may be observed in a subset of patients with SDD.
- In optical coherence tomography angiography (OCTA) B-scan overlays, SDDs frequently exhibit pseudoflow hypothesized to be secondary to intact overlying vascular plexus reflecting off the drusen or z-axial micromotion resulting in projection artifact.

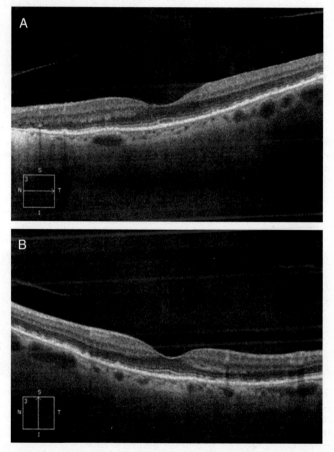

FIGURE 22.1 Optical coherence tomography (OCT) images at the fovea of a patient with reticular pseudodrusen/subretinal drusenoid deposits (SDDs). A, Note the periodic elevations of material which appear as hyperreflective material extending from the retinal pigment epithelium (RPE). B, Illustrates a B-scan of this patient near the fovea. Here, the SDDs occur temporally and are less severe.

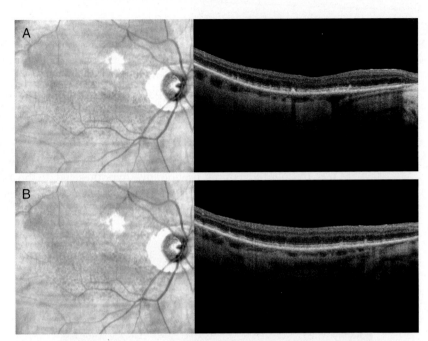

FIGURE 22.2 Optical coherence tomography (OCT) images of reticular pseudodrusen. A, Note the instances of material build-up on the retinal pigment epithelium (RPE). These aggregations appear triangular in shape and penetrate through the ellipsoid zone (EZ). This EZ penetration also causes the external limiting membrane (ELM) to slightly elevate. B, Portrays a second B-scan of this patient where subretinal drusenoid deposits (SDDs) periodically occur and extend through the EZ.

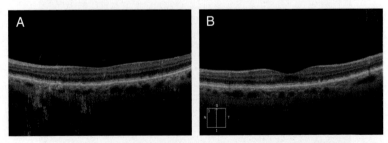

FIGURE 22.3 Optical coherence tomography (OCT) B-scans of patient with subretinal drusenoid deposits (SDDs). One noticeable SDD occurs temporally (A). Note the retinal pigment epithelium (RPE) maintains the same contour through this elevation, as the material deposit appears to rest on top of it. In this case, the SDD penetrates through the ellipsoid zone (EZ), and external limiting membrane (ELM) integrity is lost. B, Reticular pseudodrusen appears as shallower, less intense deposits of material slightly extending past the EZ.

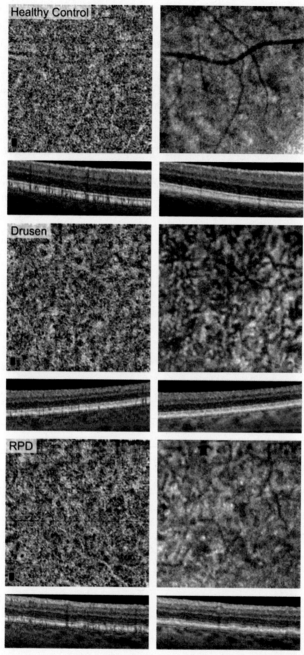

FIGURE 22.4 Optical coherence tomography angiography (OCTA) *en-face* images of choriocapillaris (left) and *en-face* structural optical coherence tomography (OCT) (right) in a healthy eye, early age-related macular degeneration (AMD) eye, and reticular pseudodrusen (subretinal drusenoid deposits [SDD]) eye demonstrating flow voids in the AMD and SDD eyes. (Reprinted with permission from Nesper PL, Soetikno BT, Fawzi AA. Choriocapillaris nonperfusion is associated with poor visual acuity in eyes with reticular pseudodrusen. *Am J Ophthalmol.* 2017;174:42-55.)

References

1. Spaide RF, Ooto S, Curcio CA. "Subretinal drusenoid deposits AKA pseudodrusen." *Surv Ophthalmol.* 2018;63(6):782-815. doi:10.1016/j. survophthal.2018.05.005.

2. Chatziralli I, Theodossiadis G, Panagiotidis D, Pousoulidi P, Theodossiadis P. Choriocapillaris' alterations in the presence of reticular pseudodrusen compared to drusen: study based on OCTA findings. *Int Ophthalmol.* 2018;38. (5):1887-1893.

3. Hou KK, Au A, Kashani AH, Freund KB, Sadda SR, Sarraf D. Pseudoflow with OCT angiography in eyes with hard exudates and macular drusen. *Transl Vis Sci Technol.* 2019;8(3):50.

4. Nesper PL, Soetikno BT, Fawzi AA. Choriocapillaris nonperfusion is associated with poor visual acuity in eyes with reticular pseudodrusen. *Am J Ophthalmol.* 2017;174:42-55.

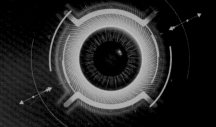

CHAPTER **23**

Neovascular Age-Related Macular Degeneration

SALIENT FEATURES

- Age-related macular degeneration (AMD) is the most common cause of visual impairment in patients older than of 55 years in industrialized countries.[1]
- Neovascular AMD (NVAMD) is characterized by growth of abnormal blood vessels (neovascularization) originating from the choroid or retina, leading to hemorrhage, exudation, and subretinal scarring and subsequent vision loss.
- The historical gold standard for initial diagnosis of choroidal neovascularization (CNV) in NVAMD is fluorescein angiography (FA). CNV may be classified as classic or occult based on the fluorescence pattern.
  - Classic CNV shows an early well-demarcated area of hyperfluorescence that progressively increases in size and intensity.
  - Occult CNV shows a mid-phase or late-phase speckled hyperfluorescence with or without progressive leakage.
- However, optical coherence tomography (OCT) has become the most common test for diagnosing NVAMD and associated exudation with optical coherence tomography angiography (OCTA) also increasing in popularity for identifying neovascularization.
- An OCT-based CNV classification system has also been described.
  - Type 1: new vessel growth from under the retinal pigment epithelium (RPE).
  - Type 2: new vessel proliferation between the RPE and neurosensory retina.
  - Type 3: new vessel proliferation originating from within the retina with anastomoses with choroidal circulation (also known as retinal angiomatous proliferation [RAP]).

OCT IMAGING

- Characteristic finding of AMD includes drusen, which are seen as RPE elevations with sub-RPE material.
- The transition to NVAMD is heralded by the development of intraretinal fluid and/or subretinal fluid, reflective of active exudation (Figures 23.1-23.3).
- NVAMD OCT findings may include RPE detachments (pigment epithelial detachment [PED]), RPE tears, subretinal fluid, intraretinal fluid, and fibrovascular scarring (Figures 23.1 and 23.2).[2]
- Type 1 CNV (occult CNV) may present as thickened elevated RPE or a PED with serous or fibrovascular sub-RPE material.
- Type 2 CNV (classic CNV) shows a hyperreflective fibrovascular lesion above the RPE typically with intraretinal cystic spaces. Borders of the lesion are irregular often with associated outer retinal hyperreflectivity.
- Type 3 CNV (RAP) often demonstrates sub-RPE CNV with intraretinal neovascularization (ie, intraretinal hyperreflectivity), associated with intraretinal cystic changes.
- OCT is the standard diagnostic tool for evaluating treatment response and need for therapy.
- Outer retinal tubulation (ORT) may also be identified as hyperreflective cystic changes that do not represent active exudation (Figure 23.4).
- OCT thickness maps may facilitate identification of abnormalities within the macula based on automated segmentation with change analysis providing comparative assessment for stability, improvement, or worsening (Figure 23.5).

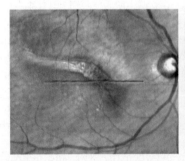
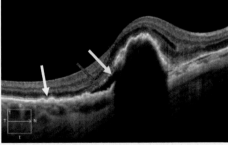

FIGURE 23.1 Patient with neovascular age-related macular degeneration (NVAMD) and defect in retinal pigment epithelium (RPE) suggesting an RPE tear (yellow arrow). The edges of the defect are scrolled. Other characteristic findings include drusen (sub-RPE material, white arrow) and subretinal fluid (SRF, red arrow).

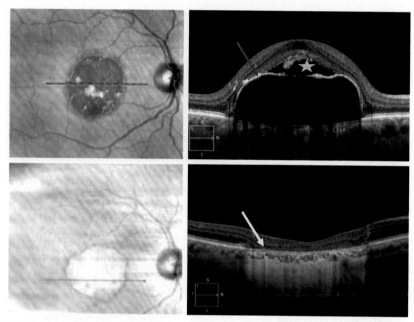

FIGURE 23.2 Patient with very large pigment epithelial detachment (PED, red arrow) and overlying subfoveal subretinal fluid (SRF, green star). Despite anti-vascular endothelial growth factor (anti-VEGF) therapy, the patient had progression of his disease over the next few years with resultant ellipsoid zone loss (yellow arrow) and atrophy of the retinal layers in the area corresponding to the prior PED.

- RPE tears may occur due to disease or as a result of anti–vascular endothelial growth factor (VEGF) therapy. OCT often shows an associated PED and a focal defect in the RPE with RPE scrolling at the defect edge (Figure 23.1). Adjacent RPE may show "pleating."
- Advanced NVAMD will show hyperreflective scarred tissue with retinal atrophy and loss of the ellipsoid zone (Figure 23.6).

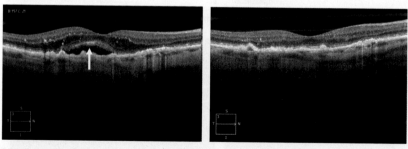

FIGURE 23.3 Left image shows subretinal fluid (SRF, white arrow) and intraretinal fluid (IRF) in a patient with neovascular age-related macular degeneration (NVAMD). The patient demonstrated a near-complete response to anti-vascular endothelial growth factor (anti-VEGF) therapy with resolution of fluid (right image).

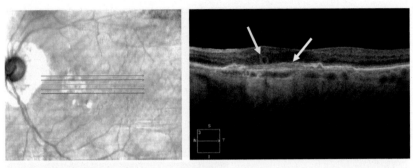

FIGURE 23.4 Outer retinal tubulation (ORT, yellow arrow) and outer retinal atrophy with irregular hyper-reflective sub–retinal pigment epithelium (RPE) material suggestive of choroidal neovascularization (CNV) (white arrow).

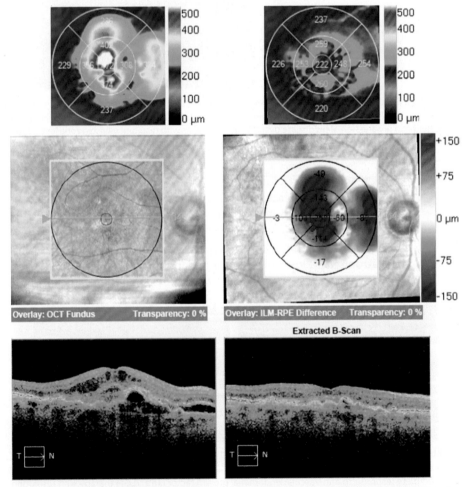

FIGURE 23.5 Change analysis map with thickness maps and corresponding B-scans demonstrating dramatic response to intravitreal anti–vascular endothelial growth factor (anti-VEGF) therapy.

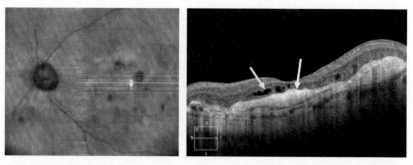

FIGURE 23.6 Large disciform subfoveal scar in a patient with end-stage neovascular age-related macular degeneration (NVAMD, white arrow). Optical coherence tomography (OCT) also shows intraretinal fluid (IRF, yellow arrow) and significant underlying atrophy.

OCTA IMAGING

- CNV may be surrounded by a "dark halo" corresponding to loss of the choriocapillaris and alterations in deep choroidal vessels (Figure 23.7).
- Appearance of CNV on OCTA may vary based on underlying type of CNV.

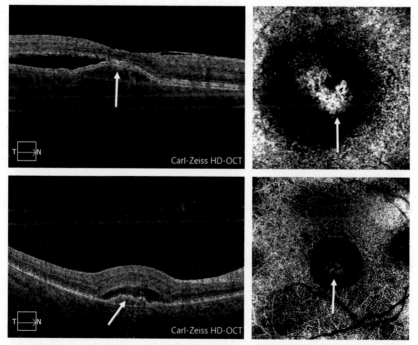

FIGURE 23.7 Optical coherence tomography angiography (OCTA) with perfusion maps of two eyes demonstrating neovascular networks corresponding to choroidal neovascularizations (CNVs) (white arrow) and surrounding dark halo corresponding to characteristic choriocapillaris alterations.

- Type 1 CNV may show a "medusa" form in which smaller vessels radiate from all sides of a main feeder vessel or a "seafan" form in which smaller vessels radiate from one side of a main feeder vessel.[3]
- Type 2 CNV may also show a "medusa" form or a "glomerulus" form. Vessels are connected to a thicker main branch that dive into the choroidal layers.[4]
- Type 3 CNV is characterized by a tuft-shaped vascular network originating from the deep capillary plexus of the outer retinal layer with adjacent telangiectatic vessels.[5]

References

1. Casaroli-Marano R, Gallego-Pinazo R, Fernández-Blanco CT, et al. Age-related macular degeneration: clinical findings following treatment with anti-angiogenic drugs. *J Ophthalmol.* 2014;2014:346-360.
2. Regatieri CV, Branchini L, Duker JS. The role of spectral-domain OCT in the diagnosis and management of neovascular age-related macular degeneration. *Ophthalmic Surg Lasers Imaging.* 2011;42(4):S56-S66.
3. Kuehlewein L, Bansal M, Lenis TL, et al. Optical coherence tomography angiography of type 1 neovascularization in age-related macular degeneration. *Am J Ophthalmol.* 2015;160:739-748.e2.
4. El Ameen A, Cohen SY, Semoun O, et al. Type 2 neovascularization secondary to age-related macular degeneration imaged by optical coherence tomography angiography. *Retina.* 2015;35:2212-2218.
5. Miere A, Querques G, Semoun O, El Ameen A, Capuano V, Souied EH. Optical coherence tomography angiography in early type 3 neovascularization. *Retina.* 2015;35:2236-2241.

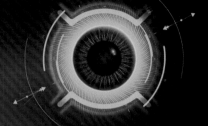

CHAPTER 24

Polypoidal Choroidal Vasculopathy

SALIENT FEATURES

- Polypoidal choroidal vasculopathy (PCV), described by Yannuzzi in 1982, manifests clinically as dilated and branching inner choroidal vessels terminating in reddish-orange aneurysm-like lesions called "polyps" of varying size.[1]
- The disease is more common in pigmented races such as Asians and commonly affects people in the sixth to seventh decade of life. Hypertension is a known systemic association.[1]
- Clinically, it presents as serous and serosanguinous detachments of the neurosensory retina and retinal pigment epithelium (RPE) in the macular and peripapillary area. The disease is broadly classified clinically into hemorrhagic and exudative variants based on the predominant clinical presentation. Spontaneous resolution of acute exudation results in subretinal fibrosis and atrophic degeneration.[1]
- PCV, owing to structural features identified by multimodal imaging, has been recently described as an aneurysmal type 1 neovascularization.[2]
- Indocyanine green angiography (ICG) is the gold standard for disease detection and characterization.
  - Early-phase ICG depicts branching vascular network (BVN) as a well-defined distinct neovascular network in the choroid (Figure 24.1A, white circle and Figure 24.2A, white circle).
  - Polyps appear within the first 6 minutes as hyperfluorescent lesions with a hypofluorescent halo (Figures 24.1B-24.3B, white boxes).

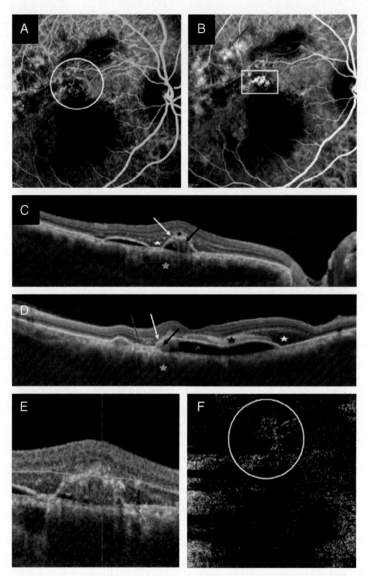

FIGURE 24.1 Multimodal imaging of a patient with polypoidal choroidal vasculopathy (PCV). Indocyanine green angiography shows a well-defined branching vascular network (white circle) in the early phase (A), while the later phase (B) shows a well-defined group of hyperfluorescent polyps (white box) with a subtle hypofluorescent halo. Note the diffuse hyperfluorescence temporally (red arrow) which denotes pachyvessels. Swept-source optical coherence tomography (C and D) depicts signs of active polypoidal choroidal vasculopathy. Horizontal scan passing above the fovea and through the polyps (C) shows a fibrovascular pigment epithelial detachment (PED—white arrow) with hyporeflective polyps under the retinal pigment epithelium (black arrow). The vertical scan (D) shows a QRS complex–shaped PED (white arrow) with fibrovascular and hemorrhagic content (red asterisk). Note the polyp (black arrow) under the PED with the adjoining double-layer sign (red arrow) with hyperreflective content. Both scans show subretinal fluid (white asterisk), subretinal hyperreflective material representing hemorrhage (black asterisk) and features of pachychoroid (blue asterisk). Manually segmented (E; blue lines) optical coherence tomography angiography (OCTA) slab (F) shows a well-defined branching vascular network (white circle) in the trunk pattern.

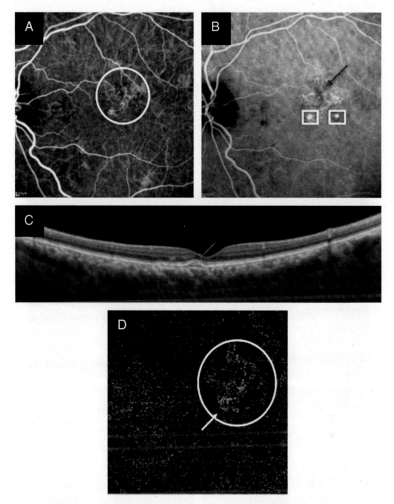

FIGURE 24.2 The fellow eye of the subject in Figure 24.1. Indocyanine green angiography demonstrates a well-defined branching vascular network (white circle) in the early phase (A) and well-defined hyperfluorescent polyps (white boxes) with a hypofluorescent halo in late phase (B). The vascular network shows increasing hyperfluorescence in the late phase, and this is defined as late geographic hyperfluorescence (red arrow). There is no activity on swept-source optical coherence tomography (C). A double-layer sign is noted (red arrow). Optical coherence tomography angiography (OCTA) (D) delineates the branching vascular pattern as glomerulus-like structure (white circle) with a subtle ring-shaped polyp (white arrow).

- In the mid-late ICG phase, choroidal hyperpermeability (Figure 24.1B, red arrow), late leakage from the polyps (Figure 24.2B, white box), and the presence of well-defined geographic hyper fluorescence (Figure 24.2B, red arrow) are noted.[3]

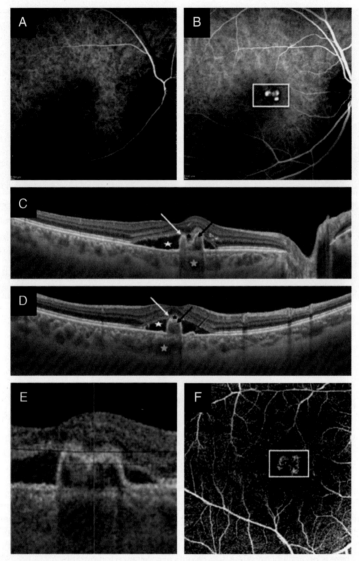

FIGURE 24.3 Multimodal imaging in polypoidal choroidal vasculopathy. Indocyanine green angiography highlights well-defined subfoveal hyperfluorescent polyps that demonstrate a progressive increase in fluorescence from early (A) to mid-phase (B, white box) and are surrounded by a distinct hypofluorescent halo. Swept-source optical coherence tomography (C and D) demonstrates characteristic fibrovascular pigment epithelial detachments (PEDs) with subretinal fluid (white asterisk). The horizontal scan (C) passing through the fovea shows an M-shaped fibrovascular PED (white arrow), while the vertical scan (D) shows a thumb-shaped PED (white arrow). Note the subtle splitting of retinal pigment epithelium from the Bruch membrane (double-layer sign) adjacent to the thumb-shaped PED denoting the branching vascular network (red arrow). Both scans detect polyps as subtle hyporeflective lesions under the PED (black arrows). Subretinal hyperreflective material is noted at the apices of the PED in both scans (black asterisk). Choroid under the PED shows thickening compared to the adjacent uninvolved area (blue asterisk). Manually segmented (E; blue lines) optical coherence tomography angiography (OCTA) slab (F) demonstrates the polyps as a cluster of increased flow-signal (white box). A peaked PED has resulted in polyps being detected in the superficial retinal slab.

OCT IMAGING

- Intraretinal and subretinal fluid (Figure 24.1C and D, white asterisk and Figure 24.3C and D, white asterisk) are seen on optical coherence tomography (OCT) and are the main indicators of disease activity. Presence of subretinal hemorrhage (Figures 24.1C,D and 24.3C,D, black asterisk) represented by subretinal hyperreflective material and hemorrhagic pigment epithelial detachments (Figure 24.1D, red asterisk) are other signs of activity in PCV.[3]
- Pigment epithelial detachments (PEDs) in PCV are characterized by atypical morphologies and content. Thumblike PED (Figure 24.3D, white arrow), sharp-peaked PED, and notched PED (Figure 24.1C, white arrow) are considered pathognomonic of PCV. The location of the notch lends an M-shape (Figure 24.3C, white arrow) or QRS complex appearance (Figure 24.1D, white arrow) to the PED. The nature of the PED in PCV is predominantly fibrovascular with hemorrhagic component typifying sub-RPE bleed.[4]
- Polyps and their associated BVN are typically located in the space between the RPE and Bruch membrane on OCT. Hyperreflective content within a split of the RPE from the Bruch membrane (referred to as a "double-layer sign") is believed to represent the BVN (Figures 24.1-24.3, red arrows in OCT images). Well-delineated round to oval low-medium reflective spaces with hyperreflective borders located on the outer surface of a PED are believed to represent polyps (Figures 24.1C,D and 24.3C,D, black arrows).[4]
- PCV is one of the disease entities included in the pachychoroid spectrum. A thickened choroid with dilated large choroidal vessels associated with Sattler layer and choriocapillaris compression typifies pachychoroid (Figures 24.1C,D and 24.3C,D, blue asterisk). The use of enhanced-depth imaging and swept-source OCT can help improve the detection and understanding of these disorders.[5]
- Type 1 neovascular membranes in the setting of a thin choroid, in contrast, is more suggestive of neovascular age-related macular degeneration (AMD).[3]

OCTA IMAGING

- Both BVN and polyps may be seen on optical coherence tomography angiography (OCTA).
- Polyps are less frequently visualized due to slower blood flow within the lesions. The relatively faster flow at the margins of the polyp results in a ring-shaped lesion with central flow void due to low decorrelation signals.[6] The outer retinal slab is better suited for polyp detection when compared to the choriocapillaris slab due to an elevated RPE.

- The presence of subretinal and sub-RPE exudation results in altered retinal anatomy, and hence, a manual segmentation may result in better polyp and BVN detection rates[6] (Figures 24.1E and 24.3E).

- Various morphological patterns of polyps have been described on OCTA. Ring (Figure 24.2D, white arrow), nodular, dot, and cluster (Figure 24.3F, white box) are a few patterns noted on the outer retinal slab on OCTA.[6]

- BVN patterns described on OCTA have similarities to various patterns of neovascular networks in AMD. This similarity supports the hypothesis of PCV being a polypoidal variant of neovascular AMD.[2,7]

- The "trunk" pattern of BVN (Figure 24.1F, white circle) represents a larger single trunk with a finer peripheral vascular network. These are large networks which respond better to a combination of anti–vascular endothelial growth factor (anti-VEGF) and photodynamic therapy when compared to the other BVN patterns. They are associated with thinner choroids and poorer visual outcomes.[7]

- The "glomeruli" pattern (Figure 24.2D, white circle) denotes a fine interconnected vascular network with no major trunk. This pattern has high recurrence rates as it is considered to represent more active networks. The choroidal thickness is greater compared to the trunk pattern and the visual outcomes are better.[7]

- The "stick" pattern consists of a fine ill-defined neovascular network. This pattern is associated with the smallest BVN area and highest choroidal thickness. Recurrences are frequent but visual outcomes are better than the trunk pattern.[7]

References

1. Imamura Y, Engelbert M, Iida T, Freund KB, Yannuzzi LA. Polypoidal choroidal vasculopathy: a review. *Surv Ophthalmol.* 2010;55(6):501-515.

2. Dansingani KK, Gal-Or O, Sadda SR, Yannuzzi LA, Freund KB. Understanding aneurysmal type 1 neovascularization (polypoidal choroidal vasculopathy): a lesson in the taxonomy of 'expanded spectra' - a review. *Clin Exp Ophthalmol.* 2018;46(2):189-200.

3. Anantharaman G, Sheth J, Bhende M, et al. Polypoidal choroidal vasculopathy: pearls in diagnosis and management. *Indian J Ophthalmol.* 2018;66(7):896-908.

4. Alshahrani ST, Al Shamsi HN, Kahtani ES, Ghazi NG. Spectral-domain optical coherence tomography findings in polypoidal choroidal vasculopathy suggest a type 1 neovascular growth pattern. *Clin Ophthalmol.* 2014;8:1689-1695.

5. Gallego-Pinazo R, Dolz-Marco R, Gomez-Ulla F, Mrejen S, Freund KB. Pachychoroid diseases of the macula. *Med Hypothesis Discov Innov Ophthalmol.* 2014;3(4):111-115.

6. Wang M, Zhou Y, Gao SS, et al. Evaluating polypoidal choroidal vasculopathy with optical coherence tomography angiography. *Invest Ophthalmol Vis Sci.* 2016;57(9):OCT526-532.

7. Huang CH, Yeh PT, Hsieh YT, Ho TC, Yang CM, Yang CH. Characterizing branching vascular network morphology in polypoidal choroidal vasculopathy by optical coherence tomography angiography. *Sci Rep.* 2019;9(1):595.

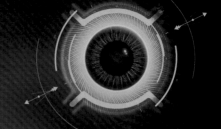

CHAPTER 25

Angioid Streaks

SALIENT FEATURES

- Angioid streaks (AS) are linear breaks in Bruch membrane that typically radiate from the optic disc and take on a deep red, brown, or gray appearance. They are usually bilateral (Figures 25.1 and 25.2).
- AS are classically associated with pseudoxanthoma elasticum (59%-87% incidence), Ehlers-Danlos syndrome, Paget disease of bone (8%-15% incidence), and sickle cell anemia and other hemoglobinopathies (0.9%-6% incidence). Half of individuals with AS have an idiopathic etiology.
- Mineralization of Bruch membrane can result in the rupture of the brittle layer with or without inciting trauma. Adjacent retinal pigment epithelium (RPE), choriocapillaris, and photoreceptors may secondarily be disrupted (Figures 25.1-25.4).
- Vision loss typically results from late complications of AS including hemorrhage, edema, and choroidal neovascularization (CNV) at the site of the breaks (42%-86% incidence, commonly subfoveal) with subsequent disciform scar (Figures 25.2, 25.4 and 25.5).

OCT IMAGING

- Optical coherence tomography (OCT) identifies focal breaks in Bruch membrane corresponding to the location of AS (Figures 25.3 and 25.4).
- OCT may also reveal hyperreflective areas of mineralized Bruch membrane.
- Intraretinal and choroidal hyperreflective foci, similar to those seen in age-related macular degeneration, may correlate to CNV activity.

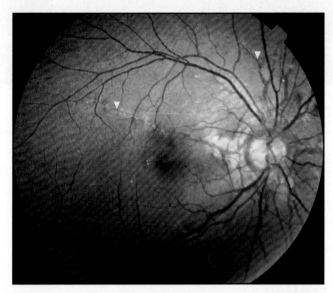

FIGURE 25.1 Color fundus photograph of the right eye of a patient with angioid streaks (AS). Numerous brown-gray streaks (white arrowheads) radiate from the optic nerve head and run deep to the retina vessels. Several demonstrate a halo of hypopigmentation which highlights the angioid streaks.

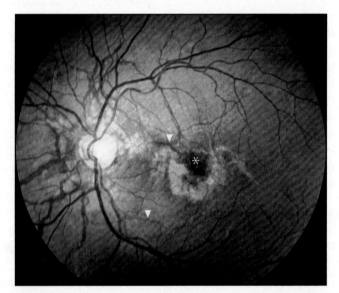

FIGURE 25.2 Color fundus photograph of the left eye of the same patient with angioid streaks (AS). Numerous prominent AS are seen extending from the optic nerve with two denoted by white arrowheads. Additionally, a pigmented, disciform scar with hemorrhage secondary to chronic choroidal neovascularization is centered in the macula at the intersection of several AS (white asterisk).

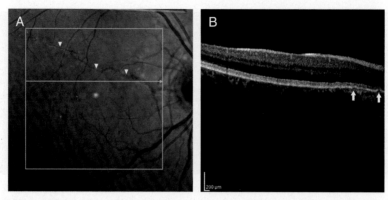

FIGURE 25.3 Spectral-domain optical coherence tomography (OCT) of the right eye of the same patient in previous figures. The near-infrared image (A) of the right eye identifies angioid streaks (AS) (white arrowheads) that radiate from the optic disc. The associated B-scan OCT (B) shows focal breaks in Bruch membrane with disruption of overlying retinal pigment epithelium (RPE) corresponding to the location of an AS (white arrows).

- CNV may appear as a hyperreflective subretinal lesion. The relationship between an AS and CNV may be best appreciated with near-infrared imaging (Figure 25.4).
- Choroid thickness is typically normal. However, the choroid is significantly thinner in patients with CNV.
- Undulations in Bruch membrane (Figure 25.4) may arise from mechanical forces on the peripapillary area and be predictive of subsequent formation or extension of AS in those areas.

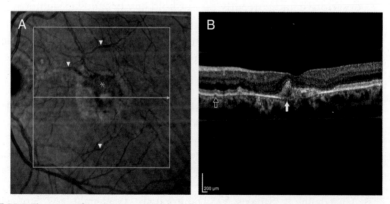

FIGURE 25.4 The near-infrared image (A) of the left eye demonstrates angioid streaks (AS) (white arrowheads) extending to a disciform fibrovascular scar in the central macula (white asterisk). B-scan optical coherence tomography (OCT) (B) reveals subfoveal disruption of the Bruch membrane/retinal pigment epithelium (RPE) complex (white arrows) with overlying subretinal hyperreflective material (white asterisk) without subretinal fluid or intraretinal edema. Undulations in Bruch membrane may predict where new AS will emerge (black arrow).

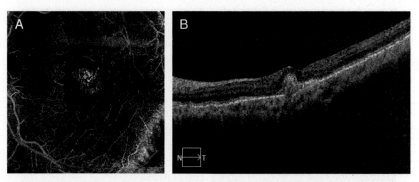

FIGURE 25.5 A, *En-face* optical coherence tomography (OCT) angiography of the same left eye as Figure 25.4 demonstrates an interlacing pattern of choroidal neovascularization at the location of the disciform scar (white asterisk). B, Structural OCT with flow overlay of the left eye demonstrates presence of blood flow in the area of fibrovascular proliferation (white asterisk) consistent with choroidal neovascularization.

OCTA IMAGING

- Optical coherence tomography angiography (OCTA) is particularly useful for identifying CNV in AS as the detection of CNV with fluorescein angiogram (FA) or indocyanine green chorioangiography (ICG) is rendered difficult due to the choriocapillaris hyperfluorescence of the window defect created by a break (Figure 25.5).
- Recent studies identified three patterns of CNV in AS: a "pruned tree" or "tangled" pattern that is associated with the absence of exudation, an "interlacing" pattern associated with active exudative CNV, and a mixed pattern (Figure 25.5). The patterns of CNV, however, are merely descriptive and currently do not hold any prognostic significance.
- In the absence of CNV, AS may show either a decreased density of choriocapillaris vessels suggesting atrophy or an irregular vascular network possibly representing the formation of fibrovascular tissue.

References

1. Ari Yaylali S, Akcakaya AA, Erbil HH, Salar S, Karakurt Y. Optical coherence tomography findings in pseudoxanthoma elasticum. *Eur J Ophthalmol.* 2010;20:397-401.
2. Chapron T, Mimoun G, Miere A, et al. Optical coherence tomography angiography features of choroidal neovascularization secondary to angioid streaks. *Eye.* 2019;33:385-391.
3. Chatziralli I, Saitakis G, Dimitriou E, Chatzirallis A, Stoungioti S, Theodossiadis G, Theodossiadis P. Angioid streaks: a comprehensive review from pathophysiology to treatment. *Retina.* 2019;39(1):1-11.
4. Chiu B, Tsui E, Hussnain SA, Barbazetto IA, Smith T. Multimodal imaging of angioid streaks associated with Turner syndrome. *Retin Cases Brief Rep.* 2018;1-4.

5. Corbelli E, Carnevali A, Marchese A, et al. Optical coherence tomography angiography features of angioid streaks. *Retina*. 2018;38:2128-2136.

6. Coscas G, De Benedetto U, Coscas F, et al. Hyperreflective dots: a new spectral-domain optical coherence tomography entity for follow-up and prognosis in exudative age-related macular degeneration. *Ophthalmologica*. 2013;229:32-37.

7. Ellabban A, Tsujikawa A, Matsumoto A, et al. Macular choroidal thickness and volume in eyes with angioid streaks measured by swept source optical coherence tomography. *Am J Ophthalmol*. 2012;153:1133-1143.

8. Gliem M, Fimmers R, Müller PL, et al. Choroidal changes associated with Bruch membrane pathology in pseudoxanthoma elasticum. *Am J Ophthalmol*. 2014;158:198-207.

9. Hanhart J, Greifner H, Rozenman Y. Locating and characterizing angioid streaks with en face optical coherence tomography. *Retina Cases Brief Rep*. 2017;11:203-206.

10. Marchese A, Parravano M, Rabiolo A, et al. Optical coherence tomography analysis of evolution of Bruch's membrane features in angioid streaks. *Eye*. 2017;31:1600-1605.

11. Parodi MB, Arrigo A, Romano F, et al. Hyperreflective foci number correlates with choroidal neovascularization activity in angioid streaks. *Invest Ophthalmol Vis Sci*. 2018;59:3314-3319.

12. Romano F, Mercuri S, Arrigo A, et al. Identification of hyperreflective foci in angioid streaks. *Eye*. 2019;33:1916-1925.

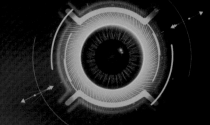

CHAPTER 26

Myopic Degeneration

SALIENT FEATURES

- Myopic degeneration may occur in eyes that typically have a refractive error exceeding -6.00D or axial length of at least 26.5 mm along with posterior pathology due to axial elongation.
- The most common retinal pathology in myopic degeneration is the development of posterior staphyloma.
- Posterior staphyloma may have two visually significant components: tractional and degenerative components.
  - Tractional component: the bulging staphyloma may result in differential stretching of the retinal layers. While the outer layers may be more elastic and expand with the staphyloma, the internal limiting membrane may become more taut resulting in stretching of the overall retina. This may progress to separation of the neurosensory and epiretinal layers (macular foveoschisis) or progress to a macular hole (see Chapter 35, Myopic Macular Schisis and Tractional Retinal Detachment).
  - Degenerative component: the bulging staphyloma results in choroidal thinning and choroidal neovascularization. This presents with lacquer cracks and retinal pigment epithelium (RPE) atrophy.
- Macular foveoschisis is best observed with optical coherence tomography (OCT).
- Fluorescein angiography (FA) in combination with OCT is the historic gold standard for detecting choroidal neovascularization in myopic degeneration.
- Optical coherence tomography angiography (OCTA) may be used as an noninvasive alternative to FA for visualizing vessels.

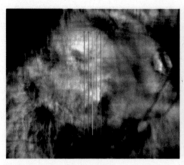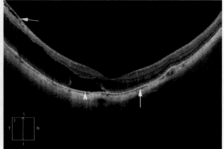

FIGURE 26.1 Myopic degeneration with associated myopic foveoschisis. Taut internal limiting membrane (ILM) and epiretinal membrane (ERM) (yellow arrow) are noted nasally with underlying myopic schisis. Subretinal fluid is also present (arrowhead). Diffuse ellipsoid zone attenuation is present with underlying choroidal thinning (white arrow). Significant curvature of the posterior eye wall is noted, consistent with high myopia.

OCT IMAGING

- Axial elongation results in steep curvature of the retina that is well-visualized on OCT (Figure 26.1).
- Depending on the location and staging of the staphyloma, posterior staphyloma may present as a steep curve with a radius that is smaller than the radius of the rest of the eye. It may also present as an inward bulge from the sclera.
- Macular foveoschisis typically presents on OCT with separation of either the outer plexiform, inner plexiform, and/or nerve fiber layers (Figure 26.1). Thin bands of retinal material bridge the tissue.
- Compound myopic macular foveoschisis may also occur, resulting in separation of multiple layers of the retina.
- Macular holes may also develop and can, in certain cases, progress too macular detachments.
- Myopic degeneration demonstrates retinal thinning, RPE irregularity, significant choroidal thinning, ellipsoid zone attenuation, and outer retinal atrophy (Figure 26.1). RPE atrophy can also develop. Spontaneous subretinal hemorrhages may develop.
- Choroidal neovascularization (CNV) may develop (Figures 26.2 and 26.3). Typically, these CNV may have less exudative fluid compared to neovascular AMD. They are often focal lesions with associated variable increased reflectivity in the outer retina with or without associated subretinal or intraretinal fluid.

OCTA IMAGING

- OCTA imaging is used to monitor myopic choroidal neovascularization (Figure 26.4).

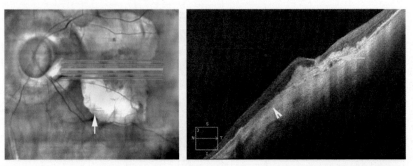

FIGURE 26.2 Severe myopic degeneration with near complete loss of the choroid nasally (arrowhead). Subfoveal inactive disciform scar is present (yellow and white arrows) with overlying retinal atrophy.

- Type 1 myopic CNV presents with neovascular coralliform complex due to formation of new vessels within the choroid.
  - These vessels present as a widely anastomosed network of numerous tiny vessels.
  - A dark halo may surround the neovascularization and separate it from normal choroid vasculature.
- Type 2 CNV is the most common presentation in myopia.
  - Appears similar to type 1 CNV, but has grown beyond RPE-Bruch membrane.

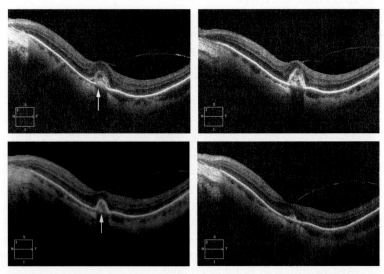

FIGURE 26.3 Myopic degeneration with choroidal neovascularization. Longitudinal optical coherence tomographies (OCTs) from presentation and following anti–vascular endothelial growth factor (VEGF) therapy. Pretreatment OCT demonstrates subfoveal heterogenous hyperreflective lesion consistent with choroidal neovascularization (CNV) (white arrow). Subretinal fluid is present with associated increased outer retinal hyperreflectivity. Following two intravitreal anti-VEGF injections, the subfoveal CNV lesion is more compact and homogenous with resolution of subretinal fluid (yellow arrow).

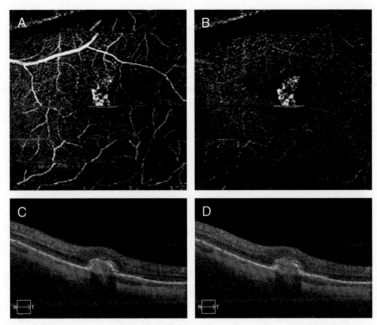

FIGURE 26.4 (A and B) 3 × 3 mm macular cube optical coherence tomography angiography (OCTA) with *en-face* projection capturing the full retina slab (A) and a deeper segmentation slab (B) isolating the choroidal neovascularization (CNV). Both segmentation slabs show neovascularization centrally with the characteristic dark halo surrounding neovasculature. (C and D) B-scans centered on the fovea show the variable segmentation lines and the decorrelation overlay, confirming flow within the CNV (red).

- Myopic CNV is typically small (compared to other forms of CNV).
- Dark halo surrounds the CNV and separates it from normal retinal material.
- While OCTA allows visualization of vessel growth, it cannot detect leakage or growth of new vessels in vessels with low blood flow.

References

1. Chung CY, Wong DSH, Li KKW. Is it necessary to cover the macular hole with the inverted internal limiting membrane flap in macular hole surgery? A case report. *BMC Ophthalmol.* 2015;15(1):115. doi: 10.1186/s12886-015-0104-1.

2. Dolz-Marco R, Fine HF, Freund KB. How to differentiate myopic choroidal neovascularization, idiopathic multifocal choroiditis, and punctate inner choroidopathy using clinical and multimodal imaging findings. *Ophthalmic Surg Lasers Imaging Retina.* 2017;48(3):196-201. doi: 10.3928/23258160-20170301-01.

3. Dansingani KK, Naysan J, Freund KB. En face OCT angiography demonstrates flow in early type 3 neovascularization (retinal angiomatous proliferation). *Eye.* 2015;29(5):703-706. doi: 10.1038/eye.2015.27.

4. Ohno-Matsui K. Patchy atrophy and lacquer cracks predispose to the development of choroidal neovascularisation in pathological myopia. *Br J Ophthalmol.* 2003;87(5):570-573. doi: 10.1136/bjo.87.5.570.

5. Adatia FA, Luong M, Munro M, Tufail A. The other CNVM: a review of myopic choroidal neovascularization treatment in the age of anti-vascular endothelial growth factor agents. *Surv Ophthalmol.* 2015;60(3):204-215. doi: 10.1016/j.survophthal.2014.10.002.

6. Wong TY, Ohno-Matsui K, Leveziel N, et al. Myopic choroidal neovascularisation: current concepts and update on clinical management. *Br J Ophthalmol.* 2014;99(3):289-296. doi: 10.1136/bjophthalmol-2014-305131.

7. Ng DSC, Cheung CYL, Luk FO, et al. Advances of optical coherence tomography in myopia and pathologic myopia. *Eye.* 2016;30(7):901-916. doi: 10.1038/eye.2016.47.

8. Itakura H, Kishi S, Li D, Nitta K, Akiyama H. Vitreous changes in high myopia observed by swept-source optical coherence tomography. *Invest Opthalmol Vis Sci.* 2014;55(3):1447. doi: 10.1167/iovs.13-13496.

9. Lim MCC, Hoh ST, Foster PJ, et al. Use of optical coherence tomography to assess variations in macular retinal thickness in myopia. *Invest Ophthalmol Vis Sci.* 2005;46(3):974. doi: 10.1167/iovs.04-0828.

10. Shimada N, Ohno-Matsui K, Baba T, Futagami S, Tokoro T, Mochizuki M. Natural course of macular retinoschisis in highly myopic eyes without macular hole or retinal detachment. *Am J Ophthalmol.* 2006;142(3):497-500. doi: 10.1016/j.ajo.2006.03.048.

11. Takano M, Kishi S. Foveal retinoschisis and retinal detachment in severely myopic eyes with posterior staphyloma. *Am J Ophthalmol.* 1999;128(4):472-476. doi: 10.1016/s0002-9394(99)00186-5.

12. Sakaguchi H, Ikuno Y, Choi JS, Ohji M, Tano T. Multiple components of epiretinal tissues detected by triamcinolone and indocyanine green in macular hole and retinal detachment as a result of high myopia. *Am J Ophthalmol.* 2004;138(6):1079-1081. doi: 10.1016/j.ajo.2004.06.078.

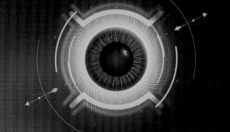

CHAPTER 27

Dome-Shaped Macula

SALIENT FEATURES

- Dome-shaped macula (DSM) is a forward macular bulging present in select patients with high myopia, with a prevalence of 20% of highly myopic eyes in Japan and 11% in Europe.[1]
- Though the pathophysiology behind DSM remains to be fully established, focal scleral thickening in the foveal area is thought to be the major factor.[1]
- DSM can lead to loss of vision secondary to subretinal fluid accumulation and increase risk for serous retinal detachments.[2] A rare cause of serous retinal detachment in DSM eyes is choroidal neovascularization (CNV), usually pachychoroid-associated (type 1) or typical myopic (type 2) CNV.[3]
- Currently, DSM is categorized by morphology: horizontal oval-shaped dome, vertical oval-shaped dome, and round dome.
- In patients with DSM, though visual acuity and central foveal thickness may be stable for years, dome height and retinal pigment epithelium (RPE) atrophy may increase.[5]

OCT IMAGING

- Optical coherence tomography (OCT) is the gold standard test for identification and monitoring DSM and its sequelae.
- To characterize DSM morphology, both vertical and horizontal OCT raster scans are needed to ensure full visualization. The horizontal-oriented oval-shaped dome can be seen on vertical spectral-domain (SD)-OCT (Figures 27.1 and 27.2).[1]

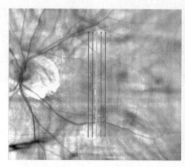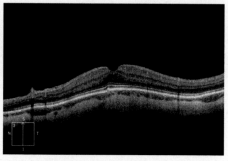

FIGURE 27.1 Spectral-domain optical coherence tomography (SD-OCT) vertical raster scan demonstrating a moderate macular bulge identifying the dome-shaped macula. Thickened subfoveal sclera is noticeable. Minimal retinal pigment epithelium (RPE) disruption is present, and overall retinal layer integrity is intact.

- DSM is typically defined by the inward bulging of the retinal pigment line of >50um above baseline connecting the RPE lines on both sides outside of the DSM (Figures 27.3 and 27.4).[4]
- Dome height greater than 400 μm on OCT has been associated with subfoveal serous retinal detachment and decreased visual acuity.[6]
- OCT is utilized to identify associated sequelae including, subretinal fluid (Figure 27.5), foveoschisis, outer retinal attenuation with ellipsoid zone loss, and choroidal neovascularization.

OCTA IMAGING

- Optical coherence tomography angiography (OCTA), in particular, swept-source (SS)-OCTA is emerging as a possible important adjunct for identification of sequelae, such as CNV (Figure 27.6) and even subclinical CNV in DSM.[3,7]
  - Type 2 CNVs are more common than type 1 CNVs secondary to DSM.

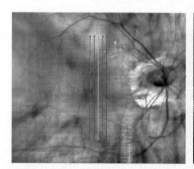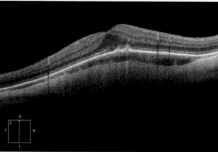

FIGURE 27.2 Spectral-domain optical coherence tomography (SD-OCT) vertical raster scan demonstrating a moderate macular bulge identifying the dome-shaped macula in the right eye. Thickened subfoveal sclera is noticeable. Minimal retinal pigment epithelium (RPE) disruption is present, and overall retinal layer integrity is intact.

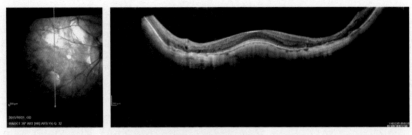

FIGURE 27.3 Swept-source optical coherence tomography (OCT) wide-field vertical scan of the left eye demonstrating dome-shaped macula with subfoveal scleral thickening (without subretinal fluid or loss of retinal layer integrity). Wide-field scan also demonstrates posterior staphyloma.

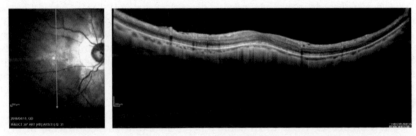

FIGURE 27.4 Swept-source optical coherence tomography (OCT) wide-field vertical scan of the right eye (of same patient in Figure 27.3) demonstrating dome-shaped macula with subfoveal scleral thickening (without subretinal fluid or loss of retinal layer integrity). Wide-field scan also demonstrates posterior staphyloma though not as prominent as the left eye.

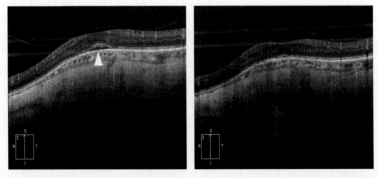

FIGURE 27.5 Subretinal fluid associated with dome-shaped macula. Vertical optical coherence tomography (OCT) of subretinal fluid (arrowhead) without associated choroidal neovascularization (CNV) in an eye with dome-shaped macula (left) that resolved spontaneously (right).

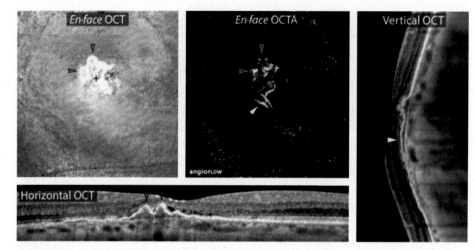

FIGURE 27.6 Optical coherence tomography (OCT) and optical coherence tomography angiography (OCTA) findings of choroidal neovascularization in dome-shaped macula (DSM). Choroidal neovascularization (CNV) lesions (pigment epithelial detachments seen on OCT) shown by red arrow heads and their respective feeding network shown by yellow arrow heads. (Reprinted with permission from Naysan J, Dansingani KK, Balaratnasingam C, Freund KB. Type 1 neovascularization with polypoidal lesions complicating dome shaped macula. *Int J Retina Vitreous*. 2015;1:8. Available at https://doi.org/10.1186/s40942-015-0008-5.)

References

1. Lorenzo D, Arias L, Choudhry N, et al. Dome-shaped macula in myopic eyes: twelve-month follow-up. *Retina*. 2017;37(4):680-686. doi:10.1097/IAE.0000000000001222.

2. Ohno-Matsui K. Pathologic myopia. *Asia Pac J Ophthalmol (Phila)*. 2016;5(6):415-423. doi:10.1097/APO.0000000000000230.

3. Marchese A, Arrigo A, Sacconi R, et al. Spectrum of choroidal neovascularisation associated with dome-shaped macula. *Br J Ophthalmol*. 2019;103(8):1146-1151. doi:10.1136/bjophthalmol-2018-312780.

4. Ellabban AA, Tsujikawa A, Matsumoto A, et al. Three-dimensional tomographic features of dome-shaped macula by swept-source optical coherence tomography. *Am J Ophthalmol*. 2013;155(2):320-328.e2. doi:10.1016/j.ajo.2012.08.007.

5. Soudier G, Gaudric A, Gualino V, et al. Long-term evolution of dome-shaped macula. *Retina*. 2016;36(5):944-952. doi:10.1097/IAE.0000000000000806.

6. Fajardo Sánchez J, Chau Ramos CE, Roca Fernández JA, Urcelay Segura JL. Clinical, fundoscopic, tomographic and angiographic characteristics of dome shaped macula classified by bulge height [in English, Spanish]. *Arch Soc Esp Oftalmol*. 2017;92(10):458-463. doi:10.1016/j.oftale.2017.07.001.

7. Agarwal A, Aggarwal K, Gupta V. Swept-source optical coherence tomography angiography of choroidal neovascularization in vertically oriented oval dome-shaped maculopathy. *Indian J Ophthalmol*. 2019;67(8):1368-1371. doi:10.4103/ijo.IJO_2077_18.

8. Naysan J, Dansingani KK, Balaratnasingam C, Freund KB. Type 1 neovascularization with polypoidal lesions complicating dome shaped macula. *Int J Retina Vitreous*. 2015;1:8. Available at https://doi.org/10.1186/s40942-015-0008-5.

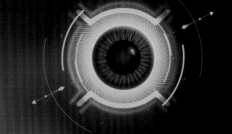

CHAPTER 28

Central Serous Chorioretinopathy

SALIENT FEATURES

- Central serous chorioretinopathy (CSCR or CSR) is associated with corticosteroid use, elevated levels of endogenous steroids, stress, and "type A" personalities.
- Acute cases are generally self-limiting with spontaneous fluid resolution (Figure 28.1).
- Chronic CSCR with periodic recurrence of subretinal fluid (SRF) may ultimately lead to complications such as retinal and retinal pigment epithelium (RPE) atrophy and choroidal neovascularization (CNV) (Figures 28.2 and 28.3).
- Primary mechanisms of disease include choroidal vasodilation and hyperpermeability, which have been demonstrated on indocyanine green (ICG) angiography.[1,2]
- Fluorescein angiography may show three patterns of leakage: "expanding dot," "smoke stack," and a "diffuse" pattern with multiple leakage points.
- Fundus autofluorescence may demonstrate increased autofluorescence in acute CSCR corresponding to areas of SRF. In chronic CSCR, autofluorescence may be decreased due to RPE atrophy.

OCT IMAGING

- Characterized by presence of pigment epithelium detachment (PED), serous neurosensory retinal detachment, and choroidal thickening with dilated deep choroidal vessels ("pachy vessels") (Figures 28.1 and 28.4).
- Choroidal abnormalities as previously mentioned may also be seen in the unaffected fellow eye.

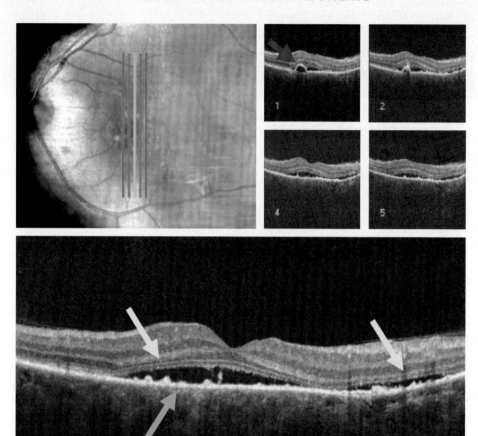

FIGURE 28.1 Foveal optical coherence tomography (OCT) of a patient with chronic, recurrent central serous chorioretinopathy (CSCR) with multifocal areas of subretinal fluid (SRF) (yellow arrows). An additional characteristic finding is the presence of a small pigment epithelium detachment (PED) (red arrow). Outer retinal changes (green arrow) are consistent with chronicity.

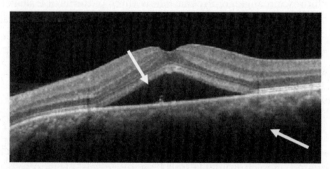

FIGURE 28.2 Optical coherence tomography (OCT) of a patient with acute central serous chorioretinopathy (CSCR). Image demonstrates significant subretinal fluid (SRF) (white arrow) with thickened choroid (yellow arrow).

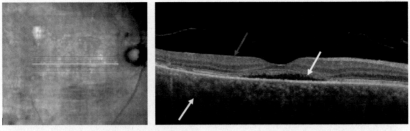

FIGURE 28.3 Optical coherence tomography (OCT) of a patient with chronic central serous chorioreti-nopathy (CSCR) illustrating multiple characteristic findings including subretinal fluid (SRF) (white arrow), thickened choroid (yellow arrow), and retinal thinning (red arrow).

- Choroidal abnormalities are best detected with enhanced depth imaging optical coherence tomography (EDI-OCT).
- OCT is helpful to track resolution of SRF over time.
- Identification of thickened choroid helps to facilitate diagnosis particularly in older individuals where neovascular AMD is in the differential.

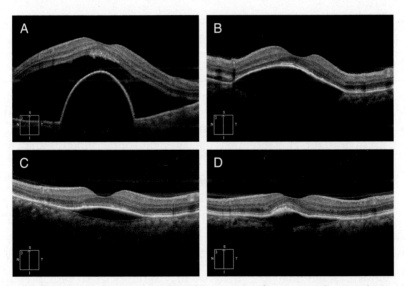

FIGURE 28.4 Optical coherence tomography (OCT) sequence of acute central serous chorioretinopa-thy (CSCR) with extensive subretinal fluid and large pigment epithelium detachment (PED) (Image A). Sequence of OCTs demonstrates spontaneous resolution of fluid and improvement of PED over time (Image B-D).

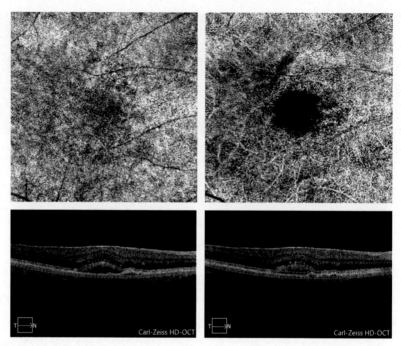

FIGURE 28.5 Optical coherence tomography angiographies (OCTAs) and corresponding perfusion maps of central serous chorioretinopathy (CSCR) showing decreased perfusion in choriocapillaris.

OCTA IMAGING

- Optical coherence tomography angiography (OCTA) of the choriocapillaris may demonstrate areas of hypoperfusion (ischemia) surrounded by areas of hyperperfusion, which may subsequently increase hydrostatic pressure that damages the outer blood-retinal barrier, resulting in SRF (Figure 28.5).[3]
- Choriocapillaris flow voids appear to correlate with areas of choriocapillaris thinning. Higher age, longer duration since diagnosis, and disease severity have been found to be associated with increased total flow void area.[4]
- OCTA may assist with detection of CNV especially in more ambiguous cases. Presence of a shallow irregular PED and intraretinal fluid with subretinal RPE material may be associated with presence of CNV (Figure 28.6).[5]

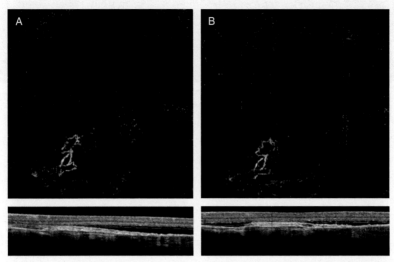

FIGURE 28.6 A, Longitudinal optical coherence tomography angiography (OCTA) images and corresponding optical coherence tomographies (OCTs) of choroidal neovascularization (CNV) secondary to central serous chorioretinopathy (CSCR). B, Same patient 5 weeks after intravitreal anti–vascular endothelial growth factor injection with no remarkable change in CNV or subretinal fluid. (Modified from de Carlo TE, Bonini Filho MA, Chin AT, et al. Spectral-domain optical coherence tomography angiography of choroidal neovascularization. *Ophthalmology.* 2015;122(6):1228-1238.)

References

1. Spaide RF, Hall L, Haas A, et al. Indocyanine green videoangiography of older patients with central serous chorioretinopathy. *Retina.* 2016;16:203-213.
2. Guyer DR, Yannuzzi LA, Slakter JS, Sorenson JA, Ho A, Orlock D. Digital indocyanine green videoangiography of central serous chorioretinopathy. *Arch Ophthalmol.* 1994;112:1057-1062.
3. Teussink MM, Breukink MB, van Grinsven MJJP, et al. Oct angiography compared to fluorescein and indocyanine green angiography in chronic central serous chorioretinopathy. *Invest Ophthalmol Vis Sci.* 2015;56:5229-5237.
4. Matet A, Daruich A, Hardy S, Behar-Cohen F. Patterns of choriocapillaris flow signal voids in central serous chorioretinopathy: an optical coherence tomography angiography study. *Retina.* 2019;39(11):2178-2188. doi: 10.1097/IAE.0000000000002271.
5. Uchida A, Manjunath D, Singh RP, et al. Optical coherence tomography angiography in eyes with indeterminate choroidal neovascularization: results from the AVATAR study. *Ophthalmol Retina.* 2018;2(11):1107-1117.

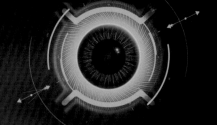

CHAPTER 29

Uveal Effusion Syndrome

SALIENT FEATURES

- Uveal effusion syndrome is defined by an idiopathic ciliochoroidal effusion, which may be accompanied by concomitant serous retinal detachment (Figure 29.1).[1]
- This typically occurs in otherwise healthy middle-aged males.[1]
- The pathophysiology suggested is a compromise of posterior segment drainage due to decreased scleral permeability and scleropathy; studies have shown an accumulation of glycosaminoglycan-like deposits and scleral thickening in patients with uveal effusion.[2,3]
- It is divided into three types[3]:
  - Type 1: Nanophthalmic eyes that are small with normal sclera
  - Type 2: Nonnanophthalmic eyes (normal axial length) with clinically abnormal sclera
  - Type 3: Nonnanophthalmic eyes (normal axial length) with clinically normal sclera
- Important to exclude secondary causes of serous choroidal detachment, such as uveitis, hypotony, hypertension, elevated uveal venous pressure (eg, Sturge-Weber, arteriovenous fistula), and neoplasm.
- Treatment consists of scleral thinning procedures such as quadrantic partial thickness sclerectomy and sclerostomy to drain suprachoroidal fluid as well as to treat the underlying scleropathy (Figure 29.2).[4] Some surgeons also combine pars plana vitrectomy with external drainage for cases with concomitant rhegmatogenous retinal detachment. Systemic steroid use is controversial; a recent

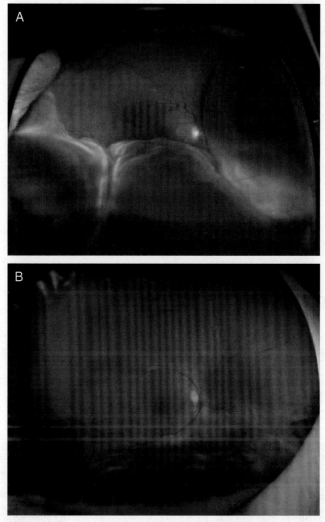

FIGURE 29.1 A, Wide-field fundus photo of a 58-year-old white male with no past medical history and negative uveitis workup and a normal axial length (22.8 mm) who presented with idiopathic choroidal effusions and exudative retinal detachment that did not improve with prednisone 60 mg/d. B, Wide-field fundus photo of the same patient showing improvement of choroidal effusions 2 weeks after partial thickness sclerotomy in the superonasal and superotemporal quadrants.

case series of type 3 uveal effusion syndrome showed improved visual acuity for patients treated with corticosteroids compared to observation.[1,5] The evidence remains weak, however, supporting the routine use of steroids for the management of uveal effusion syndrome.

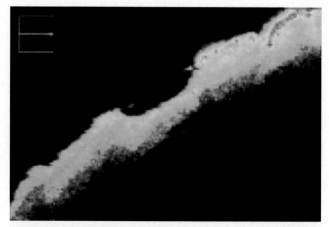

FIGURE 29.2 Intraoperative optical coherence tomography (OCT) of the sclera demonstrating the depth of a partial-thickness sclerotomy in the superotemporal quadrant.

OCT FEATURES

- Enhanced depth imaging (EDI) optical coherence tomography (OCT) is used for improved visualization of the choroid. In uveal effusion, EDI-OCT shows increased choroidal thickness.[6] Increased choroidal thickness is a nonspecific feature that, while helpful, is not diagnostic (Figure 29.3).

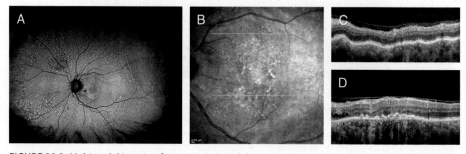

FIGURE 29.3 Multimodal imaging from a patient with long-standing history of relapsing choroidal effusions secondary to uveal effusion syndrome. A, Fundus autofluorescence (AF) reveals diffuse mottled hyper- and hypo-AF changes ("leopard spots") changes suggestive of chronic retinal pigment epithelium (RPE) damage. There are curvilinear streaks of autofluorescent changes that correspond to prior borders of choroidal effusions (blue arrow). B, Near-infrared image signifying the locations of the spectral-domain optical coherence tomography (SD-OCT) scans in C (superior green line) and D (inferior green line). C, SD-OCT scan through the superior macula shows choroidal folds (purple arrow). D, SD-OCT scan through the inferior macula shows increased choroidal thickness with large hyporeflective spaces (red asterisk); focal hypertrophy, atrophy, and small detachments of the retinal pigment epithelium (green arrow); and mild intraretinal fluid (blue asterisk).

- Low-reflective areas in the outer choroid may also be present, which may be attributed to extravascular protein, fluid in the suprachoroidal space, or enlarged choroidal veins.[6]
- OCT through "leopard spot" lesions may show focal thickening/ hypertrophy of the retinal pigment epithelium (Figure 29.3D).[7]

OCTA FEATURES

- There is currently no role for OCTA in uveal effusion syndrome.

References

1. Besirli CG, Johnson MW. Uveal effusion syndrome and hypotony maculopathy. In: Schachat A, ed. *Ryan's Retina*. Amsterdam; Elsevier; 2017:1484-1490.
2. Kawamura M, Tajima S, Azuma N, Katsura H, Akiyama K. Immunohistochemical studies of glycosaminoglycans in nanophthalmic sclera. *Graefes Arch Clin Exp Ophthalmol*. 1996; 234(1):19-24.
3. Uyama M, Takahashi K, Kozaki J, et al. Uveal effusion syndrome: clinical features, surgical treatment, histologic examination of the sclera, and pathophysiology. *Ophthalmology*. 2000;107:441-449.
4. Khatri A, Singh S, Joshi , Kharel M. Quadrantic vortex vein decompression with subretinal fluid drainage for management of nanophthalmic choroidal effusions- a review of literature and case series. *BMC Ophthalmol*. 2019;19(1):210.
5. Shields CL, Roelofs K, Di Nicola M, Sioufi K, Mashayekhi A, Shields JA. Uveal effusion syndomre in 104 eyes: response to corticosteroids – the 2017 Axel C. Hansen lecture. *Indian J Ophthalmol*. 2017;65(11):1093-1104.
6. Harada T, Machida S, Fujiwara T, Nishida Y, Kurosaka D. Choroidal findings in idiopathic uveal effusion syndrome. *Clin Ophthalmol*. 2011;5:1599-1601.
7. Okuda T, Higashide T, Wakabayashi Y, Nishimura A, Sugiyama K. Fundus autofluorescence and spectral-domain optical coherence tomography findings of leopard spots in nanophthalmic uveal effusion syndrome. *Graefes Arch Clin Exp Ophthalmol*. 2010;248:1199-1202.

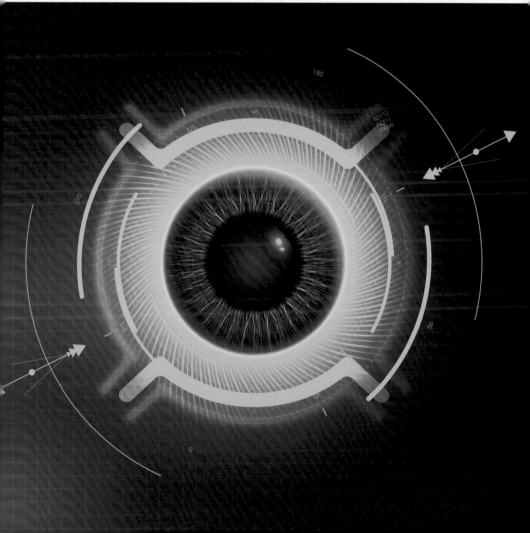

Part 4

The Vitreoretinal Interface and Peripheral Retinal Pathology

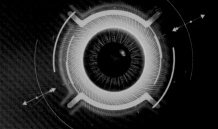

CHAPTER 30

Vitreomacular Adhesion and the Normal Vitreoretinal Interface

SALIENT FEATURES

- The vitreous includes an outer cortex of primarily type 2 collagen (ie, the posterior hyaloid) that attaches the posterior vitreous body to the internal limiting membrane (ILM).[1]
- Macromolecular attachment complexes at this interface, composed of fibronectin, laminin, and other components, form a gluelike matrix that plays a role in vitreoretinal adhesion.[2]
- This connection persists from birth through young adulthood and constitutes the normal vitreoretinal interface. With age, the vitreous gel liquifies (synchysis), collapses (syneresis), and the cortex separates from the ILM (a process known as posterior vitreous detachment [PVD]).
- Perifoveal PVD that occurs with persistent attachment at the fovea with maintenance of a normal foveal morphology is called a vitreomacular adhesion (VMA).
- VMAs are nonpathologic and asymptomatic, but persistent adhesion may lead to secondary tractional disease such as vitreomacular traction (VMT) or macular hole.
- Transition to VMT can aggravate underlying retinal conditions like diabetic macular edema or age-related macular degeneration.[3]

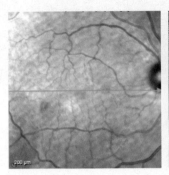
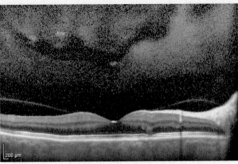

FIGURE 30.1 Enhanced vitreous imaging spectral-domain optical coherence tomography (SD-OCT) of a patient with vitreomacular adhesion (VMA) with significantly increased visualization of the vitreous interface and anatomy.

OCT IMAGING

- Optical coherence tomography (OCT) has enabled better understanding of the vitreoretinal interface and is critical to evaluate potential abnormalities.[4]
- Swept-source OCT systems and new software modifications (such as enhanced vitreous imaging) provide greater visualization detail of the vitreous anatomy (Figure 30.1).
- The International Vitreomacular Traction Study Classification System for Vitreomacular Adhesion, Traction, and Macular Hole established a clinically useful system for categorizing the different spectrum of vitreomacular traction diseases based on OCT findings.[2]
- VMA can be subclassified by anatomic features seen on OCT.
- Focal VMA has an adhesion ≤1500 μm versus broad with an adhesion >1500 μm (Figure 30.2).[2]

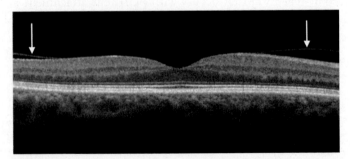

FIGURE 30.2 Optical coherence tomography (OCT) image of a patient with a broad vitreomacular adhesion (VMA). The hyperreflective material in a band courses in a somewhat conical pattern posteriorly corresponding to the attachment of the posterior hyaloid to the internal limiting membrane (ILM) in an incomplete perifoveal posterior vitreous detachment (PVD) (white arrows). Note the normal anatomical appearance of the fovea.

- Premacular release of the adhesion represents a posterior vitreous separation from the macular surface during the PVD process. If the posterior hyaloid is still visible within the OCT, it is commonly still attached to a posterior ocular structure, such as the optic nerve, and a complete PVD is often not present.
- Typically when a PVD occurs, the vitreous is no longer visible within the OCT B-scan.
- The difference in reflectivity of the parallel-fiber orientation of the ILM and acellular vitreous allows for visible differentiation of this interface on OCT (Figure 30.2).[4]

References

1. Stalmans P1, Duker JS, Kaiser PK, et al. Oct-based interpretation of the vitreomacular interface and indications for pharmacologic vitreolysis. *Retina*. 2013;33(10):2003-2011.
2. Duker JS, Kaiser PK, Binder S, et al. The International vitreomacular traction Study group classification of vitreomacular adhesion, traction, and macular hole. *Ophthalmology*. 2013;120(12):2611-2619.
3. John VJ, Flynn HW, Smiddy WE, et al. Clinical course of vitreomacular adhesion managed by initial observation. *Retina*. 2014;34(3):442-446.
4. Mirza RG, Johnson MW, Jampol LM. Optical coherence tomography use in evaluation of the vitreoretinal interface: a review. *Surv Ophthalmol*. 2007;52(4):397-421.

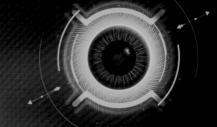

CHAPTER 31

Full-Thickness Macular Hole

SALIENT FEATURES

- Full-thickness macular hole (FTMH) is a full-thickness defect resulting in absence of all retinal layers from the internal limiting membrane to retinal pigment epithelium at the fovea (Figure 31.1).
- FTMHs have a prevalence rate of 0.02 % to 0.33% with 5% to 20% nonsimultaneous bilateral involvement.[1]
- Symptoms of FTMH include metamorphopsia, varying degrees of visual loss, and central scotoma.
- FTMHs are classified as either primary and secondary.
- The majority of FTMHs are primary, resulting from vitreomacular traction (VMT). Risk factors associated with primary FTMH are female gender and older age (Figure 31.2).
- Secondary FTMH causes include trauma, ocular inflammation, and high-degree myopia (Figure 31.3).
- Optical coherence tomography (OCT) has enabled aperture size–based classification of FTMH: small (≤250 mm), medium (>250 ≤ 400 mm), or large (>400 mm).[2]

OCT IMAGING

- OCT is the current gold standard for the diagnosis, staging, and monitoring of FTMH.
- The basic morphologic features of FTMH include hourglass-shaped loss of all retinal layers in the macula (Figures 31.2 and 31.4).

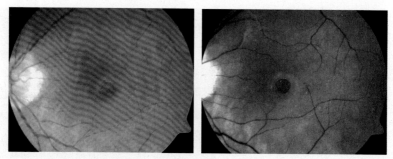

FIGURE 31.1 Color (A) and red-free (B) fundus photography of a full-thickness macular hole (FTMH). Clear, defined boundary around the dark spot in the macula indicates the boarders of the FTMH. Surrounding retinal tissue appears thickened.

- Retinal edges are usually rounded and may be thickened due to cystic intraretinal changes, which present on OCT as focal hyporeflective circular structures within the retinal tissue. A small amount of subretinal fluid, which presents as a hyporeflective space between the retina and the RPE, is often present at the hole edge (Figure 31.2).
- Aperture size of the hole is defined as the distance between two closest components of the retinal edges, measured by OCT. It is used in FTMH staging and prognostic for anatomical success after surgery[2] (Figures 31.2 and 31.3).
- Another prognostic FTMH feature is base diameter which is defined as the distance between two retinal edges at the level of RPE[2] (Figures 31.2 and 31.3).
- Both base diameter and aperture size are negatively correlated with postoperative visual outcomes.[3]

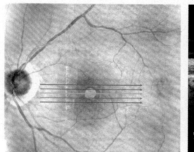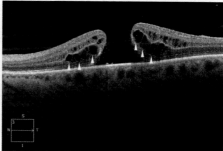

FIGURE 31.2 Large, hourglassed-shaped full-thickness macular hole (FTMH) with intraretinal cystic changes (arrowheads) and rounded retinal edges. Complete loss of layer from inner limiting membrane (ILM) to retinal pigment epithelium (RPE) is shown. Green line represents the aperture size measurement of the FTMH. Red line represents the base diameter.

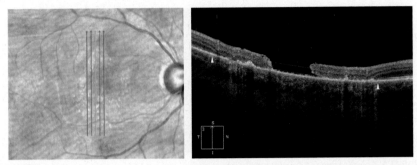

FIGURE 31.3 Large traumatic full-thickness macular hole (FTMH) with ellipsoid zone (EZ) atrophy. Green line represents the aperture size measurement of the FTMH. Red line represents the base diameter. EZ disruption can be seen in the area between two arrowheads.

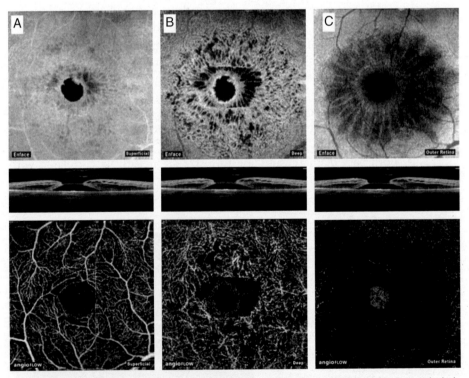

FIGURE 31.4 Optical coherence tomography angiography (OCTA) images of a full-thickness macular hole (FTMH) case with enlarged foveal avascular zone. Cystic changes surrounding the hole are best visualized on *en-face* images at deep retinal layer. (Reprinted with permission from Shahlaee A, Rahimy E, Hsu J, Gupta OP, Ho AC. Preoperative and postoperative features of macular holes on en face imaging and optical coherence tomography angiography. *Am J Ophthalmol Case Rep*. 2017;5:20-25.)

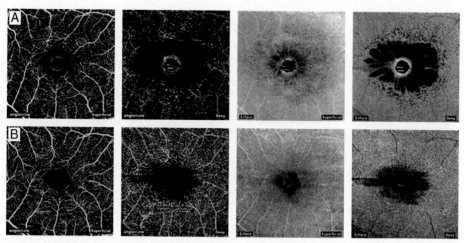

FIGURE 31.5 Optical coherence tomography angiography (OCTA) images of a surgically managed full-thickness macular hole (FTMH). Hyporeflective spaces in en-face preoperative (A) deep retina and deep capillary images represent macular hole (arrowhead) and cystic changes. Cystic changes as well as foveal avascular zone is reduced postoperatively (B). (Reprinted with permission from Shahlaee A, Rahimy E, Hsu J, Gupta OP, Ho AC. Preoperative and postoperative features of macular holes on en face imaging and optical coherence tomography angiography. *Am J Ophthalmol Case Rep*. 2017;5:20-25.)

OCTA IMAGING

- Optical coherence tomography angiography (OCTA) images demonstrate enlargement of the foveal avascular zone in FTMH, partially due to the complete absence of retinal tissue[4] (Figure 31.4).
- Intraretinal cystic changes surrounding FTMH appeared as radially elongated hyporeflective cavities in the outer plexiform layer and small, circular cavities in the inner nuclear layer. Flow surrounding the cystic cavities is shown to be preserved.[5]
- OCTA may help documentation of the resolution of cystic changes and decrease in foveal avascular zone following surgical management of FTMH[4] (Figure 31.5).

References

1. Forsaa VA, Lindtjorn B, Kvaloy JT, Froystein T, Krohn J. Epidemiology and morphology of full-thickness macular holes. *Acta Ophthalmol.* 2018;96(4):397-404.
2. Duker JS, Kaiser PK, Binder S, et al. The International Vitreomacular Traction Study Group classification of vitreomacular adhesion, traction, and macular hole. *Ophthalmology*. 2013;120(12):2611-2619.
3. Goldberg RA, Waheed NK, Duker JS. Optical coherence tomography in the preoperative and postoperative management of macular hole and epiretinal membrane. *Br J Ophthalmol*. 2014;98(suppl 2):ii20-ii23.

4. Shahlaee A, Rahimy E, Hsu J, Gupta OP, Ho AC. Preoperative and postoperative features of macular holes on en face imaging and optical coherence tomography angiography. *Am J Ophthalmol Case Rep.* 2017;5:20-25.

5. Rizzo S, Savastano A, Bacherini D, Savastano MC. Vascular features of full-thickness macular hole by OCT angiography. *Ophthalmic Surg Lasers Imaging Retina.* 2017;48(1):62-68.

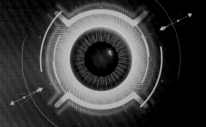

CHAPTER **32**

Epiretinal Membrane

SALIENT FEATURES

- Epiretinal membrane (ERM), also termed "macular pucker," is a common condition that arises from fibrocellular proliferation at the vitreoretinal interface.[1]
- ERM is most commonly idiopathic and associated with aging. Secondary causes include retinal vascular disease, uveitis, retinal detachment, or iatrogenic from laser or surgical intervention.[2]
- Clinical presentation can vary from asymptomatic to complaints of visual distortion, metamorphopsia, and loss of central vision.
- On examination, early ERMs appear as a cellophane sheen with blunted foveal reflex. In advanced cases, the ERM appears as preretinal fibrosis and causes retinal distortion and tractional folds.[1]
- The majority of ERMs are nonprogressive and asymptomatic and thus can be observed.
- Management of visually significant epiretinal membranes is surgical and involves pars plana vitrectomy with ERM peeling. Concurrent internal limiting membrane peeling is often performed to decrease the risk of ERM recurrence.[3]

OCT IMAGING

- Optical coherence tomography (OCT) is the diagnostic imaging test of choice to assess epiretinal membranes, which appear as a hyperreflective band on the retinal surface[4] (Figure 32.1).
- Several OCT-based ERM classification systems have been proposed and take into account clinically relevant anatomic changes that occur

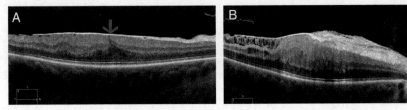

FIGURE 32.1 A, Optical coherence tomography (OCT) showing an epiretinal membrane (red arrow) causing traction on the retina with loss of the foveal contour. B, OCT of the same patient 1 year later showing progression of the epiretinal membrane. There is disruption of the inner retinal layers and ectopic inner foveal layers present (red star).

as a result of membrane contracture. One scheme includes the following four stages[5]:

- Stage 1: Presence of foveal pit with well-defined retinal layers
- Stage 2: Absence of foveal pit with well-defined retinal layers
- Stage 3: Absence of foveal pit with well-defined retinal layers and presence of ectopic inner foveal layers
- Stage 4: Absence of foveal pit with disrupted retinal layers and presence of ectopic inner foveal layers (Figure 32.1)
- Other OCT findings associated with ERM include increased central foveal thickness, intraretinal fluid, retinal folding, ellipsoid zone (EZ) attenuation, subfoveal material, lamellar, and macular hole.[4,5]
- Surgical removal of ERM can release traction and improve foveal contour (Figure 32.2). Most frequently, some architectural alterations remain even after surgical removal.

OCTA IMAGING

- There may be an emerging role for OCT angiography (OCTA) in assessment of epiretinal membranes.[6-9]
- Tangential forces from ERM contracture result in retinal vessel dragging visible on OCTA.

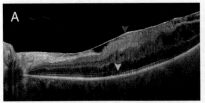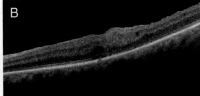

FIGURE 32.2 A, Optical coherence tomography (OCT) showing an epiretinal membrane (red arrow) with cystoid macular edema and loss of foveal contour. There is also attenuation of the external limiting membrane (ELM) and ellipsoid zone (EZ) secondary to tractional forces (green arrow). B, OCT following pars plana vitrectomy with epiretinal membrane peeling. The retinal contour is improved, and there is ellipsoid zone reconstitution (red arrow).

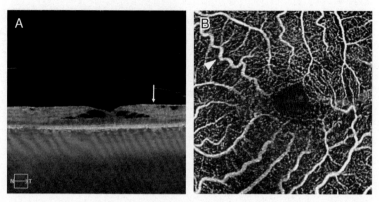

FIGURE 32.3 A, Epiretinal membrane (arrow) with intraretinal fluid on optical coherence tomography (OCT). B, Optical coherence tomography angiography 3 × 3 mm slab of the retinal microvasculature. There is increased tortuosity with vascular dragging (arrowhead).

- OCTA can be used to visualize the extent of retinal vascular displacement from ERM and has also shown a decreased foveal avascular zone[7,9] (Figure 32.3).
- The prognostic and visual significance of microvasculature changes in ERM is still under investigation.

References

1. Fraser-Bell S, Guzowski M, Rochtchina E, Wang JJ, Mitchell P. Five-year cumulative incidence and progression of epiretinal membranes: the Blue Mountains Eye Study. *Ophthalmology*. 2003;110:34-40.
2. Yazici AT, Alagoz N, Celik HU, et al. Idiopathic and secondary epiretinal membranes: do they differ in terms of morphology? An optical coherence tomography-based study. *Retina*. 2011;31:779-784.
3. Sandali O, El Sanharawi M, Basli E, et al. Epiretinal membrane recurrence: incidence, characteristics, evolution, and preventive and risk factors. *Retina*. 2013;33:2032-2038.
4. Stevenson W, Prospero Ponce CM, Agarwal DR, Gelman R, Christoforidis JB. Epiretinal membrane: optical coherence tomography-based diagnosis and classification. *Clin Ophthalmol*. 2016;10:527-534.
5. Govetto A, Lalane RA III, Sarraf D, Figueroa MS, Hubschman JP. Insights into epiretinal membranes: presence of ectopic inner foveal layers and a new optical coherence tomography staging scheme. *Am J Ophthalmol*. 2017;175:99-113.
6. Muftuoglu IK, Amador M, Meshi A, Nudleman E, Lin T, Freeman WR. Foveal avascular zone distortion in epiretinal membrane by optical coherence tomography angiography. *Ophthalmic Surg Lasers Imaging Retina*. 2019;50:295-301.
7. Yoon YS, Woo JM, Woo JE, Min JK. Superficial foveal avascular zone area changes before and after idiopathic epiretinal membrane surgery. *Int J Ophthalmol*. 2018;11:1711-1715.

8. Nelis P, Alten F, Clemens CR, Heiduschka P, Eter N. Quantification of changes in foveal capillary architecture caused by idiopathic epiretinal membrane using OCT angiography. *Graefes Arch Clin Exp Ophthalmol.* 2017;255: 1319-1324.

9. Kim YJ, Kim S, Lee JY, Kim JG, Yoon YH. Macular capillary plexuses after epiretinal membrane surgery: an optical coherence tomography angiography study. *Br J Ophthalmol.* 2018;102:1086-1091.

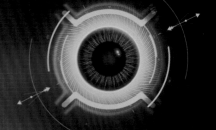

CHAPTER 33

Lamellar Macular Hole and Epiretinal Proliferation

SALIENT FEATURES

- Lamellar macular holes are partial-thickness defects of the macula with intraretinal separation between retinal layers causing loss of the foveal inner retinal layers.
- Various subtypes of lamellar holes have been described, including those associated with the tractional epiretinal membrane, lamellar hole–associated epiretinal proliferation (LHEP), or degenerative changes associated with worse prognoses.
- The clinical presentation is similar to those of full-thickness macular holes with blurriness and distortion of vision though usually to a lesser extent.
- Surgical management is controversial. In symptomatic cases of lamellar holes with epiretinal membrane–related traction, surgical intervention may be successful in improving visual acuity. In those eyes with significant tissue loss, LHEP, and foveal atrophy with ellipsoid zone loss, surgical intervention is less commonly performed. Internal limiting membrane (ILM) peeling should be considered in surgical intervention due to the risk of postoperative full-thickness macular holes.
- Lamellar holes have retinal tissue loss differentiating this entity from macular pseudoholes.

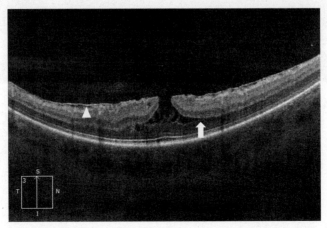

FIGURE 33.1 Tractional lamellar hole with epiretinal membrane (arrowhead) and a distinct separation of layers between the outer nuclear layer (ONL) and outer plexiform layer (OPL) (arrow).

OCT IMAGING

- The hallmark optical coherence tomography (OCT) findings are the irregular foveal contour, loss of retinal tissue, intraretinal separation between the inner and outer retina, and intact foveal photoreceptors.
- Tractional lamellar holes secondary to the epiretinal membrane typically have elevated foveal edges with most separation occurring between the outer nuclear and outer plexiform layers and including vertical hyperreflective bridges between spaces of hyporeflectivity, often with minimal actual tissue loss (Figure 33.1).
- Degenerative lamellar macular holes (Figure 33.2) with associated LHEP often present with wide round-edged intraretinal cavitation devoid of vertical hyperreflective bridges and lacking a clear tractional element.
- Intraretinal pathology can affect all layers including the ellipsoid zone with atrophy and thinning. Foveal edges are generally not elevated in contrast to tractional holes.
- LHEP can be distinguished from the epiretinal membrane by its comparatively decreased reflectivity, limited tractional quality, and continuity between the inner retina and the proliferative tissue.

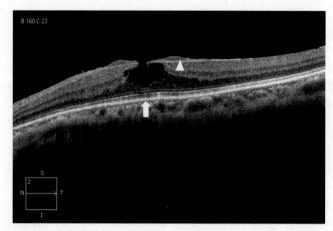

FIGURE 33.2 Degenerative lamellar hole with epiretinal proliferation (arrow) and intraretinal defects affecting the outer retina including thinning and ellipsoid zone disruption (arrow).

OCTA IMAGING

- Optical coherence tomography angiography (OCTA) may demonstrate increased vascular density in the superior capillary plexus in the perifoveal avascular zone in degenerative lamellar macular hole eyes and fellow eyes relative to healthy controls (Figure 33.3).
- Lamellar macular holes compared to healthy controls demonstrate no significant changes in the deep capillary plexus and choriocapillaris (Figure 33.4).

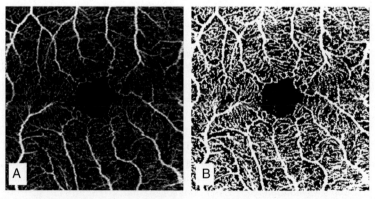

FIGURE 33.3 Optical coherence tomography angiography (OCTA) of the superficial capillary plexus (A) in a lamellar macular hole patient with a binarized version of the same image (B). (Reprinted with permission from Pierro L, Iuliano L, Gagliardi M, Arrigo A, Bandello F. Higher vascular density of the superficial retinal capillary plexus in degenerative lamellar macular holes. *Ophthalmic Surg Lasers Imaging Retina.* 2019;50(4):e112-e117.)

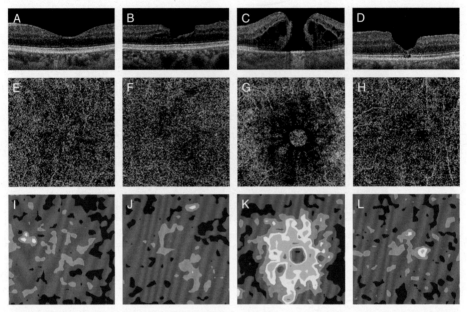

FIGURE 33.4 Optical coherence tomography (OCT) foveal B-scan (top row), choriocapillaris optical coherence tomography angiography (OCTA) (middle row) with corresponding choriocapillaris perfusion density map (lower row) of a normal patient (first column), lamellar macular hole patient (second column), full-thickness macular hole patient pre- (third column) and postsurgical repair (fourth). The choriocapillaris of the lamellar macular hole is equivalent to the normal patient, while the full-thickness macular hole is significantly less perfused preoperatively. (Reprinted with permission from Ahn J, Yoo G, Kim JT, Kim SW, Oh J. Choriocapillaris layer imaging with swept-source optical coherence tomography angiography in lamellar and full-thickness macular hole. *Graefes Arch Clin Exp Ophthalmol.* 2018;256(1):11-21.)

References

1. Haritoglou C, Tadayoni R, Hubschman JP. Lamellar macular hole surgery – current concepts, future prospects. *Clin Ophthalmol.* 2019;13:143-146.

2. Reibaldi M, Parravano M, Varano M, et al. Foveal microstructure and functional parameters in lamellar macular hole. *Am J Opthalmol.* 2012;154(6):974-980.

3. Ahn J, Yoo G, Kim JT, Kim SW, Oh J. Choriocapillaris layer imaging with swept-source optical coherence tomography angiography in lamellar and full-thickness macular hole. *Graefes Arch Clin Exp Ophthalmol.* 2018;256(1):11-21.

4. Pierro L, Iuliano L, Gagliardi M, Arrigo A, Bandello F. Higher vascular density of the superficial retinal capillary plexus in degenerative lamellar macular holes. *Ophthalmic Surg Lasers Imaging Retina.* 2019;50(4):e112-e117.

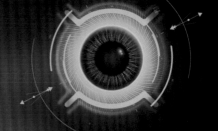

CHAPTER 34

Vitreomacular Traction Syndrome

SALIENT FEATURES

- Incomplete separation of the posterior hyaloid from the macula during the posterior vitreous detachment process with resulting traction is defined as vitreomacular traction (VMT).
- VMT syndrome is defined as VMT with associated epiretinal membrane.
- VMT frequency increases with age and is estimated at a prevalence of 1.6% in the population. It is present in 23% of exudative (wet) age-related macular degeneration (AMD) eyes and 29% of diabetic macular edema (DME) eyes.[1]
- VMT may be symptomatic with metamorphopsia, photopsia, blurred vision, and decreased visual acuity, affecting quality of life.[2]
- VMT is associated with a range of vision-impairing macular diseases such as epiretinal membrane (ERM), macular hole (MH), age-related macular degeneration, diabetic retinopathy, and diabetic macular edema.
- Prognosis, especially following treatment, depends on a variety of factors including concurrent macular disease, baseline visual acuity, age, ERM presence, and vitreomacular adhesion (VMA) diameter.[3]

OCT IMAGING

- Optical coherence tomography (OCT) is the gold standard for diagnosis, surveillance, and posttreatment monitoring of VMT.
- Traction between the posterior hyaloid and the foveal center results in the key OCT findings associated with VMT (Figures 34.1-34.3):
  - Altered foveal contour with anterior traction on the inner retinal surface.

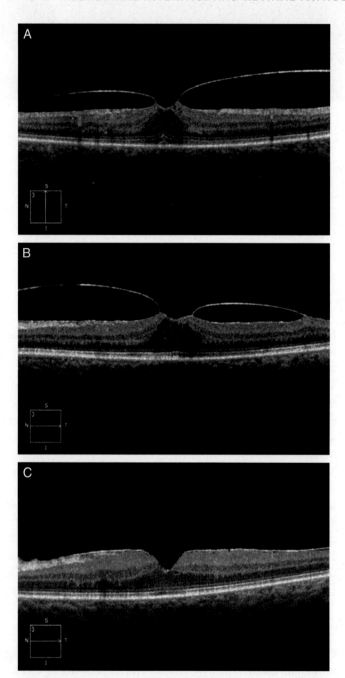

FIGURE 34.1 A, Optical coherence tomography (OCT) image demonstrating vitreomacular traction (VMT) with trace epiretinal membrane (ERM) with loss of foveal contour and small amount of intraretinal fluid. B, Progression of VMT with additional intraretinal fluid accumulation. C, Postoperative OCT scan showing resolution of VMT but persistent ERM.

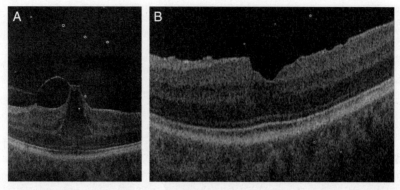

FIGURE 34.2 A, Optical coherence tomography (OCT) image of a patient with vitreomacular traction inducing cyst formation and focal ellipsoid zone (EZ) attenuation prior to surgery. B, One year following surgery, OCT demonstrates resolved vitreomacular traction (VMT) and EZ restoration with mild epiretinal membrane formation.

- Intraretinal fluid
- Subretinal fluid
- Outer retinal defects
- Pseudocysts and macular holes secondary to VMT may also be identified with OCT.
- Potential retinal morphology features for functional outcomes of interest include ellipsoid zone (EZ) integrity, central foveal thickness, and central subfield thickness.
- Lack of ERM, greater EZ integrity, and smaller VMA diameter are more favorable prognostic characteristics.

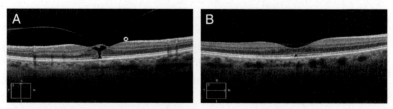

FIGURE 34.3 Optical coherence tomography (OCT) image in vitreomacular traction (VMT) case that demonstrates outer retinal defect with near full-thickness macular hole (A). Following spontaneous VMT release, fovea contour is restored with mild ellipsoid zone defect and minimal residual subretinal fluid (B).

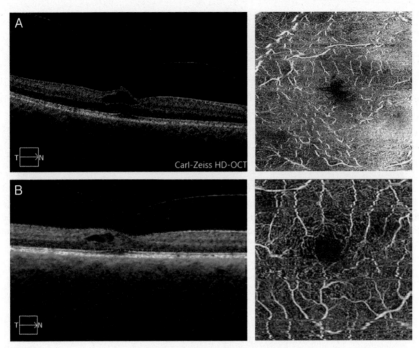

FIGURE 34.4 Optical coherence tomography angiography (OCTA) in two vitreomacular traction (VMT) cases. Motion artifact is noted on the first OCTA with limited quality of the scan (A). The second case demonstrates higher quality OCTA image with flow voids corresponding to areas of cystic alterations (B).

OCTA IMAGING

- Optical coherence tomography angiography (OCTA) is emerging as a modality for evaluating the retinal vascular impact of VMT that may have prognostic value (Figure 34.4).[4]
- There are variable findings in the current limited literature on OCTA in VMT. Findings reported include:
  - Decreased vascular perfusion in regions of VMT and surrounding retina which was reversible with vitrectomy.[5]
  - Lack of change in perfusion densities within all three plexuses, but that foveal avascular zone in the superficial capillary plexus (SCP) was reduced compared to healthy eyes.[4]
- Foveal traction and anatomic distortion may limit OCTA quality and increase potential for artifacts.

References

1. Meuer SM, Myers CE, Klein BEK, et al. The epidemiology of vitreoretinal interface abnormalities as detected by spectral-domain optical coherence tomography: the Beaver Dam Eye study. *Ophthalmology.* 2015;122(4):787-795. doi:10.1016/j.ophtha.2014.10.014.

2. Steel DHW, Lotery AJ. Idiopathic vitreomacular traction and macular hole: a comprehensive review of pathophysiology, diagnosis, and treatment. *Eye.* 2013;27(suppl 1):S1-S21. doi:10.1038/eye.2013.212.

3. Singh RP, Li A, Bedi R, et al. Anatomical and visual outcomes following ocriplasmin treatment for symptomatic vitreomacular traction syndrome. *Br J Ophthalmol.* 2014;98(3):356-360. doi:10.1136/bjophthalmol-2013-304219.

4. Iuliano L, Fogliato G, Colombo R, et al. Reduced perfusion density of superficial retinal capillary plexus after intravitreal ocriplasmin injection for idiopathic vitreomacular traction. *BMC Ophthalmol.* 2019;19(1):1-11. doi:10.1186/s12886-019-1119-9.

5. Kashani AH, Zhang Y, Capone A, et al. Impaired retinal perfusion resulting from vitreoretinal traction: a mechanism of retinal vascular insufficiency. *Ophthalmic Surg Lasers Imaging Retina.* 2016;47(3):1-11. doi:10.3928/23258160-20160229-03.

6. Duker JS, Kaiser PK, Binder S, et al. The international vitreomacular traction study group classification of vitreomacular adhesion, traction, and macular hole. *Ophthalmology.* 2013;120(12):2611-2619.

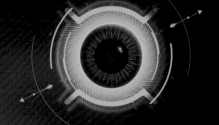

CHAPTER **35**

Myopic Macular Schisis and Tractional Retinal Detachment

SALIENT FEATURES

- Myopia is a risk factor for retinal detachment, macular holes, choroidal neovascularization, and retinoschisis.
- In the myopic environment, traction on the retina induced by the posterior hyaloid can cause splitting of the inner retinal layers, known as macular schisis or myopic foveoschisis.
- Myopic macular schisis and macular hole can progress to retinal detachment, which is relatively rare and occurs most commonly in association with posterior staphyloma.[1]

OPTICAL COHERENCE TOMOGRAPHY IMAGING

- Common findings on optical coherence tomography (OCT) include macular schisis, vitreoretinal abnormalities, and posterior staphyloma (Figure 35.1).
- Macular schisis is the most common OCT finding in highly myopic eyes.[2]
- Other anatomic findings on OCT associated with macular schisis include (Figures 35.2-35.4):
  - Dome-shaped macula
  - Photoreceptor detachment
  - Defects in the ellipsoid zone (EZ) in the fovea
  - Disruption of the internal limiting membrane (ILM)
  - Lamellar hole (LH) or full-thickness macular hole (FTMH)
  - Retinal detachment with FTMH

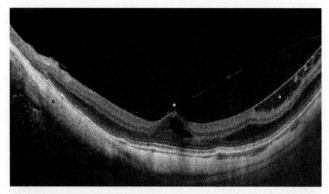

FIGURE 35.1 Optical coherence tomography (OCT) image from a patient with high myopia demonstrating vitreomacular traction (white asterisk), retinoschisis (A), and posterior staphyloma (B). The choroid is remarkably thin and the posterior sclera is visualized.

- There is likely a progression from retinoschisis to FTMH and, rarely, to macular-hole associated retinal detachment, although the rate of progression and incidence of each stage is not well understood or studied (Figures 35.2 and 35.3).
- Epiretinal traction from epiretinal membrane (ERM), vitreomacular traction (VMT), or both is thought to be the underlying process for myopic schisis and tractional retinal detachment. It is found in just under half of eyes with high myopia (Figure 35.2).[3]

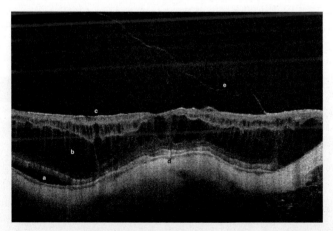

FIGURE 35.2 Optical coherence tomography (OCT) image from a patient with high myopia shows neurosensory retinal detachment (a), retinoschisis (b), trace epiretinal membrane (c), dome-shaped macula (d), and incomplete posterior vitreous detachment (PVD) (e).

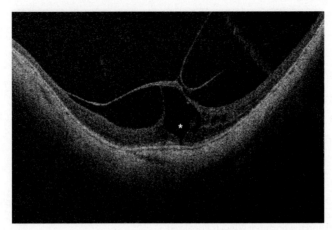

FIGURE 35.3 Optical coherence tomography (OCT) image from a patient with high myopia highlights a full-thickness macular hole associated with vitreomacular traction. A posterior staphyloma is present and the choroidal vasculature is severely thinned within the staphyloma.

- Highly myopic eyes with posterior vitreous detachment (PVD) are significantly less likely to develop complications and vision loss as compared to eyes with posterior vitreous schisis.[4] Frequently, it is difficult to assess for true PVD versus vitreoshisis in these eyes as there is extensive vitreous condensations over the nerve mimicking a Weiss ring (Figure 35.2).
- Posterior staphyloma, an increased arc of curvature of the posterior wall of the eye, is readily visible on examination and OCT.
- Choroidal thickness can be measured on OCT and is inversely correlated with age and myopic refractive error.[5]

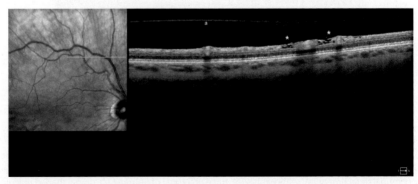

FIGURE 35.4 Optical coherence tomography (OCT) image from a patient with high myopia highlighting perivascular cystoid spaces and lamellar holes. The posterior hyaloid (a) is visualized just above the retinal surface indicative of an incomplete posterior vitreous detachment (PVD).

- Many eyes with high myopia exhibit paravascular abnormalities (PVAs) visible on OCT including paravascular microfolds, paravascular cysts, paravascular lamellar holes. These are more common along the inferior and superior temporal vascular arcade than along the nasal vascular arcade (Figure 35.4).[6]

OCT ANGIOGRAPHY IMAGING

- Myopia increases the risk for vascular fundus lesions including macular hemorrhage and choroidal neovascularization.[7]
- Retinal vascular alterations in high myopia include decreased retinal vessel density, which can be detected by OCT angiography (OCTA) (Figure 35.5).[8]
- On OCTA, choroidal dysfunction may be visualized as flow deficits in the choriocapillaris.[9]
- Myopic eyes with staphyloma are difficult to segment which decreases the accuracy of OCT and OCTA imaging. Understanding the limitations of the imaging technology and artifacts from segmentation are very important (Figures 35.2-35.5).[10]

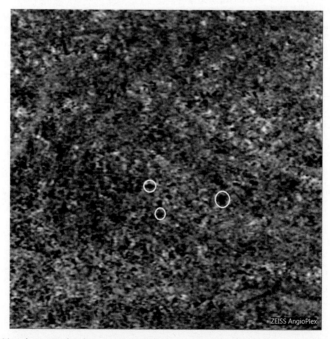

FIGURE 35.5 Macular optical coherence tomography angiography (OCTA) image with choriocapillaris segmentation demonstrating small foci of flow deficit (circles). Careful evaluation of the segmentation is critical to differentiate artifact from true flow deficits.

References

1. Mura M, Iannetta D, Buschini E, de Smet MD. T-shaped macular buckling combined with 25G pars plana vitrectomy for macular hole, macular schisis, and macular detachment in highly myopic eyes. *Br J Ophthalmol.* 2017;101(3):383-388. doi:10.1136/bjophthalmol-2015-308124.

2. You QS, Peng XY, Xu L, Chen CX, Wang YX, Jonas JB. Myopic maculopathy imaged by optical coherence tomography: the Beijing Eye Study. *Ophthalmology.* 2014;121(1):220-224.

3. Ripandelli G, Coppe AM, Parisi V, Stirpe M. Fellow eye findings of highly myopic subjects operated for retinal detachment associated with a macular hole. *Ophthalmology.* 2008;115:1489-1493.

4. Panozzo G, Mercanti A. Optical coherence tomography findings in myopic traction maculopathy. *Arch Ophthalmol.* 2004;122:1455-1460.

5. Alkabes M, Pichi F, Nucci P, et al. Anatomical and visual outcomes in high myopic macular hole (HM-MH) without retinal detachment: a review. *Graefe's Arch Clin Exp Ophthalmol.* 2014;252(2):191-199. doi:10.1007/s00417-013-2555-5.

6. Nishida Y, Fujiwara T, Imamura Y, et al. Choroidal thickness and visual acuity in highly myopic eyes. *Retina.* 2012;32:1229-1236.

7. Li T, Wang X, Zhou Y, et al. Paravascular abnormalities observed by spectral domain optical coherence tomography are risk factors for retinoschisis in eyes with high myopia. *Acta Ophthalmol.* 2018;96(4):e515-e523. doi:10.1111/aos.13628.

8. Yang Y, Wang J, Jiang H, et al. Retinal microvasculature alteration in high myopia. *Invest Ophthalmol Vis Sci.* 2016;57(14):6020-6030. doi:10.1167/iovs.16-19542.

9. Venkatesh R, Sinha S, Gangadharaiah D, et al. Retinal structural-vascular-functional relationship using optical coherence tomography and optical coherence tomography-angiography in myopia. *Eye Vis (Lond).* 2019;6(1):8. doi:10.1186/s40662-019-0133-67.

10. Al-Sheikh M, Phasukkijwatana N, Dolz-Marco R, et al. Quantitative OCT angiography of the retinal microvasculature and the choriocapillaris in myopic eyes. *Invest Ophthalmol Vis Sci.* 2017;58(4):2063-2069.

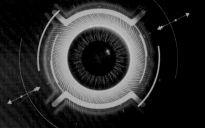

CHAPTER 36

Rhegmatogenous Retinal Detachment

SALIENT FEATURES

- Rhegmatogenous retinal detachment (RRD) is the most common form of retinal detachment and results from fluid gaining access to the subretinal space due to a retinal break (eg, retinal hole, retinal tear).
- RRD is defined as the separation of the neurosensory retina from the underlying retinal pigment epithelium (RPE) due to fluid influx from the vitreous cavity into the subretinal space secondary to a retinal break.
- Common causes and risk factors for retinal breaks include posterior vitreous detachment, lattice degeneration, and trauma.
- Involvement of the macula is a major determinant of the urgency of surgical repair. In addition, the status of the macula plays an important role in visual prognosis.

OCT IMAGING

- Detachment of the retina from the RPE can be clearly visualized by retinal elevation on optical coherence tomography (OCT) in both macula-off and macula-on RRDs with hyporeflective subretinal fluid (SRF) (Figures 36.1-36.3).
- Features that may be noted on OCT prior to surgical repair include outer retinal corrugations, intraretinal fluid, and retinal folds (Figures 36.1 and 36.3).
- If proliferative vitreoretinopathy (PVR) is present, preretinal and/or subretinal membranes may be identified with OCT (Figures 36.1 and 36.2).

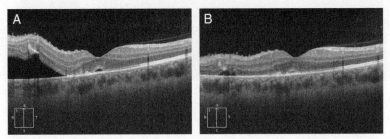

FIGURE 36.1 Predominantly fovea-sparing but macula-involving rhegmatogenous retinal detachment (RRD) with small cuff of subfoveal fluid. Subretinal membrane is noted as a hyperreflective lesion in the area of detachment (A). Following surgical repair, a small focal area of subretinal fluid remains in area of the subretinal membrane. Persistent ellipsoid zone attenuation/loss is noted (B).

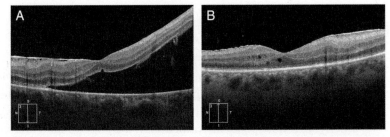

FIGURE 36.2 Macula-involving rhegmatogenous retinal detachment (RRD) with associated epiretinal membrane (A). Following surgical repair, intraretinal fluid is noted with significant ellipsoid zone attenuation. Subretinal fluid has completely resolved. Epiretinal membrane persists (B).

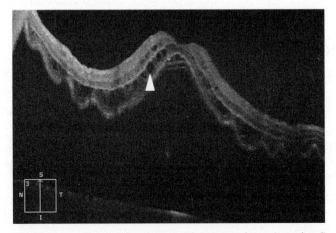

FIGURE 36.3 Total retinal detachment with intraretinal cysts (arrowhead).

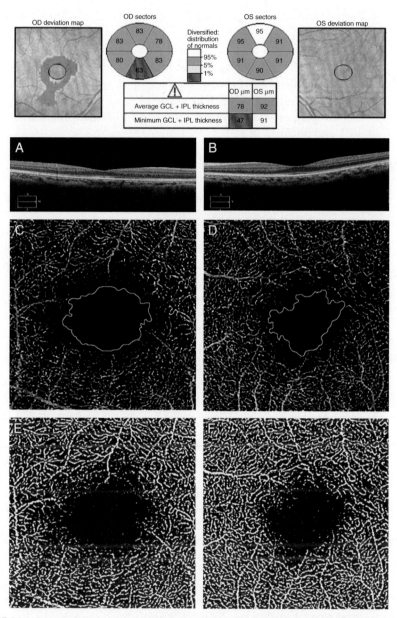

FIGURE 36.4 Comparative assessment of retinal vasculature in postoperative rhegmatogenous retinal detachment (RRD) in right eye treated with silicone oil tamponade and normal fellow eye imaging with macular optical coherence tomography (OCT) (A and B), optical coherence tomography angiography (OCTA) (C and D), converted binary images (E and F) showing an enlarged foveal avascular zone and reduced vascular density in the RRD eye. (Reprinted with permission from Lee JY, Kim JY, Lee SY, Jeong JH, Lee EK. Foveal microvascular structures in eyes with silicone oil tamponade for rhegmatogenous retinal detachment: a swept-source optical coherence tomography angiography study. *Sci Rep.* 2020;10(1):1-9.)

- Postoperatively, OCT can confirm complete reattachment and resolution of SRF.
- In addition, OCT can be utilized to evaluate for chronic sequelae related to RRD, including cystoid macular edema (CME) and epiretinal membrane (ERM) (Figure 36.2).
- Postoperative features, such as ellipsoid zone integrity and outer retinal atrophy, provide information related to visual prognosis (Figures 36.1 and 36.2).

OCTA IMAGING

- Macula-on RRD does not appear to alter the macular microvasculature compared to fellow eye analyses.
- Increased superficial and deep foveal avascular zone (FAZ) areas are observed in macula-on RRD after surgery compared to macula-off RRD. The extent of the avascular zones in macula-off RDs correlates with postoperative visual outcomes.
- In RRD eyes with silicone oil tamponade, FAZ was higher and vascular density lower postoperatively in the deep plexus compared to healthy fellow eyes (Figure 36.4).
  - Silicone oil tamponade duration correlates with increased FAZ enlargement and vascular density loss.

References

1. Auger G, Winder S. Spectral domain OCT: an aid to diagnosis and surgical planning of retinal detachments. *J Ophthalmol.* 2011;2011:725362.
2. Hagimura N, Suto K, Iida T, Kishi S. Optical coherence tomography of the neurosensory retina in rhegmatogenous retinal detachment. *Am J Ophthalmol.* 2000;129(2):186-190.
3. Hajari JN, Kyhnel A, Bech-Azeddine J, la Cour M, Kiilgaard JF. Progression of foveola-on rhegmatogenous retinal detachment. *Br J Ophthalmol.* 2014;98(11):1534-1538.
4. Nakanishi H, Hangai M, Unoki N, et al. Spectral-domain optical coherence tomography imaging of the detached macula in rhegmatogenous retinal detachment. *Retina.* 2009;29(2):232-242.
5. Woo JM, Yoon YS, Woo JE, Min JK. Foveal avascular zone area changes analyzed using OCT angiography after successful rhegmatogenous retinal detachment repair. *Curr Eye Res.* 2018;43(5):674-678.
6. Yoshikawa Y, Shoji T, Kanno J, et al. Evaluation of microvascular changes in the macular area of eyes with rhegmatogenous retinal detachment without macular involvement using swept-source optical coherence tomography angiography. *Clin Ophthalmol.* 2018;12:2059.
7. Lee JY, Kim JY, Lee SY, Jeong JH, Lee EK. Foveal microvascular structures in eyes with silicone oil tamponade for rhegmatogenous retinal detachment: a swept-source optical coherence tomography angiography study. *Sci Rep.* 2020;10(1):1-9.

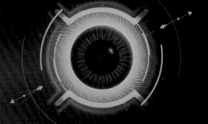

CHAPTER 37

Degenerative Retinoschisis

SALIENT FEATURES

- Usually presents as a dome-shaped retinal elevation with uniform convexity that is commonly bilateral and interotemporal in location.
- Prevalence is 7% of people older than 40 years.
- Most commonly characterized by splitting of the neurosensory retina at the outer plexiform layer; occasionally, inner plexiform layer splitting is present.
- Lacks retinal tears, vitreous pigment cells, or a demarcation line seen in rhegmatogenous retinal detachment.
- Blanches with laser due to reaction in the outer layer that remains in apposition to the retinal pigment epithelium (RPE).
- An absolute visual field defect is seen due to irreversible interruptions of the neuronal pathway between the photoreceptors and the ganglion cells.
- Patients are most commonly asymptomatic.
- Outer retinal holes can be seen.
- Retinoschisis-associated rhegmatogenous retinal detachment may occur when both inner and outer retinal breaks are present.

OCT IMAGING

- Optical coherence tomography (OCT) is helpful in differentiating retinoschisis and rhegmatogenous retinal detachment.
- OCT of retinal periphery shows retinoschisis as a split in the neurosensory retina: the outer leaf is a distinct separate layer lying in apposition to the hyperreflective band of the RPE (Figure 37.1).

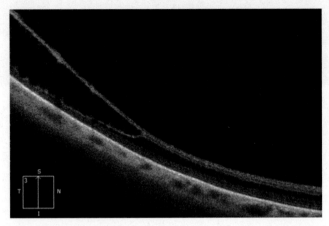

FIGURE 37.1 Peripheral OCT (optical coherence tomography) of the edge of retinoschisis cavity exhibiting a split in the neurosensory retina: the outer leaf is a distinct separate layer lying in apposition to the hyperreflective band of the retinal pigment epithelium (RPE).

- Retinal detachment, on the other hand, is seen as a complete detachment of the neurosensory retina from the RPE surface (Figure 37.2).
- Outer retinal holes can be imaged with OCT.
- Outer retinal holes can be flat with 360 degrees of apposition between the edges of the outer retinal hole and the RPE (Figure 37.3A).
- The edges of the outer retinal hole could be elevated partially or in 360° configuration (Figure 37.3B).
- With the elevation of the outer retinal hole edges, the OCT of the edge of retinoschisis can appear similar to that of rhegmatogenous retinal detachment (Figure 37.3C).

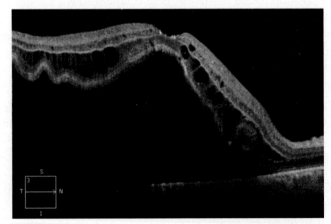

FIGURE 37.2 Optical coherence tomography (OCT) of the edge of rhegmatogenous retinal detachment with complete detachment of the neurosensory retina from the retinal pigment epithelium (RPE) surface.

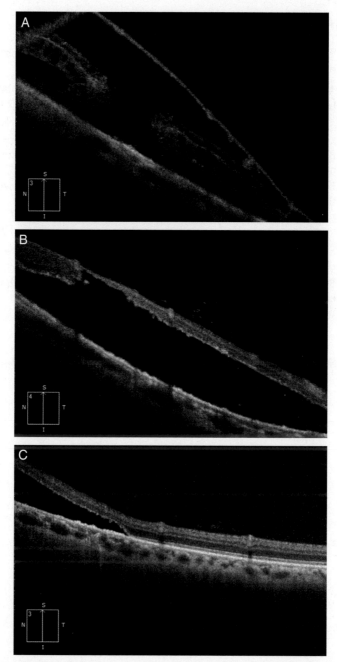

FIGURE 37.3 Peripheral optical coherence tomography (OCT) of the outer retinal holes seen in retinoschisis patients. Various configurations can be observed: (A) the edges of the outer retinal hole are attached to the retinal pigment epithelium (RPE) circumferentially, (B) the edges of the outer retinal hole are elevated from the RPE, and (C) the edge of retinoschisis appears similar to that of rhegmatogenous retinal detachment.

OCTA IMAGING

- There are currently no reports on optical coherence tomography angiography (OCTA) findings in degenerative retinoschisis.
- The peripheral location of retinoschisis makes OCTA imaging challenging, but might become feasible with wide-field OCTA imaging.

References

1. Byer NE. Perspectives on the management of the complications of senile retinoschisis. *Eye (Lond)*. 2002;16(4):359-364.
2. Byer NE. Long-term natural history study of senile retinoschisis with implications for management. *Ophthalmology*. 1986;93(9):1127-1137.
3. Byer NE. Clinical study of senile retinoschisis. *Arch Ophthalmol*. 1968;79(1): 36-44.
4. Shea M, Schepens CL, Von Pirquet SR. Retionoschisis. I. senile type: a clinical report of one hundred seven cases. *Arch Ophthalmol*. 1960;63:1-9.
5. Rachitskaya AV, Yuan A, Singh RP, Sears JE, Schachat AP. Optical coherence tomography of outer retinal holes in senile retinoschisis and schisis-detachment. *Br J Ophthalmol*. 2017;101(4):445-448.

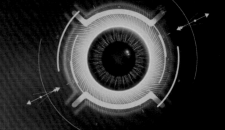

CHAPTER 38

Lattice Degeneration

SALIENT FEATURES

- Lattice degeneration (LD) is characterized by asymptomatic focal peripheral funduscopic lesions which are associated with retinal holes, retinal traction, and retinal detachment.
- Lattice lesions are generally peripheral, circumferentially oriented, sharply demarcated, round or oval atrophic retinal lesions that may have associated pigmentary change on funduscopic examination (Figures 38.1A, 2A, and 3A, teal arrows).
- There may be associated overlying vitreous liquefaction and vitreoretinal adhesions at the margins of LD.
- LD is present in 6% to 8% of the general population and 30% of phakic retinal detachments. Prevalence of lattice in the fellow eye of patients with retinal detachment is estimated to be 35%.

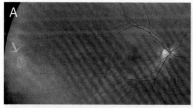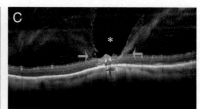

FIGURE 38.1 A, Color photograph with teal arrow highlighting a small focus of lattice degeneration. B, Higher magnification image through the lattice lesion with green arrow signifying location of spectral-domain optical coherence tomography (SD-OCT) scan. C, SD-OCT image through the lattice shows a small focus of disorganized, atrophic retina (red arrow), a hyporeflective focus of liquefied vitreous overlying the lesion (yellow asterisk), and condensed, hyperreflective vitreous adhered to the margins of the lesions (green arrows).

- Pathophysiology of these lesions is considered multifactorial including genetic and environmental elements. Theories have suggested developmental anomalies of the internal limiting membrane, abnormal vitreoretinal traction, and choroidal abnormalities may contribute to the development of LD.
- Studies utilizing fluorescein angiography have demonstrated that lattice degeneration lesions exist within zones of peripheral nonperfusion. The vasculature within or around the lattice degeneration can often be seen to be atrophic or sclerotic.
- Therefore, some have suggested a primary ischemic insult with subsequent reparative gliosis may be the etiology of development of lattice degeneration.
- Laser photocoagulation of these lesions as prophylaxis for retinal tears is considered, although evidence for this practice is only significant in the case of symptomatic flap tears.

OCT IMAGING

- Focal retinal thinning on optical coherence tomography (OCT) is often evident and can be appreciated throughout the entire area of lattice with poor distinction between inner and outer retinal layers, photoreceptor loss, and retinal pigment epithelium (RPE) disruption (Figures 38.2C, blue asterisks and Figure 38.3C, purple arrow). The inner retinal layers are more prominently affected. Thinned neural retina may appear hyperreflective.
- U-shaped vitreous traction defects may be present. Hyporeflective areas overlying central portions of lattice degeneration are believed to represent areas of liquefied vitreous (Figures 38.1 and 38.2C, yellow asterisks) in contrast to the hyperreflective, firmly adherent vitreous gel at the margins of the lesion (Figures 38.1 and 38.2C, green arrows). These adhesions may be associated with underlying retinal detachment (Figure 38.2C, red arrows).

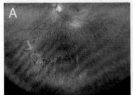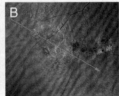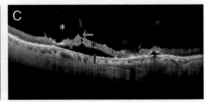

FIGURE 38.2 A, Color photograph with teal arrow demonstrating a linear pigmented patch of lattice degeneration. B, Higher magnification image through the lattice lesion with green arrow signifying location of the spectral-domain optical coherence tomography (SD-OCT) scan. There is a small retinal hole within the temporal edge of the lattice lesion (green asterisk). C, SD-OCT image through the lattice shows a strip of atrophic retina (blue asterisk), a hyporeflective focus of liquefied vitreous overlying the lesion (yellow asterisk), and condensed, hyperreflective vitreous adhered to the margins of the lesions (green arrows). There are two foci of neurosensory retinal detachment (red arrows) and small vitreous hyperreflective dots (pink asterisks).

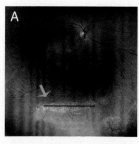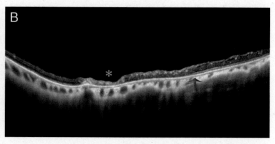

FIGURE 38.3 A, Color photograph with teal arrow demonstrating a small focus of lattice degeneration. The black line identifies the location of the spectral-domain optical coherence tomography (SD-OCT) image. B, SD-OCT through the lattice lesion demonstrates thinned, atrophic retina (blue asterisk). The ellipsoid layer reconstitutes at the temporal edge of the lesions (purple arrow).

- Retinal breaks include atrophic holes and subclinical retinal detachment and may occur in the absence of vitreous traction, peripheral vascular disease (PVD), or flap. Retinoschisis may be present.
- OCT may demonstrate vitreous membrane formation in the posterior hyaloid and retina seen as a band of hyperreflectivity. Hyperreflective deposits within the detached vitreous may represent accumulation of glial cells secondary to extracellular cell product breakdown and fibrosis (Figure 38.2C, pink asterisks).
- Prior focal sectorial laser photocoagulation around areas of lattice degeneration will appear as focal areas of RPE hypertrophy with overlying retinal atrophy.

OCTA IMAGING

- There is currently no role for optical coherence tomography angiography (OCTA) in lattice degeneration.

References

1. Wilkinson CP. Interventions for asymptomatic retinal breaks and lattice degeneration for preventing retinal detachment. *Cochrane Database Syst Rev.* 2014;2014(9):CD003170. doi: 10.1002/14651858.CD003170.pub4.
2. Byer NE. Rethinking prophylactic therapy of retinal detachment. In: Stirpe M, eds. *Advances in Vitreoretinal Surgery.* New York, NY: Ophthalmic Communications Society; 1992:399-411.
3. Madjarov B, Hilton GF, Brinton DA, Lee SS. A new classification of the retinoschises. *Retina.* 1995;15:282-285.
4. Meguro A, Ideta H, Ota M, et al. Common variants in the COL4A4 gene confer susceptibility to lattice degeneration of the retina. *PLoS One.* 2012;7(6):e39300. doi:10.1371/journal.pone.0039300.
5. Manjunath V, Taha M, Fujimoto JG, Duker JS. Posterior lattice degeneration characterized by spectral domain optical coherence tomography. *Retina.* 2011;31(3):492-496.

6. Choudhry N, Golding J, Manry MW, Rao RC. Ultra-widefield steering-based spectral-domain optical coherence tomography imaging of the retinal periphery. *Ophthalmology*. 2016;123(6):1368-1374. doi:10.1016/j.ophtha.2016.01.045.

7. Tsai CY, Hung KC, Wang SW, Chen MS, Ho TC. Spectral-domain optical coherence tomography of peripheral lattice degeneration of myopic eyes before and after laser photocoagulation. *J Formos Med Assoc*. 2019;118(3):679-685.

8. Chen SN, Hwang JF, Wu WC. Peripheral retinal vascular patterns in patients with rhegmatogenous retinal detachment in taiwan. *PLoS One*. 2016;11(2):e0149176. Available at https://doi.org/10.1371/journal.pone.0149176.

Part 5
Inflammation and Infection

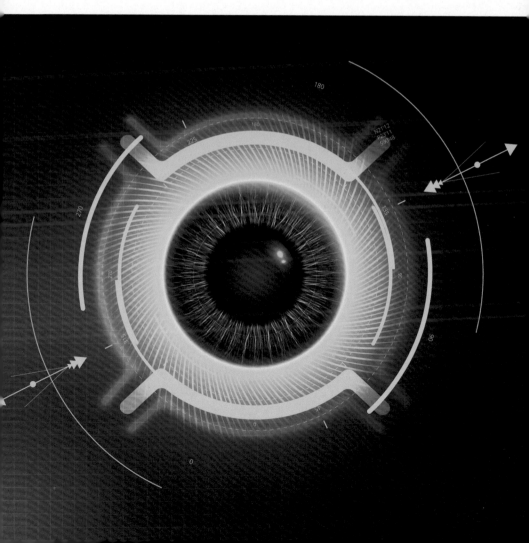

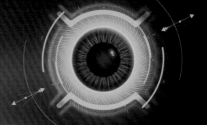

CHAPTER **39**

Cystoid Macular Edema

SALIENT FEATURES

- Cystoid macular edema (CME) occurs as a common sequel of various pathological conditions such as intraocular inflammation, vitreomacular traction, retinal vascular disease, postoperative-related inflammation, choroidal neovascularization, and retinal degenerative disorders.
- CME presenting as multiple cystlike areas of fluid causing retinal swelling.
- The pathophysiology of macular edema is not fully understood but involves loss of homeostasis between the blood retinal barriers of the retinal pigment epithelium (RPE), choroid, and retinal vasculature such that fluid is allowed to accumulate in the extracellular retinal spaces. In uveitis, this is thought to be due to dysregulation of inflammatory mediators.
- Macular edema and its sequelae are common causes of decreased vision in uveitis patients.
- Patients with macular edema, and in particular CME, complain of decreased vision, metamorphopsia, micropsia, and central scotoma.
- Examination classically reveals retinal thickening and cystoid spaces, which may be highlighted better with a green filter.
- Fluorescein angiography is seen atypical petalloid pattern formed by leakage from perifoveal capillaries.

- Although clinical diagnosis has previously been the historical gold standard for diagnosis of CME, the advent of optical coherence tomography (OCT), and particularly spectral-domain (SD)-OCT, allows for more sensitive and detailed identification of CME.
- Generally, treatment is targeted toward the inciting pathology that resulted in CME development, such as:
  - Topical, periocular, or intravitreal steroids for inflammatory-related CME
  - Intravitreal anti–vascular endothelial growth factor (VEGF) for retinal vascular disease–related CME.
  - Topical nonsteroidal anti-inflammatory drugs (NSAIDs) are also used for inflammatory-related CME, often in combination with steroids.

OCT IMAGING

- OCT imaging of CME reveals hyporeflective intraretinal cystoid spaces which may often be associated with a small amount of subretinal fluid.
- Cystoid spaces are often clearly defined hyporeflective cystic spaces that are separated by thin, hyperreflective retinal tissues (Figure 39.1A, Figure 39.2).
- Chronic CME may result in retinal atrophy and photoreceptor degeneration, leading to permanent loss of vision.
- Concurrent disease should be carefully considered, including sub-RPE compartment disease, such as CNV that may dictate treatment course.

OCTA IMAGING

- Optical coherence tomography angiography (OCTA) imaging of CME reveals large cystoid spaces that lack flow signal (Figure 39.2).
- These flowless cystoid spaces are often associated with an increase in size of the foveal avascular zone (FAZ) (Figure 39.3).[3]
  - The enlargement of the FAZ is likely due to peripheral displacement of retinal capillaries owing to large cystoid spaces or cysts developing in preferentially nonperfused areas.[3]

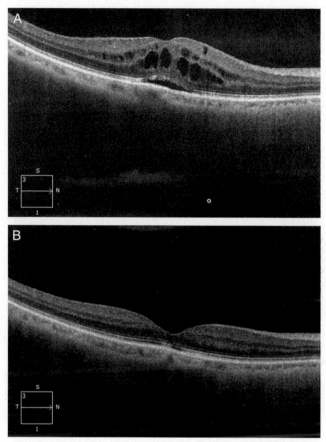

FIGURE 39.1 Optical coherence tomography (OCT) B-scan of patient presenting with large foveal cysts and a small cuff of subretinal fluid following cataract surgery (A) and the same eye with complete fluid resolution following topical anti-inflammatory treatment (B).

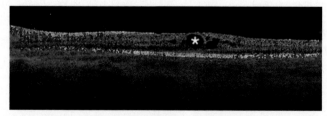

FIGURE 39.2 Optical coherence tomography (OCT) B-scan with overlaid optical coherence tomography angiography (OCTA) flow signal. OCT reveals large hyporeflective cystoid spaces that lack flow signal on the overlaid OCTA (white asterisk).

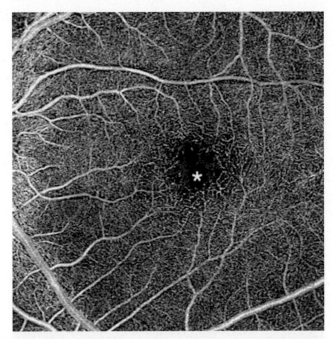

FIGURE 39.3 *En-face* optical coherence tomography angiography (OCTA) image demonstrating absence of flow signal in the large cystoid spaces and enlargement of the foveal avascular zone (FAZ) (white asterisk).

References

1. Grajewski RS, Boelke AC, Adler W, et al. Spectral-domain optical coherence tomography findings of the macula in 500 consecutive patients with uveitis. *Eye (Lond)*. 2016;30(11):1415-1423.
2. Gupta S, Shah DN, Joshi SN, Aryal M, Puri LR. Patterns of macular edema in uveitis as diagnosed by optical coherence tomography in tertiary eye center. *Nepal J Ophthalmol*. 2018;10(19):39-46.
3. Waizel M, Todorova MG, Terrada C, LeHoang P, Massamba N, Bodaghi B. Superficial and deep retinal foveal avascular zone OCTA findings of non-infectious anterior and posterior uveitis. *Graefes Arch Clin Exp Ophthalmol*. 2018;256(10):1977-1984.

CHAPTER 40

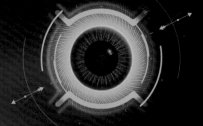

Syphilitic Chorioretinitis

SALIENT FEATURES

- Ocular syphilis is a masquerade syndrome that can have a wide variety of manifestations.
- The best described form of posterior segment involvement is acute syphilitic posterior placoid chorioretinitis (ASPPC) which presents with one or more characteristic yellow placoid lesions in the posterior pole.
- The choriocapillaris is thought to be the primary site of infection, with subsequent spread of inflammation to the retinal pigment epithelium (RPE) and photoreceptors.
- Ocular syphilis may occur in immunocompetent or immunocompromised patients. Workup should include testing for human immunodeficiency virus (HIV).
- The mainstay for treatment for all forms of ocular syphilis is 2 weeks of intravenous penicillin G.

OCT IMAGING

- The acute phase is characterized by a focal bleb of subretinal fluid (Figure 40.1A) that tends to self-resolve within a week of symptom onset and prior to antibiotic treatment[1-3] (Figure 40.1B).
- Punctate hyperreflective dots may be present in the choroid which may reflect the extent of choroidal inflammation[2,4] (Figure 40.2A).
- Loss of choroidal vascular detail, segmental loss of the ellipsoid zone (EZ), and external limiting membrane disruption are often present[2] (Figure 40.2A).

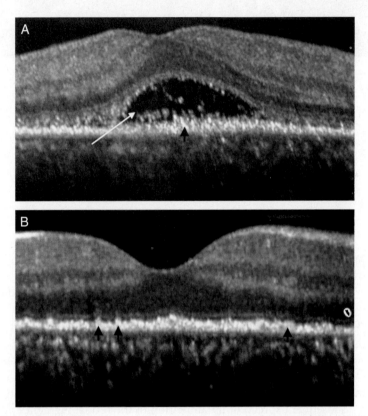

FIGURE 40.1 A, Optical coherence tomography (OCT) of a patient with acute syphilitic posterior placoid chorioretinitis demonstrating foveal subretinal fluid (white arrow). Diffuse granular hyperreflectivity of the retinal pigment epithelium (RPE) is present (black arrow). This photo was taken 5 days after symptom onset. B, Spectral-domain OCT of the same eye 2 days after presentation shows spontaneous resolution of subretinal fluid prior to initiation of antibiotics. Irregular granular thickening of the RPE is still present (black arrows). The ellipsoid zone (EZ) is notably absent, but the external limiting membrane (ELM) remains intact.

- After treatment, ellipsoid zone changes completely resolve in the majority of patients[1,2] (Figure 40.2B).
- Optical coherence tomography OCT) reveals focal nodular thickening of the RPE (Figure 40.1A) and granular hyperreflectivity of the EZ (Figure 40.2A) which colocalize to yellow-white punctate lesions seen on fundus examination.

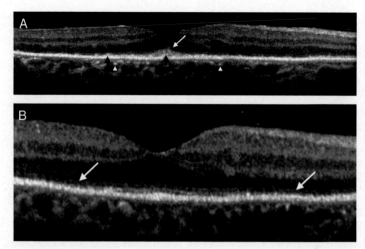

FIGURE 40.2 A, Optical coherence tomography (OCT) of a patient with syphilitic chorioretinitis 1 week after symptom onset. Multiple focal areas of retinal pigment epithelium (RPE) thickening can be seen (black arrows). Loss of the external limiting membrane is also present in the fovea (white arrow). Hyperreflective dots can be seen in the choroid (white arrowhead). Note this patient has concurrent proliferative diabetic retinopathy with diabetic macular edema. B, OCT of the same patient 1 month after treatment with intravenous penicillin G. The RPE changes and the subfoveal external limiting membrane/ellipsoid zone disruption have improved. The ellipsoid zone is still not well delineated in the extrafoveal regions (white arrows). The hyperreflective dots in the choroid have also resolved.

OCTA IMAGING

- Reduced choriocapillaris flow is seen within the area of the placoid lesion and improves post treatment[1] (Figure 40.3).
- The area of choriocapillaris nonperfusion tends to be larger in ASPPC than in other placoid disorders, such as acute posterior multifocal placoid pigment epitheliopathy.[1]
- Rarely, choroidal neovascularization may complicate syphilitic chorioretinitis, which would present on optical coherence tomography angiography (OCTA) as a fine branching network of vessels in the subretinal space or between the RPE and Bruch membrane.[5]

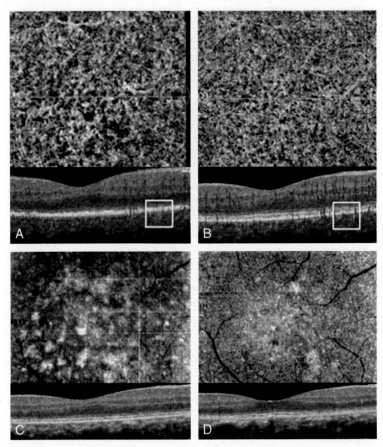

FIGURE 40.3 En-face optical coherence tomography (OCT) angiography (A and B) and en-face structural OCT (C and D) of the patient from Figure 40.1 2 days after presentation (A and C) and 2 months after treatment (B and D). Segmentation at the level of the choriocapillaris demonstrates areas of decreased choriocapillaris flow (A—white box, red circle). After treatment, there is resolution of the flow void (B—white box, red circle). En-face structural OCT at the level of the ellipsoid zone demonstrates hyperreflective clumps (C). After treatment, the en-face OCT shows marked improvement in these areas of hyperreflectivity (D). (Reprinted with permission from Tsui E, Gal-Or O, Ghadiali Q, Freund KB. Multimodal imaging adds new insights into acute syphilitic posterior placoid chorioretinitis. *Retin Cases Brief Rep.* 2018;12(suppl 1):S3-S8.)

References

1. Tsui E, Gal-Or O, Ghadiali Q, Freund KB. Multimodal imaging adds new insights into acute syphilitic posterior placoid chorioretinitis. *Retin Cases Brief Rep.* 2018;12:S3-S8.
2. Burkholder BM, Leung TG, Ostheimer TA, Butler NJ, Thorne JE, Dunn JP. Spectral domain optical coherence tomography findings in acute syphilitic posterior placoid chorioretinitis. *J Ophthalmic Inflamm Infect.* 2014;4(1):2.

3. Pichi F, Ciardella AP, Cunningham ET, et al. Spectral domain optical coherence tomography findings in patients with acute syphilitic posterior placoid chorioretinopathy. *Retina*. 2014;34(2):373-384.

4. Zett C, Lima LH, Vianello S, et al. En-face optical coherence tomography of acute syphilitic posterior placoid chorioretinopathy. *Ocul Immunol Inflamm*. 2018;26(8):1264-1270.

5. Giuffrè C, Marchese A, Cicinelli MV, et al. Multimodal imaging and treatment of syphilitic choroidal neovascularization. *Retin Cases Brief Rep*.2019:1.

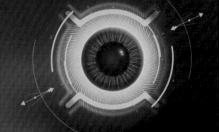

CHAPTER 41

Vogt-Koyanagi-Harada Disease

SALIENT FEATURES

- Vogt-Koyanagi-Harada (VKH) disease is a systemic disease with characteristic intraocular manifestations of bilateral nonnecrotizing granulomatous panuveitis with associated exudative retinal detachments.
- Its extraocular manifestations are numerous, including the presence of cerebrospinal fluid pleocytosis with meningismus, dysacusis, tinnitus, sensorineural hearing loss, alopecia, vitiligo, and poliosis.[1]
- While bilateral panuveitis and exudative retinal detachments are the most characteristic ocular findings in the acute phase of the disease, the late or convalescent phase demonstrates a classic "sunset glow fundus" due to diffuse depigmentation of the retina pigment epithelium (RPE).[1,2]
- Ocular manifestations of VKH are nearly identical to sympathetic ophthalmia (SO), and the two entities are considered to be "sister diseases." Therefore, the presence of prior penetrating ocular trauma or surgery is required for a diagnosis of SO.
- While the exact pathogenesis remains unknown, evidence suggests the disease is driven by a systemic autoimmune response involving T-lymphocytes targeting the uveal tract.
- The mainstay of treatment includes systemic corticosteroids with some patients requiring additional immunomodulatory agents such as cyclosporine. Systemic and visual prognosis depend on early diagnosis and initiation of systemic treatment, ideally during the acute stage of the disease.

- Local ocular corticosteroid treatment is also utilized as a supplement for suppression of inflammation.
- Multimodal imaging is often critical for making the diagnosis of VKH. Fluorescein angiography (FA), indocyanine green angiography (ICGA), B-scan ultrasonography, and optical coherence tomography (OCT) are useful for substantiating the clinical diagnosis and monitoring response to treatment (Figures 41.1-41.5).[3-5]

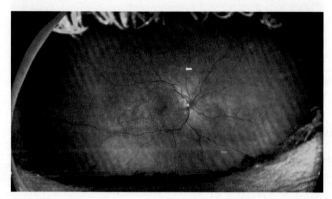

FIGURE 41.1 Wide-field fundus photograph of acute uveitic phase Vogt-Koyanagi-Harada (VKH) disease, demonstrating characteristic optic disc edema and hyperemia, multiple small focal yellow deposits at the level of the retina pigment epithelium (RPE) (termed Dalen-Fuchs nodules; white arrow), and a focal exudative retinal detachment (green arrow).

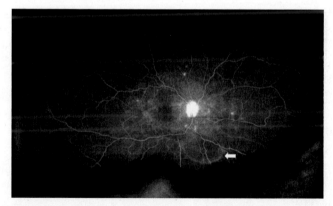

FIGURE 41.2 Wide-field fluorescein angiography (FA) of acute uveitic phase Vogt-Koyanagi-Harada (VKH) disease corresponding to Figure 41.1, demonstrating multifocal small pinpoint areas of leakage scattered throughout the posterior pole with focal exudative retinal detachment seen inferior to the optic disc (white arrow).

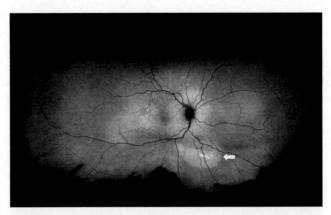

FIGURE 41.3 Wide-field fundus autofluorescence (FAF) of acute uveitic phase Vogt-Koyanagi-Harada (VKH) disease corresponding to Figure 41.1, demonstrating multiple discrete and coalescing areas of mottled hyperautofluorescence and a well-demarcated area of hyperautofluorescence inferior to the disc corresponding to area of localized retinal detachment (white arrow).

OCT IMAGING

Acute Uveitic Phase Features

- Singular or multifocal serous neurosensory retinal detachments are common[3,4] (Figure 41.4).
- Fibrinous membranes in the subretinal space, often contiguous with the ellipsoid zone (EZ) of attached retina with RPE attachments and forming septa that divide the subretinal space into multiple compartments[3,4] (Figure 41.4). A foveal bacillary detachment may be present which typically appears as neurosensory detachment with splitting of the photoreceptors, septae may be present within the hyporeflective space and the EZ appears to still appose the RPE (Figure 41.4).
- Other features include intraretinal cystoid spaces, focal retinoschisis, RPE and choroidal undulations, and folds and inward bulging alongside excavation[4] (Figure 41.4).
- Thickened choroid is seen best with enhanced depth imaging (EDI).[5]

Chronic/Convalescent Phase

- Serous retinal detachments resolve[4] (Figure 41.5).
- EZ and internal limiting membrane (ILM) may remain irregular for months after treatment with eventual reconstitution of these layers.[4]
- Focal areas of RPE thinning/irregularity overlying irregular Bruch membrane (BM) can persist.[6]
- In some cases, EZ attenuation and outer retinal atrophy may develop without layer reconstitution.

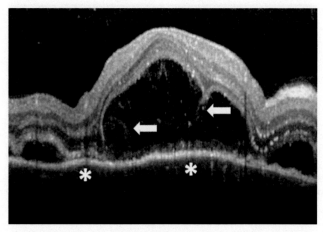

FIGURE 41.4 Optical coherence tomography (OCT) of the fovea in acute uveitic phase Vogt-Koyanagi-Harada (VKH) disease, demonstrating characteristic multifocal neurosensory retinal detachments with subretinal fibrinous membranes (white arrows), creating the appearance of a septate subretinal space likely consistent with a bacillary detachment. Note the undulated appearance of the underlying choroid and retina pigment epithelium (RPE) (white asterisks) and irregular disruption of the RPE and ellipsoid zone (EZ).

OCTA IMAGING

Acute Uveitic Phase Features

- Multiple foci of choriocapillaris flow voids, corresponding with ICGA, can be seen that decrease in number and size with treatment.[7]
- Hypoperfusion in Sattler layer (Figure 41.6), corresponding with ICGA, resolve with treatment.[8]

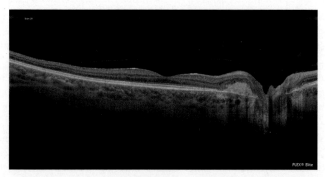

FIGURE 41.5 Optical coherence tomography (OCT) of the same eye after successful treatment of Vogt-Koyanagi-Harada (VKH) disease, demonstrating complete resolution of neurosensory retinal detachments, return of the normal foveal architecture, resolution of choroidal and retina pigment epithelium (RPE) undulations, and reconstitution of the ellipsoid zone (EZ).

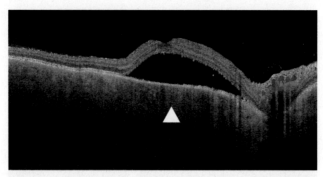

FIGURE 41.6 Decorrelation overlay from optical coherence tomography angiography (OCTA) of Vogt-Koyanagi-Harada (VKH) patient showing serous retinal detachment and hypoperfusion of Sattler layer (arrowhead).

References

1. Moorthy RS, Inomata H, Rao NA. Vogt-Koyanagi-Harada syndrome. *Surv Ophthalmol.* 1995;39(4):265-292. doi:10.1016/S0039-6257(05)80105-5.

2. Read RW, Holland GN, Rao NA, et al. Revised diagnostic criteria for Vogt-Koyanagi-Harada disease: report of an international committee on nomenclature. *Am J Ophthalmol.* 2001;131(5):647-652. doi:10.1016/S0002-9394(01)00925-4.

3. Yamaguchi Y, Otani T, Kishi S. Tomographic features of serous retinal detachment with multilobular dye pooling in acute vogt-koyanagi-harada disease. *Am J Ophthalmol.* 2007;144(2):260-265. doi:10.1016/j.ajo.2007.04.007.

4. Ishihara K, Hangai M, Kita M, Yoshimura N. Acute vogt-koyanagi-harada disease in enhanced spectral-domain optical coherence tomography. *Ophthalmology.* 2009;116(9):1799-1807. doi:10.1016/j.ophtha.2009.04.002.

5. Fong AHC, Li KKW, Wong D. Choroidal evaluation using enhanced depth imaging spectral-domain optical coherence tomography in Vogt-Koyanagi-Harada disease. *Retina.* 2011;31(3):502-509. doi:10.1097/IAE.0b013e3182083beb.

6. Vasconcelos-Santos DV, Sohn EH, Sadda S, Rao NA. Retinal pigment epithelial changes in chronic vogt-koyanagi-harada disease: fundus autofluorescence and spectral domain-optical coherence tomography findings. *Retina.* 2010;30(1):33-41. doi:10.1097/IAE.0b013e3181c5970d.

7. Aggarwal K, Agarwal A, Mahajan S, et al. The role of optical coherence tomography angiography in the diagnosis and management of acute vogt–koyanagi–harada disease. *Ocul Immunol Inflamm.* 2018;26(1):142-153. doi:10.1080/09273948.2016.1195001.

8. Wintergerst MWM, Herrmann P, Finger RP. Optical coherence tomography angiography for evaluation of Sattler's layer in Vogt-Koyanagi-Harada disease. *Ophthalmic Surg Lasers Imaging Retina.* 2018;49(8):639-642. doi:10.3928/23258160-20180803-14.

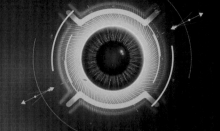

CHAPTER 42

Ocular Tuberculosis

SALIENT FEATURES

- Ocular tuberculosis (TB) is an extrapulmonary form of systemic tuberculosis resulting from hematogenous dissemination of the organism, *Mycobacterium tuberculosis*. It may be seen with or without concurrent, clinically apparent pulmonary involvement.
- In the eye, the disease has protean manifestations including granulomatous and nongranulomatous anterior uveitis, broad-based posterior synechiae, iris granuloma, intermediate uveitis (IU), posterior uveitis in the form of choroidal tubercle, choroidal tuberculoma, subretinal abscess, serpiginous-like choroiditis (multifocal serpiginoid choroiditis [MSC]), retinal vasculitis, neuroretinitis, and optic neuropathy. It is also known to cause endophthalmitis and panophthalmitis.
- The presence of chorioretinal scars underlying a blood vessel in the setting of IU is suggestive of TB uveitis (Figure 42.1).
- On fluorescein angiography (FA), choroidal tubercles show early hypofluorescence with late hyperfluorescence (Figure 42.2). Choroidal granulomas (tuberculomas) show early hyperfluorescence with increase in hyperfluorescence in the late phase and pooling in the surrounding exudative retinal detachment.
- MSC shows early hypofluorescence and late hyperfluorescence of active lesions on FA (Figure 42.3), while on indocyanine green angiography, early and late hypofluorescence, indicating a choroidal disease.

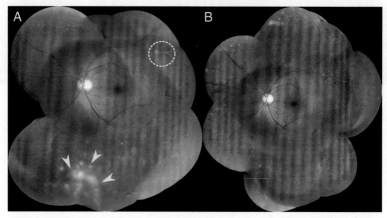

FIGURE 42.1 A, Fundus photograph of a patient with tuberculosis-related intermediate uveitis (IU). Snowballs are seen inferiorly (yellow arrowheads). Superotemporally, a sclerosed vessel with underlying chorioretinal scar is noted (dashed white circle). This is an important sign suggestive of tubercular etiology in this patient. B, Fundus photograph of the same patient showing resolution of IU.

- Fundus autofluorescence (FAF) can monitor response to therapy in cases of MSC. Various stages of healing on FAF have been described (Figure 42.4):
  - Stage I (acute): an ill-defined halo of hyperautofluorescence surrounds the lesion.
  - Stage II (active): stippled hyperautofluorescence of the lesions accompany well-defined hypoautofluorescence at the borders.
  - Stage III (healing): stippled hypoautofluorescence throughout the lesion.
  - Stage IV (completely healed): uniform hypoautofluorescence.

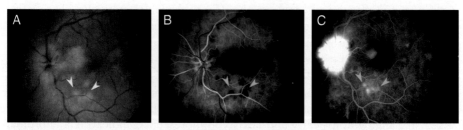

FIGURE 42.2 A, Fundus photograph of a patient with optic disc edema and choroidal tubercles seen as multifocal deep yellowish lesions (yellow arrowheads). B, Choroidal tubercles appear hypofluorescent (green arrowheads) in the early phase of fluorescein angiography (FA). C, Late phase shows hyperfluorescence of the lesions (blue arrowheads).

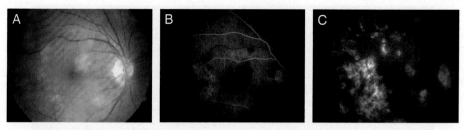

FIGURE 42.3 A, Fundus photograph of a patient with multifocal serpiginoid choroiditis (MSC). B, In the early-phase FA, active lesions show hypofluorescence. C, Active lesions become hyperfluorescent in the late phase.

OCT IMAGING

- Optical coherence tomography (OCT) is routinely used to identify and monitor uveitic macular edema in the form of cystoid macular edema (CME) with or without neurosensory detachment (Figure 42.5).
- Although CME is a common feature of IU, snowballs are more frequently seen in tuberculosis-associated IU.
- In acute and active MSC (stage I and II on FAF), OCT demonstrates choroidal thickening plus irregular hyperreflective elevations of the RPE and interdigitation zone (IZ), ellipsoid zone (EZ), external limiting membrane (ELM) disruption with minimal distortion of inner retinal layers (Figure 42.6A). The hyperreflectivity in the RPE and outer retina causes an underlying shadowing effect.

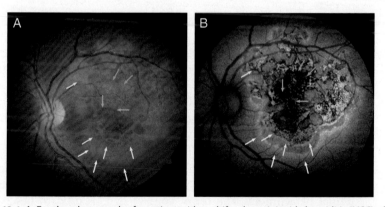

FIGURE 42.4 A, Fundus photograph of a patient with multifocal serpiginoid choroiditis (MSC), showing various stages of healing. B, The acute stage or active edge, clinically seen as a creamy lesion, shows an ill-defined, diffuse halo of hyperautofluorescence on fundus autofluorescence (FAF) photograph (stage I) (white arrows). Yellow arrows depict areas in stage II seen as stippled hyperautofluorescence with well-defined hypoautofluorescent margins. Lesions in stage III clinically appear as grayish well-defined lesions and show stippled hypoautofluorescence on FAF (green arrows). Completely resolved lesions with scarring and pigmentation appear as areas of uniform hypoautofluorescence (stage IV) (blue arrows).

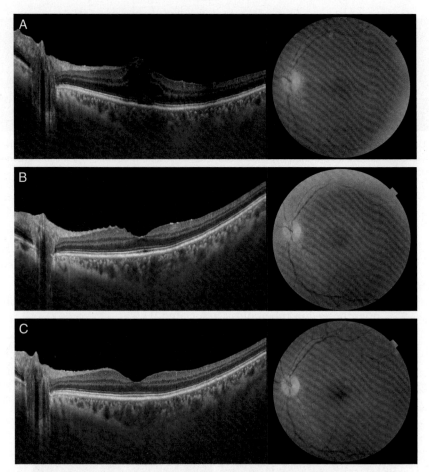

FIGURE 42.5 A, Optical coherence tomography (OCT) of a patient with tuberculosis-associated interme-diate uveitis (IU) shows cystoid macular edema (CME). B, OCT at 3-month follow-up shows resolution of CME. C, OCT at 1-year follow-up shows progressive resolution of associated diffuse choroidal thickening.

- In the healing stages (stage III and IV on FAF), RPE shows knoblike elevations and atrophy with IZ, EZ, and ELM atrophy and attenuation with increased signal transmission (Figure 42.6B).
- A TB choroidal granuloma (tuberculoma) appears as a single round area of hyporeflectivity within the choroid with dome-shaped ele-vation of the overlying RPE with or without surrounding exudative retinal detachment. The term "contact sign" is used to describe the localized adhesion between the RPE choriocapillaris and neurosen-sory retina (Figure 42.7A).
- A tuberculoma may resemble a large choroidal vessel. However, the increased signal transmission effect underlying the area of hyporeflec-tivity in a granuloma helps to differentiate it from a large choroidal vessel (Figure 42.7A, white asterisk). This important feature helps in detecting even small choroidal granulomas.

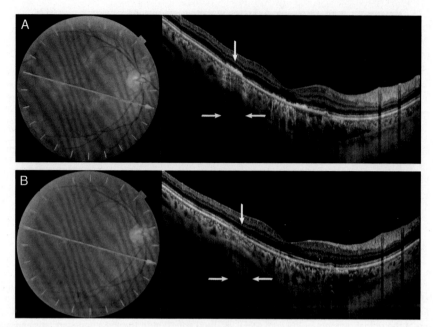

FIGURE 42.6 A, Optical coherence tomography (OCT) of a patient with multifocal serpiginoid choroiditis (MSC) shows disruption of interdigitation zone (IZ), ellipsoid zone (EZ) and external limiting membrane (ELM), and hyperreflective irregular elevations of the retinal pigment epithelium (RPE) (white arrow) with underlying shadowing effect (yellow arrow). B, OCT of the same patient following resolution of lesions shows attenuation of outer retinal layers and RPE with increased signal transmission.

- A tuberculoma may be differentiated from acute VKH disease by the presence of massive, diffuse choroidal thickening in the latter (Figure 42.8A) and from toxoplasma retinochoroiditis where there is a focal thickening of choroid with hyperreflectivity of all retinal layers (Figure 42.8B).

OCTA IMAGING

- In acute and active MSC (stage I and II on FAF), optical coherence tomography angiography (OCTA) demonstrates areas of flow voids with surrounding diffusely increased signal at the choriocapillaris layer.
- The areas of flow void in the choriocapillaris slab of active MSC show irregular hyperreflectivity of the RPE and outer retina on corresponding B-scan image (Figure 42.9A). These hyperreflective areas cause an underlying reduced signal transmission. In the active/acute stage, it is difficult to determine whether these areas of flow void represent true nonperfusion or reduced signal transmission.

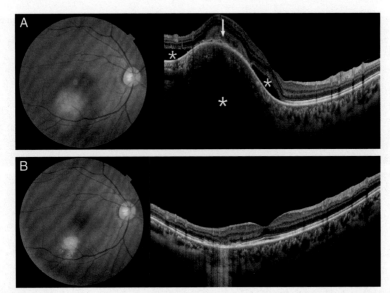

FIGURE 42.7 A, Optical coherence tomography (OCT) of a choroidal granuloma shows the lesion as a well-defined round area of hyporeflectivity within the choroid (white asterisk) with dome-shaped elevation of the retinal pigment epithelium (RPE), localized adhesion of the RPE choriocapillaris and neurosensory retina (contact sign) (white arrow) with surrounding subretinal fluid (yellow asterisk). B, OCT appearance of the same lesion on resolution shows outer retinal atrophy and attenuation with increased signal transmission and reduced choroidal thickness.

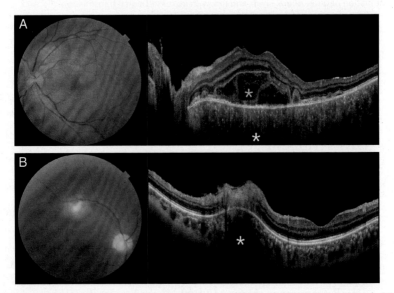

FIGURE 42.8 A, Optical coherence tomography (OCT) of a patient with Vogt-Koyanagi-Harada (VKH) disease shows massive, diffuse thickening of choroid (white asterisk) with outer retinal blebs (bacillary layer detachment). Note the typical hyperreflective content of the fluid (blue asterisk). B, OCT of a patient with toxoplasma retinochoroiditis shows focal thickening of choroid (yellow asterisk) and hyperreflectivity and disruption of retinal layers with reduced signal transmission.

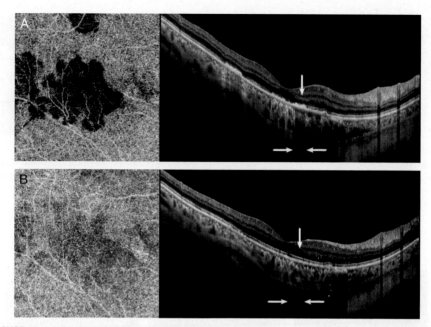

FIGURE 42.9 A, Swept-source optical coherence tomography angiography (SS-OCTA) of the same patient with multifocal serpiginoid choroiditis (MSC) as in Figure 42.6 shows areas of flow void in the choriocapillaris layer. Corresponding B-scan shows interdigitation zone (IZ), ellipsoid zone (EZ), external limiting membrane (ELM) disruption and hyperreflective elevations of the retinal pigment epithelium (RPE) (white arrow) with underlying reduced signal transmission (yellow arrows). B, SS-OCTA of the same patient following resolution of lesions shows reduced density (true nonperfusion) at the choriocapillaris layer. Corresponding B-scan shows partial anatomical restoration of photoreceptor layers and RPE (white arrow) with increased signal transmission (yellow arrows).

- The increased signal surrounding the areas of flow void corresponds to the hyperautofluorescence seen on FAF in active lesions. This might represent increased vascular flow due to increased metabolic activity of RPE versus an unmasking effect from overlying EZ attenuation.
- In the healing stages (stage III and IV on FAF), increased flow signal of the borders is absent. Islands of preserved choriocapillaris are seen along with visibility of underlying medium and large choroidal vessels. In this stage, the attenuated outer retina does not obstruct signal transmission and the areas of flow void represent true loss (Figures 42.9B and 42.10).
- OCTA may detect areas of nonperfusion and neovascularization if TB-associated occlusive vasculitis is present (Figure 42.11).
- Diffuse low flow signal surrounding an inflamed blood vessel seen in the choriocapillaris layer on OCTA is due to retinal edema causing reduced signal transmission. This must be interpreted with caution while looking for areas of nonperfusion (Figure 42.11).

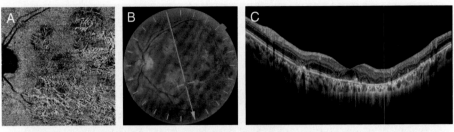

FIGURE 42.10 A, Swept-source optical coherence tomography angiography (SS-OCTA) of a patient with healed multifocal serpiginoid choroiditis (MSC) showing islands of preserved choriocapillaris with visualization of medium and large choroidal vessels. B and C, Corresponding fundus photo and B-scan show severe loss of outer retinal structures with increased signal transmission.

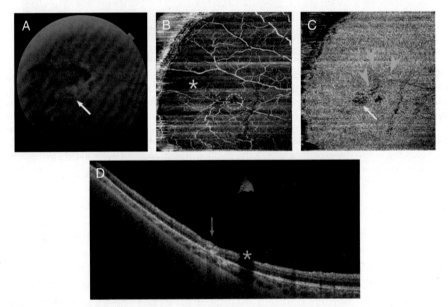

FIGURE 42.11 A, Color fundus photograph of the superotemporal periphery of the right eye of a patient with tuberculosis-related retinal vasculitis shows perivascular exudates, retinal hemorrhages, and a chorioretinal (CR) scar underlying the inflamed blood vessel (white arrow). B, The superficial vascular plexus on swept-source optical coherence tomography angiography (SS-OCTA) shows an area of nonperfusion (yellow asterisk). C, The choriocapillaris layer shows an area of apparent flow void (yellow arrow) corresponding to the CR scar. A shadowing effect is seen from a vitreous opacity (dashed blue circle). Note this shadow in the superficial layer as well. Inflamed blood vessels appear as linear areas of reduced signal (blue arrowheads) due to projection artifacts. D, B-scan shows hyperreflectivity at the retinal pigment epithelium (RPE) choriocapillaris and outer retina corresponding to the CR scar, with an underlying shadowing effect (pink arrow). An adjacent shadowing effect is also seen from a vitreous opacity (blue asterisk).

ACKNOWLEDGMENT

Abhilasha Baharani acknowledges Mr. Beeram Madhusudhan Reddy's contribution in retrieving the images.

References

1. Gupta A, Bansal R, Gupta V, Sharma A. Fundus autofluorescence in serpiginous like choroiditis. *Retina.* 2012;32(4):814-825.
2. Bansal R, Basu S, Gupta A, Rao N, Invernizzi A, Kramer M. Imaging in tuberculosis-associated uveitis. *Indian J Ophthalmol.* 2017;65(4):264-270.
3. Gupta V, Gupta A, Rao NA. Intraocular tuberculosis – an update. *Surv Ophthalmol.* 2007;52(6):561-587.
4. Agarwal A, Mahajan S, Khairallah M, Mahendradas P, Gupta A, Gupta V. Multimodal imaging in ocular tuberculosis. *Ocul Immunol Inflamm.* 2017;25(1):134-145.
5. Mandadi SKR, Agarwal A, Aggarwal K, et al. Novel findings on optical coherence tomography angiography in patients with tubercular serpiginous-like choroiditis. *Retina.* 2017;37(9):1647-1659.
6. Gupta A, Bansal R, Gupta V, Sharma A, Bambery P. Ocular signs predictive of tubercular uveitis. *Am J Ophthalmol.* 2010;149(4):562-570.
7. Invernizzi A, Cozzi M, Staurenghi G. Optical coherence tomography and optical coherence tomography angiography in uveitis: a review. *Clin Exp Ophthalmol* 2019;47(3):357-371.

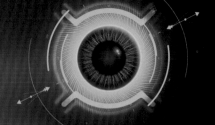

CHAPTER 43

Sympathetic Ophthalmia

SALIENT FEATURES

- Sympathetic ophthalmia (SO) is a rare bilateral nonnecrotizing granulomatous panuveitis that occurs a few days to several decades following a penetrating ocular injury or surgery.
- Most cases present, within the first 3 months after ocular injury, with worsening panuveitis of both the traumatized ("exciting") and fellow ("sympathizing") eye.[1,2]
- Ophthalmic manifestations of SO are variable and include numerous sequela that arise from the worsening granulomatous panuveitis with eventual development of bilateral exudative retinal detachments, choroidal granulomas, and Dalen-Fuchs nodules.[1-4]
- Ocular features may be clinically indistinguishable from Vogt-Koyanagi-Harada (VKH) disease. In fact, most experts consider SO and VKH to be "sister diseases." However, the presence of an antecedent penetrating ocular surgery or trauma distinguishes the two entities.[2]
- The exact pathogenesis of SO is unknown, but the most recent investigations suggest a VKH-like immunologic basis with T-cell–mediated autoimmune response against antigenic proteins from the uvea, particularly tyrosinase peptide.[5-8]
- Treatment consists of high-dose systemic corticosteroids with the addition of immunomodulatory agents as needed for sustainable long-term immunosuppression.
- Anti-inflammatory local therapy is often also utilized in concert with systemic therapy to reduce disease activity.

- Diagnosis of SO is clinical, based on history and physical examination.
- Multimodal imaging with fluorescein angiography (FA), indocyanine green angiography (ICGA), B-scan ultrasonography, optical coherence tomography (OCT), and OCT angiography (OCTA) may be utilized to support the diagnosis and follow treatment response.

OCT IMAGING

- OCT can show singular or multifocal serous neurosensory retinal detachments (Figure 43.1).[10,11]
- Subretinal fibrinous membranes, often contiguous with the ellipsoid zone (EZ) of attached retina, with retina pigment epithelium (RPE) attachments and formation of septa dividing the subretinal space into multiple compartments (Figure 43.1).[11]
- Disruption of the external limiting membrane (ELM), ellipsoid zone (EZ), and RPE is common (Figures 43.1 and 43.2).[9-12]
- Choroidal thickening (seen best with enhanced depth imaging [EDI] or swept-source systems) during acute phase resolves after treatment and choroidal undulations and folds are also visible on OCT (Figures 43.1 and 43.2).[9,12,13]
- Dalen-Fuchs nodules can be observed as hyperreflective lesions at the level of the RPE with overlying disruption of the EZ that improve with treatment but may persist (Figure 43.3).[11]

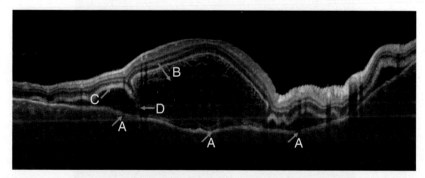

FIGURE 43.1 Optical coherence tomography (OCT) of acute sympathetic ophthalmia demonstrating thickened choroid with choroidal folds/undulations (A), multiple serous retinal detachments and a possible central bacillary detachment with splitting of the photoreceptors. (B), elongation of photoreceptors (C), and hyperreflective septa (D) dividing the subretinal space into multiple fluid-filled compartments. (Reprinted with permission from Agrawal R, Jain M, Khan R, et al. Choroidal structural changes in sympathetic ophthalmia on swept-source optical coherence tomography. *Ocul Immunol Inflamm.* 2019:1-6. doi:1 0.1080/09273948.2019.1685110 with features marked with additional arrows.)

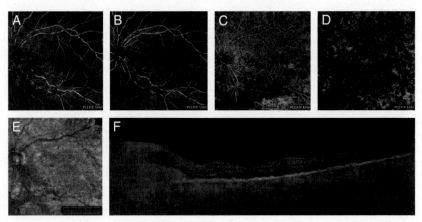

FIGURE 43.2 Swept-source optical coherence tomography angiography (OCTA) images of a 36-year-old male with acute-phase sympathetic ophthalmia. The top row demonstrates 12 × 12 mm scans at the level of the superficial (A) and deep (B) capillary plexuses, the outer retina (C), and choriocapillaris (D). There are no notable structural vascular changes at the levels of the superficial (A) and deep (B) capillary plexuses. Multiple dark spots are seen scattered across the posterior pole at the levels of the outer retina (C) and choriocapillaris (D). En-face imaging (E) shows no abnormalities other than shadowing artifact from vitritis, which is also present in A-D. Enhanced-depth imaging OCT (F) reveals peripapillary subretinal hyperreflective material and thickened choroid with overlying retinal pigment epithelium (RPE) irregularity and drusenoid-like changes. (Reprinted with permission from Brar M, Sharma M, Grewal SPS, Grewal DS. Treatment response in sympathetic ophthalmia as assessed by widefield OCT angiography. *Ophthalmic Surg Lasers Imaging Retina*. 2018;49(9):726-730. doi:10.3928/23258160-20180831-13.)

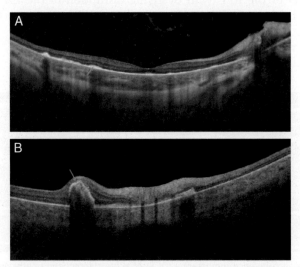

FIGURE 43.3 Optical coherence tomography (OCT) of acute sympathetic ophthalmia demonstrating two presentations of Dalen-Fuchs nodules (orange arrows). The top image (A) demonstrates round irregular-shaped hyperreflective areas at the level of the retinal pigment epithelium (RPE) with disruption of the overlying RPE (orange arrows). The bottom image (B) demonstrates an alternative appearance with medium-reflectivity with underlying shadowing and disruption of the overlying Bruch membrane and RPE (orange arrow). (Reprinted with permission from Agrawal et al. Agrawal R, Jain M, Khan R, et al. Choroidal structural changes in sympathetic ophthalmia on swept-source optical coherence tomography. *Ocul Immunol Inflamm*. 2019:1-6. doi:10.1080/09273948.2019.1685110.)

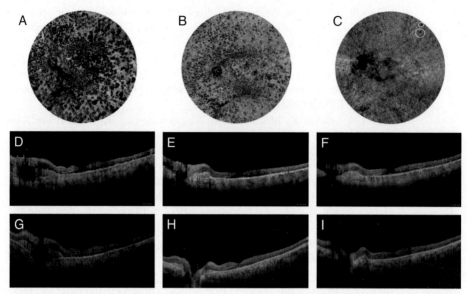

FIGURE 43.4 Serial montage swept-source optical coherence tomography angiography (OCTA) images at the level of the choriocapillaris (top row A-C) and corresponding OCT with flow overlays (bottom row D-F) of a 36-year-old male with acute-phase sympathetic ophthalmia (A and D) and 3 months (B and E) and 6 months (C and F) after treatment. At presentation, there are multiple diffuse dark foci of flow voids (A and D), suspected to represent areas of choriocapillaris hypoperfusion. At 3 months after initiation of systemic immunosuppression, there is significant reduction in the size and number of these dark lesions on imaging (B) and increased choriocapillaris flow on OCT overlay (E). At 6 months of treatment, there is nearly complete resolution of these dark foci (C) and again improved OCT flow overlay (F). (Reprinted with permission from Brar M, Sharma M, Grewal SPS, Grewal DS. Treatment response in sympathetic ophthalmia as assessed by widefield OCT angiography. *Ophthalmic Surg Lasers Imaging Retina.* 2018;49(9):726-730. doi:10.3928/23258160-20180831-13.)

OCTA IMAGING

- Multiple small areas of choriocapillaris flow voids may be identified during the acute phase that diminish during treatment and may potentially resolve months after treatment (Figures 43.2 and 43.4).[12]
- OCTA also demonstrates increased choroidal vascular index (CVI).[11]

References

1. Duke-Elder S. Sympathetic ophthalmitis. In: Duke-Elder S, ed. *System of Ophthalmology.* Vol 9. St. Louis: Mosby; 1966:558-593.
2. Goto H, Rao NA. Sympathetic ophthalmia and Vogt-Koyanagi-Harada syndrome. *Int Ophthalmol Clin.* 1990;30(4):279-285. doi:10.1097/00004397-199030040-00014.
3. Castiblanco CP, Adelman RA. Sympathetic ophthalmia. *Graefe's Arch Clin Exp Ophthalmol.* 2009;247(3):289-302. doi:10.1007/s00417-008-0939-8.

4. Lubin JR, Albert DM, Weinstein M. Sixty-five years of sympathetic ophthalmia: a clinicopathologic review of 105, cases (1913-1978). *Ophthalmology.* 1980;87(2):109-121. doi:10.1016/S0161-6420(80)35270-6.

5. Rao NA, Robin J, Marak GE, Hartmann D, Sweeney JA. The role of the penetrating wound in the development of sympathetic ophthalmia: experimental observations. *Arch Ophthalmol.* 1983;101(1):102-104. doi:10.1001/archopht.1983.01040010104019.

6. Sugita S, Sagawa K, Mochizuki M, Shichijo S, Itoh K. Melanocyte lysis by cytotoxic T lymphocytes recognizing the MART-1 melanoma antigen in HLA-A2 patients with Vogt-Koyanagi-Harada disease. *Int Immunol.* 1996;8(5):799-803. doi:10.1093/intimm/8.5.799.

7. Hammer H. Cellular hypersensitivity to uveal pigment confirmed by leucocyte migration tests in sympathetic ophthalmitis and the Vogt-Koyanagi-Harada syndrome. *Br J Ophthalmol.* 1974;59(9):773-776. doi:10.1136/bjo.58.9.773.

8. Rao NA, Wong VG. Aetiology of sympathetic ophthalmitis. *Trans Ophthalmol Soc UK.* 1981;101(pt 3):357-360.

9. Agrawal R, Jain M, Khan R, et al. Choroidal structural changes in sympathetic ophthalmia on swept-source optical coherence tomography. *Ocul Immunol Inflamm.* 2019:1-6. doi:10.1080/09273948.2019.1685110.

10. Gupta V, Gupta A, Dogra MR, Singh I. Reversible retinal changes in the acute stage of sympathetic ophthalmia seen on spectral domain optical coherence tomography. *Int Ophthalmol.* 2011;31(2):105-110. doi:10.1007/s10792-011-9432-1.

11. Muakkassa NW, Witkin AJ. Spectral-domain optical coherence tomography of sympathetic ophthalmia with dalen-fuchs nodules. *Ophthalmic Surg Lasers Imaging Retina.* 2014;45(6):610-612. doi:10.3928/23258160-20141008-01.

12. Brar M, Sharma M, Grewal SPS, Grewal DS. Treatment response in sympathetic ophthalmia as assessed by widefield OCT angiography. *Ophthalmic Surg Lasers Imaging Retina.* 2018;49(9):726-730. doi:10.3928/23258160-20180831-13.

13. Behdad B, Rahmani S, Montahaei T, Soheilian R, Soheilian M. Enhanced depth imaging OCT (EDI-OCT) findings in acute phase of sympathetic ophthalmia. *Int Ophthalmol.* 2015;35(3):433-439. doi:10.1007/s10792-015-0058-6.

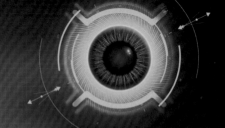

CHAPTER 44

Toxoplasmosis Chorioretinitis

SALIENT FEATURES

- Toxoplasmosis chorioretinitis is the most common cause of posterior uveitis worldwide.[1]
- Affected patients are generally young and immunocompetent. The infection can be asymptomatic, or patients may complain of photophobia, floaters, and decreased vision. Vision loss may vary dramatically depending on location of infection and the severity of intraocular inflammation (Figure 44.1).
- Risk factors include male gender, ingestion of raw or undercooked meat, and cohabitation with felines.[1]
- Most commonly, ocular toxoplasmosis presents as recurrence from prior or congenital infection as a focus of chorioretinitis with overlying vitritis arising from the edge of a chorioretinal scar (Figure 44.2A). Adjacent or distant segmental retinal periarteritis may be noted (Figure 44.2E, blue arrow).[2] The diagnosis is typically made clinically. Anterior segment inflammation and ocular hypertension may be present.
- Primary infection can be seen as a focus of retinitis or chorioretinitis without the adjacent scar.
- The diagnosis in atypical infection, or infection in those at risk of multiple opportunistic infections, can be supported by polymerase chain reaction (PCR) positivity in aqueous samples. Serologies are more useful if negative to help rule out the disease.
- Caution must be taken in immunocompromised individuals, especially those with acquired immune deficiency syndrome, as concurrent intracranial involvement may be seen.

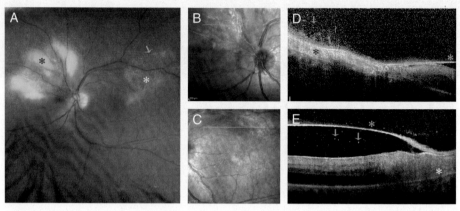

FIGURE 44.1 Multimodal imaging with primary ocular toxoplasmosis in an immunocompromised individual. The patient presented with photophobia, floaters, and decreased vision. A, Fundus photograph reveals a multifocal area of bright retinitis nasally (red asterisk) and a duller area of retinitis along the superotemporal arcade extending into the macula (yellow asterisk). B and C, Near-infrared images showing locations of the spectral-domain optical coherence tomography (SD-OCT) images in (D and E) through the nasal and temporal areas of retinitis, respectively. D and E, SD-OCTs reveal full-thickness retinal hyperreflectivity that is brighter in the nasal lesion (red asterisk) than the temporal lesion (yellow asterisk). There is also severe thinning and full-thickness disruption of the retina (more prominent nasal relative to the temporal lesion). There are vitreous hyperreflective dots (green arrows) and a densely hyperreflective posterior hyaloid (green asterisk) in both images. Polymerase chain reaction (PCR) of the aqueous humor revealed positive *toxoplasmosis gondii* nucleotide and undetectable viral nucleotides. Serologies were positive for antitoxoplasmosis gondii IgM and IgG. The patient responded favorably to oral trimethoprim and sulfamethoxazole and prednisone. Central nervous system imaging was within normal limits.

- Toxoplasmosis chorioretinitis is generally a self-limited disease process; however, vision loss may occur secondary to optic nerve or macular involvement or due to sequelae of severe ocular inflammation.
- Antimicrobial therapy and steroid therapy may be employed to limit the destructive process and is especially important in immunocompromised individuals.
- Classic therapy consists of pyrimethamine, sulfadiazine, and folinic acid with the addition of oral prednisone 24 to 48 hours after. More frequently used alternatives include trimethoprim and sulfamethoxazole, azithromycin, clindamycin, and atovaquone. Intravitreal clindamycin with and without intravitreal dexamethasone may be employed in macular or optic nerve threatening disease.[3]
- Azithromycin, atovaquone, and clindamycin along with intravitreal clindamycin may be used in pregnancy.
- Visual prognosis is dependent on the primary location of disease and complications resultant of intraocular inflammation. Recurrences may occur.

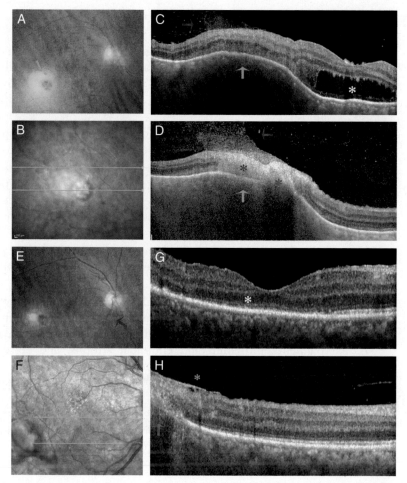

FIGURE 44.2 Multimodal imaging of a patient with ocular toxoplasmosis. A, Fundus photo of a 45-year-old female with decreased vision and floaters with a focal area of retinal whitening adjacent to a hyperpigmented chorioretinal scar (blue arrow). Media opacity is comprised due to mild vitritis. B, Near-infrared image of the active area showing locations for the spectral-domain optical coherence tomography (SD-OCT) scans in C (superior green arrow) and D (inferior green arrow). C and D, A focal area of choroidal expansion is seen under the area of the greatest retinal involvement (green arrows). There is full-thickness retinal hyperreflectivity in the inferior scan (red asterisk). There is a pocket of cystic outer retinal fluid in the macula with a hyperreflective line inner to the retinal pigment epithelium, recently described as a bacillary layer detachment (yellow asterisk). The chorioretinal scar is evidence on SD-OCT as nodule of hyperreflectivity (blue asterisk). There is a condensed hyperreflective vitreous adhesion to the affected retina with overlying diffuse hyperreflective foci corresponding clinically to vitritis (red arrows). E, Fundus photo taken 2 months after initial presentation status post treatment with oral trimethoprim and sulfamethoxazole, oral prednisone, and a single intravitreal clindamycin injection. The media is clearer, and the retinal lesion has decreased in size. Blue arrow indicates an arteriole with persistent segmental retinal arteritis. F, Near-infrared image of the active area showing locations for the SD-OCT scans in G (superior green arrow) and H (inferior green arrow). G and H, The bacillary detachment has resolved, but there remains loss of the ellipsoid zone and attenuation of the external limiting membrane (ELM) (yellow asterisk). There is a small epiretinal membrane (green asterisk), and there is full-thickness disruption of the retina and loss of the ellipsoid zone (EZ), ELM, and retinal pigment epithelium (RPE) (purple arrow). The choroidal expansion has also decreased.

OCT FEATURES

- Characteristic optical coherence tomography (OCT) findings in ocular toxoplasmosis include focal choroidal expansion and full-thickness retinal thickening and hyperreflectivity with overlying vitreous hyperreflectivity and adhesions adjacent to an chorioretinal scar (Figures 44.2C and D).[4,5]
- Intraretinal fluid, subretinal fluid, and focal outer retinal cystic spaces termed bacillary detachments may be seen (Figure 44.2C).[6,7]
- Preretinal vitreous hyperreflective aggregations, presumed to be clumps of inflammatory debris, are also more common in ocular toxoplasmosis than viral retinitis. A greater degree of choroidal thickness and involvement can help distinguish ocular toxoplasmosis from viral retinitis as well.[8]
- Nevertheless, primary ocular toxoplasmosis, not arising from a prior chorioretinitis scar, can be limited to the retina initially and can mimic viral retinitis.
- In the chronic, resolved phase of the infection, OCT findings include disruption of the retinal laminations and full-thickness thinning in prior site of chorioretinitis, clearance of vitreous hyperreflective foci, retinal pigment epithelium and choroidal atrophy, and epiretinal membrane formation (Figures 44.2G and H).

OCTA FEATURES

- There is currently no role for optical coherence tomography angiography (OCTA) in ocular toxoplasmosis.

References

1. Kijlstra A, Petersen E. Epidemiology, pathophysiology, and the future of ocular toxoplasmosis. *Ocul Immunol Inflamm.* 2014;22(2):138-147. doi:10.3109 /09273948.2013.823214.
2. Tsui E, Leong BCS, Mehta N, et al. Evaluation of segmental retinal arteritis with optical coherence tomography angiography. *Retina Cases Brief Rep.* 2019. doi:10.1097/ICB.0000000000000900.
3. Ozgonul C, Besirli CG. Recent developments in the diagnosis and treatment of ocular toxoplasmosis. *Ophthalmic Res.* 2017;57(1):1-12. doi:10.1159/000449169.
4. Ouyang Y, Li F, Shao Q, et al. Subretinal fluid in eyes with active ocular toxoplasmosis observed using spectral domain optical coherence tomography. *PLoS One.* 2015;10(5):e0127683. doi:10.1371/journal.pone.0127683.
5. Ouyang Y, Pleyer U, Shao Q, et al. Evaluation of cystoid change phenotypes in ocular toxoplasmosis using optical coherence tomography. *PLoS One.* 2014;9(2):e86626. doi:10.1371/journal.pone.0086626.

6. Mehta N, Chong J, Tsui E, et al. Presumed foveal bacillary layer detachment IN a patient with toxoplasmosis chorioretinitis and pachychoroid disease. *Retina Cases Brief Rep.* 2018. doi:10.1097/ICB.0000000000000817.

7. Lujan BJ. Spectral domain optical coherence tomography imaging of punctate outer retinal toxoplasmosis. *Saudi J Ophthalmol.* 2014;28(2):152-156. doi:10.1016/j.sjopt.2014.03.010.

8. Invernizzi A, Agarwal AK, Ravera V, et al. Comparing optical coherence tomography findings in different aetiologies of infectious necrotising retinitis. *Br J Ophthalmol.* 2018;102(4):433-437. doi:10.1136/bjophthalmol-2017-310210.

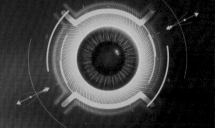

CHAPTER 45

Sarcoidosis

SALIENT FEATURES

- Sarcoidosis is a systemic noncaseating granulomatous inflammatory disease that can manifest itself in virtually any organ system.
- Signs
  - Intraocular sarcoidosis can manifest with a myriad of different signs on ocular examination including granulomatous anterior uveitis, iris or trabecular meshwork granulomas, vitritis, multifocal chorioretinal lesions, macular edema with associated uveitis, periphlebitis (with or without classically described "candle wax drippings"), choroidal granulomas, and optic disc infiltration.
- Symptoms
  - Wide-ranging, including asymptomatic, blurred vision, photophobia, floaters, red eye, and pain.
  - Patients should be screened for systemic manifestations when sarcoid is suspected including shortness of breath, difficulty breathing, cough, arthritis, myalgias, and rash (classically erythema nodosum).
- Indocyanine green (ICG) has been considered the gold standard for monitoring choroidal lesions in sarcoid granulomatous disease, classically demonstrating multifocal hypocyanescent lesions (Figure 45.1).
- Advancements in optical coherence tomography (OCT) and optical coherence tomography angiography (OCTA) technology have made them useful diagnostic tools in the diagnosis of sarcoid granulomas and for monitoring their activity.

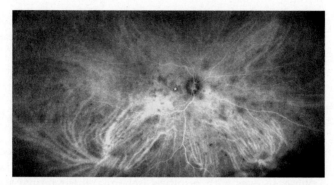

FIGURE 45.1 Late-phase indocyanine green (ICG) demonstrating multifocal hypocyanescent lesions throughout the posterior pole (white asterisk) and midperiphery consistent with choroidal granulomas in a patient with known sarcoidosis.

OCT IMAGING

- Choroidal findings
  - Small sarcoid choroidal granulomas that begin in the inner choroidal stroma are oftentimes difficult to resolve on OCT (Figure 45.2).[1]
  - As the granulomas increase in size, they become apparent as large, oftentimes, full-thickness, hyporeflective lesions within the choroid (Figure 45.3).[1-4]
  - The granulomas are associated with an increased signal transmission and shadowing effects.[3,4]
  - A disproportionately enlarged Sattler medium vessel layer compared to Haller large vessel layer is associated with a diagnosis of sarcoidosis compared to similar tuberculosis choroidal granulomatous disease.[2]

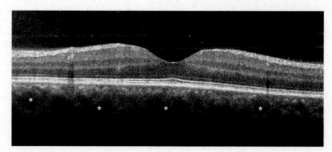

FIGURE 45.2 Optical coherence tomography (OCT) of the same patient from Figure 45.1 with generalized choroidal thickening and multiple, large hyporeflective lesions within the choroid (white asterisks) that correspond to the hypocyanescent lesions on indocyanine green (ICG).

- Active granulomatous choroidal disease is associated with increased choroidal thickening when compared to quiescent disease.[2]
- Retinal and vitreous findings
  - Vitritis is usually associated with decreased signal strength and increased hyperreflective foci within the vitreous, representing inflammatory cells.
  - Cystoid macular edema (CME) may be present concurrently with active inflammation.
  - In eyes with sarcoid-associated vasculitis, areas of increased reflectivity due to inner retinal ischemia may be identified in the acute phase. In eyes with resulting ischemia, inner retinal atrophy may also be noted.
  - Eyes demonstrating large active granulomas with concurrent intraocular inflammation may also have associated CME and subretinal fluid.
- Treatment of ocular sarcoidosis results in distinctive healing pattern with decreased anteroposterior dimension followed by decreased lateral extension. This characteristic healing pattern allows for earlier detection of response to therapy by enhanced-depth imaging (EDI)-OCT when compared to ICG.[4]

OCTA IMAGING

- Small sarcoid choroidal granulomas of Sattler layer, which may be seen as small hypocyanescent lesions on ICG, are typically not identifiable on with OCTA.[1]
- As the granulomas grow, they compress the surrounding choroidal vasculature and appear as areas of no flow on OCTA that can be colocalized with ICG (Figures 45.3 and 45.4).[1]

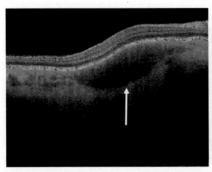 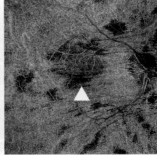

FIGURE 45.3 Optical coherence tomography (OCT) B-scan showing large granuloma (arrow) with decorrelation overlay (left). Optical coherence tomography angiography (OCTA) of the choroid with resulting flow void (arrowhead).

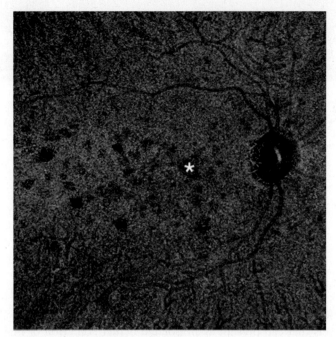

FIGURE 45.4 En-face optical coherence tomography angiography (OCTA) demonstrating flow voids within the choriocapillaris (white asterisk) that can be colocalized with the hypocyanescent lesions on indocyanine green (ICG).

- In eyes with retinal vascular involvement, OCTA may demonstrate perifoveal capillary arcade disruptions, area of decrease capillary perfusion, and capillary abnormalities.
  - In addition, capillary vessel density of the deep capillary plexus and the choriocapillaris was significantly lower in eyes with ocular sarcoidosis than normal controls.[5]

References

1. Pichi F, Sarraf D, Morara M, Mazumdar S, Neri P, Gupta V. Pearls and pitfalls of optical coherence tomography angiography in the multimodal evaluation of uveitis. *J Ophthalmic Inflamm Infect.* 2017;7(1):20.
2. Mehta H, Sim DA, Keane PA, et al. Structural changes of the choroid in sarcoid- and tuberculosis-related granulomatous uveitis. *Eye (Lond).* 2015;29(8):1060-1068.
3. Invernizzi A, Mapelli C, Viola F, et al. Choroidal granulomas visualized by enhanced depth imaging optical coherence tomography. *Retina.* 2015;35(3):525-531.
4. Invernizzi A, Agarwal A, Mapelli C, Nguyen QD, Staurenghi G, Viola F. Longitudinal follow-up of choroidal granulomas using enhanced depth imaging optical coherence tomography. *Retina.* 2017;37(1):144-153.
5. Cerquaglia A, Iaccheri B, Fiore T, et al. New insights on ocular sarcoidosis: an optical coherence tomography angiography study. *Ocul Immunol Inflamm.* 2019;27(7):1057-1066.

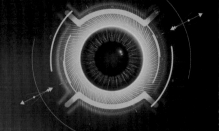

CHAPTER 46

Retinal Vasculitis

SALIENT FEATURES

- Retinal vasculitis is characterized by inflammation of the retinal vessels that can present as an isolated ocular condition or may be associated with systemic inflammatory disorders.
- Symptoms of retinal vasculitis may include blurred vision, flashes, floaters, metamorphopsia, and pain.
- Clinical examination classically reveals areas of continuous or segmental vascular sheathing. Associated findings may include cotton wool spots, hemorrhage, focal retinitis, retinal ischemia, vitritis, anterior uveitis, and its subsequent neovascular sequalae.
- The differential diagnosis for retinal vasculitis is large and can be narrowed by identifying the vessels predominantly involved: arteritis, phlebitis, or both.
- Fluorescein angiography (FA) is the gold standard for diagnosis and monitoring retinal vasculitis. It is also used in staging retinal vasculitis.[1]
  - Stage 1—active inflammation—perivascular retinal infiltrates, retinal edema, hemorrhages, and occlusions (Figure 46.1)
  - Stage 2—ischemia—sclerosing vessels and tortuous collaterals
  - Stage 3—neovascularization—peripheral neovascularization and/or iris neovascularization
  - Stage 4—neovascular complications—tractional retinal detachment and neovascular glaucoma

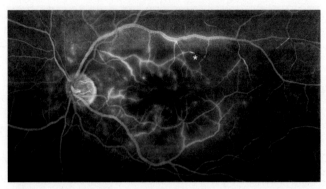

FIGURE 46.1 Late fluorescein angiography of a patient with known lupus demonstrating severe perivascular staining and leakage, in addition to a segmental retinal artery occlusion (white asterisk).

- Although FA remains essential to the diagnosis and monitoring of retinal vasculitis, optical coherence tomography (OCT) and optical coherence tomography angiography (OCTA) have demonstrated significant utility in monitoring for complications of vasculitis (ie, macular edema, inner retinal atrophy, capillary nonperfusion) and have evolved to serve as surrogates for disease activity.

OCT IMAGING

- OCT imaging is a useful modality in detecting anatomic changes caused by retinal vasculitis such as retinal thickening, increased retinal hyperreflectivity, or macular edema caused by incompetent, inflamed vessels (Figure 46.2) with associated ischemia. In chronic cases, retinal atrophy caused by chronic ischemia or inflammatory infarcts may be identified (Figure 46.3).

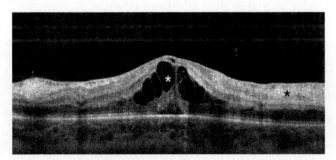

FIGURE 46.2 Optical coherence tomography (OCT) of an occlusive vasculitis patient soon after onset of visual symptoms with inner retinal hyperreflectivity (black asterisk), loss of lamination, retinal thickening (black asterisk), cystoid macular edema (white asterisk), and subretinal fluid (red asterisk).

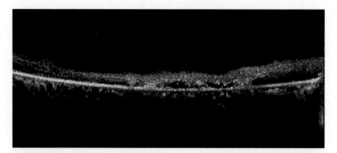

FIGURE 46.3 Optical coherence tomography (OCT) of an occlusive vasculitis patient 3 months after the onset of symptoms with generalized atrophy and loss of retinal organization.

- OCT is also useful in detecting anatomic changes that cannot be picked up on fundus examination. OCT in regions of active vasculitis found there was adjacent retinal thickening and loss of normal retinal lamination on OCT. Treatment resulted in atrophy and thinning of the previously affected retina on OCT.[2]
- Perivascular thickening is associated with worsening vasculitis and has been advocated as a surrogate for vasculitis activity (Figures 46.4 and 46.5). In fact, incremental decrease in perivascular thickening on OCT scans after systemic corticosteroid therapy that correlated with decreased vascular leakage on FA has been demonstrated.[3]
- Perivascular thickening, macular thickening, and generalized thickening on swept-source wide-field OCT imaging have been positively correlated with peripheral capillary leakage on FA with, suggesting that these OCT findings may also be used as biomarkers for disease activity.[4]

OCTA IMAGING

- OCTA can provide high-resolution images of vascular flow networks and gives us a noninvasive means of detecting perfusion status which may be altered in areas of active vasculitis.

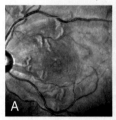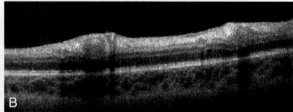

FIGURE 46.4 A, Near-infrared scanning laser ophthalmoscopy image and associated optical coherence tomography (OCT). B, B-scan through the superior arcade of a patient with occlusive vasculitis which showed perivascular retinal thickening and increased inner retinal hyperreflectivity (white asterisks).

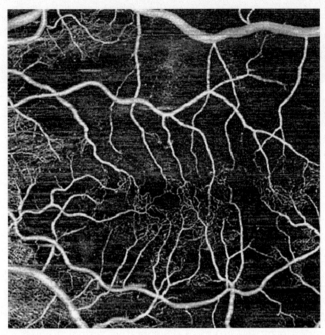

FIGURE 46.5 En-face optical coherence tomography angiography (OCTA) of a patient with occlusive vasculitis revealing diffuse loss of capillary flow signal throughout the macula.

- OCTA imaging of vessels with perivascular infiltration have been demonstrated to lack of flow signal in the adjacent capillary bed. Treatment did not result in return of capillary flow to the affected areas.[2]
- Areas of OCTA capillary nonperfusion and reduced perfusion are present in up to 49% of patients with intermediate uveitis and vasculitis.[4]
- In addition, nonperfusion of the superficial and deep capillary plexus on swept-source wide-field OCTA has been associated with peripheral ischemia on FA.[4]

References

1. Agarwal A, Afridi R, Agrawal R, Do DV, Gupta V, Nguyen QD. Multimodal imaging in retinal vasculitis. *Ocul Immunol Inflamm.* 2017;25(3):424-433.
2. Spaide RF. Microvascular flow abnormalities associated with retinal vasculitis: a potential of mechanism of retinal injury. *Retina.* 2017;37(6):1034-1042.
3. Knickelbein JE, Tucker W, Kodati S, Akanda M, Sen HN. Non-invasive method of monitoring retinal vasculitis in patients with birdshot chorioretinopathy using optical coherence tomography. *Br J Ophthalmol.* 2018;102(6):815-820.
4. Tian M, Tappeiner C, Zinkernagel MS, Huf W, Wolf S, Munk MR. Evaluation of vascular changes in intermediate uveitis and retinal vasculitis using swept-source wide-field optical coherence tomography angiography. *Br J Ophthalmol.* 2019;103(9):1289-1295.

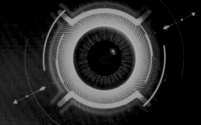

CHAPTER 47

Autoimmune Retinopathy

SALIENT FEATURES

- Autoimmune retinopathies (AIRs) are a heterogenous and often underdiagnosed group of degenerative retinal diseases causing vision loss, photopsias, scotomas, and visual field constriction without evidence of inherited retinal disease or overt inflammation.
- The fundus often appears normal; however vascular attenuation, retinal atrophy, pigmentary abnormalities, and waxy disc pallor may be present.
- Given the challenges of diagnosing AIR clinically, it is important to use multimodal testing (both structural and functional) to properly identify and monitor patients afflicted by this condition.
- There are three main AIR subtypes:
  - Cancer-associated retinopathy (CAR)
    - CAR is associated with small-cell lung cancer (most commonly); cervical, ovarian, endometrial and breast carcinoma; mixed Mullerian tumors; uterine sarcoma; and invasive thymoma.[1]
    - Visual symptoms precede diagnosis of malignancy in nearly 50% of cases, thus, a systemic workup for malignancy should be completed once there is reasonable suspicion.[2-4]
    - CAR is most commonly associated with the photoreceptor-affecting antirecoverin and antienolase retinal antibodies.
  - Melanoma-associated retinopathy (MAR)
    - MAR is mostly observed in patients who have a previous diagnosis of cutaneous or uveal melanoma.[2]
    - Nyctalopia is the most common symptom, and MAR autoantibodies target rod bipolar cells.[5]

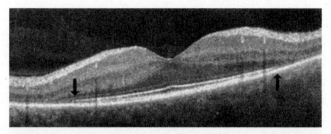

FIGURE 47.1 Spectral-domain optical coherence tomography (SD-OCT) in a patient with nonneoplastic autoimmune retinopathy showing subfoveal preservation of the outer nuclear layer (ONL) and ellipsoid zone (EZ) with parafoveal loss of these layers (black arrows) and more peripheral loss of the external limiting membrane (ELM). This is known as "flying-saucer" sign. There is also peripheral retinal pigment epithelium (RPE) atrophy.

- Nonparaneoplastic autoimmune retinopathy (npAIR)
  - This is the most common subtype and is frequently associated with an underlying autoimmune disease.[2]
  - Acute zonal occult outer retinopathy is a considered subtype of npAIR and is often characterized by a trizonal pattern of retinal and retinal pigment epithelium (RPE) degeneration (see Chapter 53).

SPECTRAL-DOMAIN OPTICAL COHERENCE TOMOGRAPHY IMAGING

- A pathognomonic finding on OCT is parafoveal attenuation of the outer nuclear layer (ONL), external limiting membrane (ELM), and ellipsoid zone (EZ) in the presence of subfoveal preservation (Figures 47.1 and 47.2).[2,6]

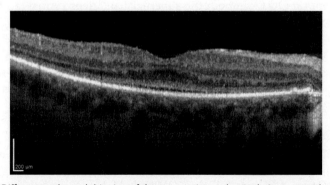

FIGURE 47.2 Diffuse atrophy and thinning of the outer retina and retinal pigment epithelium (RPE) in a case of nonparaneoplastic autoimmune retinopathy (npAIR). Note shed photoreceptors, primarily seen centrally.

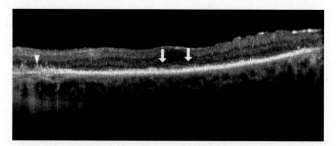

FIGURE 47.3 Severe dropout of outer nuclear layer (ONL), external limiting membrane (ELM), and ellipsoid zone (EZ), with minimal, residual anatomic preservation of these elements subfoveally, as well as extensive external limiting membrane (RPE) atrophy in a patient with cancer-associated retinopathy (CAR). Note the presence of a "flying-saucer sign" (arrows), ERM and RPE clumping with migration into the peripheral outer retina (arrowhead).

- Intraretinal cystic spaces (nonleaking), RPE atrophy, choriocapillaris atrophy, and decreased overall macular thickness have also been described.[8]
- Diffuse outer retinal atrophy, decreased overall macular thickness, and RPE atrophy can be seen in advanced cases (Figure 47.3).
- Normal OCT findings have been documented in 18% of cases,[2] making the use of multimodal imaging important for the proper diagnosis and monitoring of clinical course.

OCTA IMAGING

- Very little is known about the optical coherence tomography angiography (OCTA) features, given the rarity of this disease group, with only few images available from isolated case reports.
- OCTA of one case of npAIR showed an area void of perfusion in the choriocapillaris of the central macula.[8]
- MAR has been associated with perifoveal small-vessel capillary dropout on OCTA in both the superficial and deep retinal layers.[9]
- Preliminary, unpublished results from manually segmented scans of a small series of patients with AIR seen at the University of Wisconsin-Madison reveal decreased vessel density of the deep capillary plexus as well as perifoveal thinning (corresponding to the "flying-saucer" sign seen on OCT) compared to healthy, age-matched controls.

References

1. Grewal D, Fishman G, Jampol L. Autoimmune retinopathy and antiretinal antibodies: a review. *Retina.* 2014;34(5):827-845. doi:10.1097/IAE.0000000000000119.
2. Khanna S, Martins A, Oakey Z, Mititelu M. Non-Paraneoplastic autoimmune retinopathy: multimodal testing characteristics of 13 cases. *J Ophthalmic Inflamm Infect.* 2019;9(1):6. doi:10.1186/s12348-019-0171-1.

3. Canamary A, Takahashi W, Sallum J. Autoimmune retinopathy: a review. *Int J Retina Vitreous*. 2018;4:1. doi:10.1186/s40942-017-0104-9.

4. Rahimy E, Sarraf D. Paraneoplastic and non-paraneoplastic retinopathy and optic neuropathy: evaluation and management. *Surv Ophthalmol*. 2013;58(5):430-458. doi:10.1016/j.survophthal.2012.09.001.

5. Dhingra A, Fina M, Beinstein A, et al. Autoantibodies in melanoma-associated retinopathy target TRPV1 cation channels of retinal on bipolar cells. *J Neurosci*. 2011;31(11):3962-3967. doi:10.1523/JNEUROSCI.6007-10.2011.

6. Abazari A, Allam S, Adamus G, Ghazi N. Optical coherence tomography findings in autoimmune retinopathy. *Am J Ophthalmol*. 2012;153(4):750-756, 756.e1. doi:10.1016/j.ajo.2011.09.012.

7. Pepple K, Cusick M, Jaffe G, Mruthyunjaya P. SD-OCT and autofluorescence characteristics of autoimmune retinopathy. *Br J Ophthalmol*. 2013;97(2): 139-144. doi:10.1136/bjophthalmol-2012-302524.

8. Kasogole D, Raval V, Mruthyunjaya P, Narayanan R. Multimodal imaging in non-paraneoplastic autoimmune retinopathy. *Indian J Ophthalmol*. 2019;67(7):1171-1173. doi:10.4103/ijo.IJO_1416_18.

9. Patel S, Moysidis SN, Koulisis N, et al. Is it melanoma-associated retinopathy or drug toxicity? Bilateral cystoid macular edema posing a diagnostic and therapeutic dilemma. *Am J Ophthalmol Case Rep*. 2018;10:77-80. doi:10.1016/j.ajoc.2018.01.030.

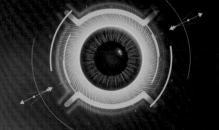

CHAPTER 48

Viral Retinitis: Acute Retinal Necrosis and CMV Retinitis

SALIENT FEATURES

- Acute retinal necrosis (ARN)
  - The most common manifestation of posterior uveitis caused by a herpes virus is acute necrotizing retinitis.
  - ARN typically presents as vision loss, floaters, and variable levels of conjunctival injection in an immunocompetent patient.
  - Examination classically reveals a granulomatous anterior uveitis, vitritis, initially patchy, then confluent, areas of retinal whitening, and associated arteritis that begins peripherally and spreads centripetally.
- Progressive outer retinal necrosis (PORN)
  - PORN occurs in immunocompromised patients presenting with painless vision loss that oftentimes affects the macula.
  - PORN presents with multifocal deep white retinal lesions that begin in the posterior pole and spread peripherally.
  - As PORN occurs in severely immunocompromised patients, limited vitritis and decreased vasculitis are present compared to their ARN counterparts.
- Cytomegalovirus (CMV) retinitis
  - CMV retinitis occurs in immunocompromised patients and classically presents with painless vision loss and floaters.
  - Examination demonstrates areas of granular retinal whitening and associated retinal hemorrhage that typically begins peripherally and follows the retinal arteries as it spreads centrally (Figure 48.1).

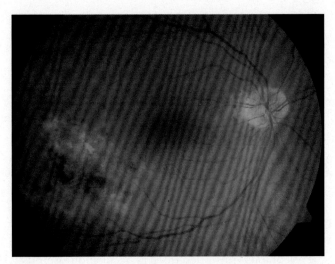

FIGURE 48.1 Fundus photograph demonstrating granular retinal whitening in the inferotemporal macula with associated retinal hemorrhage and arterial sheathing in CMV retinitis.

- The visual prognosis of viral necrotizing retinitis is dependent on disease location but is often times poor due to both direct retinal necrosis and high risk of long-term sequelae including ischemic optic neuropathy and rhegmatogenous retinal detachment.

OCT IMAGING

- ARN
  - Early optical coherence tomography (OCT) imaging demonstrates thickening and increased hyperreflectivity between the nerve fiber layer and the outer plexiform layer that progresses to full-thickness involvement and loss of discernible features of the ellipsoid zone.[1,2]
  - With resolution of active retinitis on clinical examination, there is concurrent thinning of the retina without recovery of the ellipsoid zone.[2]
- PORN
  - Active lesions show thickening of the retina and increased hyperreflectivity of the inner retinal layers with secondary shadowing of the outer layers.[3,4]
  - Associated retinal schisis and hyperreflective foci in the preretinal space (ie, vitreous) have also been reported.[3]
  - OCT imaging of inactive lesions demonstrate retinal thinning and total loss of identifiable retinal layers that correspond clinically to areas of necrosis and atrophy.[4]

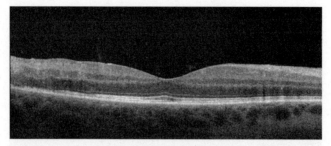

FIGURE 48.2 Optical coherence tomography (OCT) of early cytomegalovirus (CMV) retinitis through the clinical lesion seen in Figure 48.1 showing early increased hyperreflectivity of the inner retinal layers.

- Cytomegalovirus retinitis
  - Active lesions[5]
    - Nebulous vitritis described as peculiar diffuse, dusty, background with generalized increased reflectivity studded with hyperreflective dots.
    - Foci of vitreous attachment to necrotic retina were common findings on OCT.
    - Epiretinal membranes are common.
    - Retinal thickening and increased hyperreflectivity of the inner retina were hallmark patterns of active CMV viral retinitis (Figure 48.2).
      - There were two specific patterns of active retinitis seen on OCT:
        - Full-thickness pattern—hyperreflectivity affecting all layers of the retina with loss of lamination, associated retinal pigment epithelium (RPE) thickening, and loss of choriocapillaris detail (Figure 48.3).

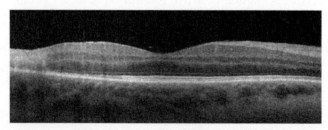

FIGURE 48.3 Interval optical coherence tomography (OCT) of the same lesion seen in Figure 48.1 showing progression to full-thickness hyperreflectivity of the affected retina with development of retinal thinning.

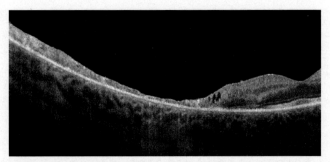

FIGURE 48.4 Follow-up optical coherence tomography (OCT) of the now-inactive cytomegalovirus (CMV) retinitis showing severe retinal atrophy, generalized hyperreflectivity compared to adjacent healthy retina, loss of retinal organization, and few adjacent cystoid spaces.

- Cavernous pattern—inner retinal hyperreflectivity, large empty spaces in the outer nuclear layer with overlying bridges of inner retinal tissue, and sparing of the RPE and choriocapillaris.
    - The cavernous pattern is associated with a higher rate of retinal detachment.
- OCT findings in inactive lesions[5]
    - The hallmark of inactive retinitis is uniformly atrophic retina with loss of lamination, that is thinner than surrounding, healthy retina (Figure 48.4).
    - Previously described nebulous vitritis typically resolves.
    - Epiretinal membranes persist in all patients.

OCTA IMAGING

- ARN
    - Decreased macular vascular density in the superficial and deep vascular plexuses adjacent to the necrotizing retinal lesion.[6]
    - Treatment results in return of flow signal to areas that do not become necrotic.[6]
    - The choriocapillaris is not affected.[6]
- CMV retinitis
    - Appears to display similar optical coherence tomography angiography (OCTA) findings as in ARN with decreased macular vascular density in the superficial and deep vascular plexuses adjacent to the active retinitis (Figure 48.5).

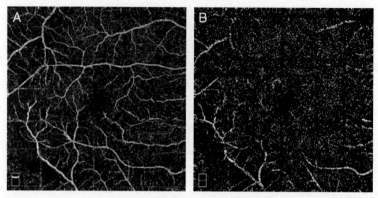

FIGURE 48.5 En-face optical coherence tomography angiography (OCTA) of the superficial and deep retinal vasculature showing loss of flow signal in the inferotemporal macula that corresponds to the clinical CMV lesion in Figure 48.1.

References

1. Murata K, Yamada W, Nishida T, et al. Sequential optical coherence tomography images of early macular necrosis caused by acute retinal necrosis in nonhuman immunodeficiency virus patients. *Retina*. 2016;36(7):e55-e57.

2. Ohtake-Matsumoto A, Keino H, Koto T, Okada AA. Spectral domain and swept source optical coherence tomography findings in acute retinal necrosis. *Graefes Arch Clin Exp Ophthalmol*. 2015;253(11):2049-2051.

3. Chawla R, Tripathy K, Gogia V, Venkatesh P. Progressive outer retinal necrosis-like retinitis in immunocompetent hosts. *BMJ Case Rep*. 2016;2016:bcr2016216581.

4. Almony A, Dhalla MS, Feiner L, Shah GK. Macular optical coherence tomography findings in progressive outer retinal necrosis. *Can J Ophthalmol*. 2007;42(6):881.

5. Invernizzi A, Agarwal A, Ravera V, Oldani M, Staurenghi G, Viola F. Optical coherence tomography findings in cytomegalovirus retinitis: a longitudinal study. *Retina*. 2018;38(1):108-117.

6. Costa de Andrade G, Marchesi Mello LG, Martines GC, Maia A. Optical coherence tomography angiography findings in acute retinal necrosis. *Retin Cases Brief Rep*. 2018.

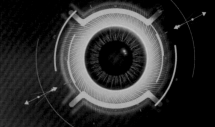

CHAPTER 49

Birdshot Chorioretinopathy

SALIENT FEATURES

- Birdshot chorioretinopathy (BCR) challenges even the most experienced clinician in the management of patients who frequently carries a guarded visual prognosis.[1]
- The course of patients with BCR—which makes up 6% to 8% of posterior uveitis—most commonly features gradual deterioration of vision, even when properly treated.[2]
- BCR is frequently found in middle-aged individuals[3] and manifests bilaterally (often asymmetrically).
- Strongly associated with HLA-A29, the fundi of BCR patients feature centripetal white spots and can demonstrate cystoid macular edema, retinal vasculitis, and—less uniformly—optic disc edema.[4]
- The disease frequently produces retinal inflammation with vitreous haze, afflicting patients with blurred vision, photopsias, paracentral scotomas, and floaters.[5]

OCT IMAGING

- Perivascular thickening, as measured by optical coherence tomography (OCT), was noted to correlate with increased vitreous haze as well as retinal vascular leakage as noted by fluorescein angiography, particularly in eyes with active inflammation from birdshot (Figures 49.1).[6]
- Peripapillary edema, cystoid macular edema, and choroidal thinning have been noted on OCT evaluation of patients with birdshot chorioretinopathy, as well as thinning of the outer retina (Figures 49.2).[7]

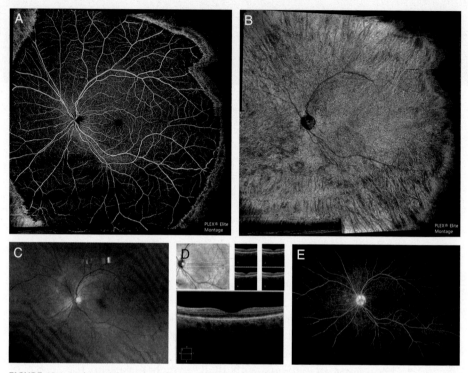

FIGURE 49.1 Multimodal imaging of a retina featuring birdshot chorioretinopathy patient. A, Deep slab of montage of demonstrating vascular flow detail. B, Choroidal slab demonstrating punched out lesions traditionally seen on indocyanine green (ICG). C, Corresponding wide-field color photograph of retina showing characteristic birdshot lesions. D, Optical coherence tomography (OCT) of retina demonstrating outer retinal changes. E, Fluorescein angiography of retina showing hyperfluorescent areas in periphery which correspond with lesions seen on OCT angiography (OCTA) and color fundus photos.

OCTA IMAGING

- Deep vascular plexus capillary loops, telangiectatic vessels, and increased capillary spaces have been noted on OCTA.[8]
- Decreased choroidal blood flow was noted, as well as choroidal thinning and larger choroidal vessels.[9]

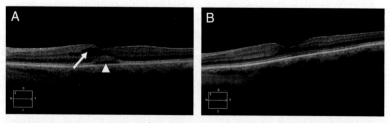

FIGURE 49.2 Optical coherence tomography (OCT) of birdshot chorioretinopathy pretreatment (A) with cystoid macular edema (CME) (arrow) and subretinal fluid (arrowhead) that both resolve post therapy (B).

References

1. Menezo V, Taylor SR. Birdshot uveitis: current and emerging treatment options. *Clin Ophthalmol.* 2014;8:73-81. doi:10.2147/opth.s54832.

2. Shah KH, Levinson RD, Yu F, et al. Birdshot chorioretinopathy. *Surv Ophthalmol.* 2005;50(6):519-541. doi:10.1016/j.survophthal.2005.08.004.

3. Levinson RD, Monnet D. Imaging in birdshot chorioretinopathy. *Int Ophthalmol Clin.* 2012;52(4):191-198. doi:10.1097/IIO.0b013e318265d4b1.

4. Levinson RD, Brezin A, Rothova A, Accorinti M, Holland GN. Research criteria for the diagnosis of birdshot chorioretinopathy: results of an international consensus conference. *Am J Ophthalmol.* 2006;141(1):185-187. doi:10.1016/j.ajo.2005.08.025.

5. Gasch AT, Smith JA, Whitcup SM. Birdshot retinochoroidopathy. *Br J Ophthalmol.* 1999;83(2):241-249.

6. Thomas AS, Hatef AL, Stinnett SS, Keenan RT, Jaffe GJ. Perivascular thickening on optical coherence tomography as a marker of inflammation in birdshot retinochoroiditis. *Retina.* 2019;39(5):956-963. doi:10.1097/iae.0000000000002038.

7. Pichi F, Invernizzi A, Tucker WR, Munk MR. Optical coherence tomography diagnostic signs in posterior uveitis. *Prog Retin Eye Res.* 2019:100797. doi:10.1016/j.preteyeres.2019.100797.

8. Pohlmann D, Macedo S, Stubiger N, Pleyer U, Joussen AM, Winterhalter S. Multimodal imaging in birdshot retinochoroiditis. *Ocul Immunol Inflamm.* 2017;25(5):621-632. doi:10.1080/09273948.2017.1375532.

9. de Carlo TE, Bonini Filho MA, Adhi M, Duker JS. Retinal and choroidal vasculature IN birdshot chorioretinopathy analyzed using spectral domain optical coherence tomography angiography. *Retina.* 2015;35(11):2392-2399. doi:10.1097/iae.0000000000000744.

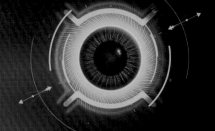

CHAPTER 50

Punctate Inner Choroidopathy

SALIENT FEATURES

- Patients with punctate inner choroidopathy (PIC) are typically myopic young women.[1]
- Patients complain of scotomas and photopsias.
- Small, round, yellow to white, well-defined punctate lesions are typical.
- Frank absence of other intraocular inflammation.[1]
- Hypocyanescent spots are seen on indocyanine green angiography.[2]

OCT IMAGING

- Optical coherence tomography (OCT) imaging in PIC is a key component for disease evaluation and surveillance over time.[2]
  - Features in outer retina include a disrupted external limiting membrane.
  - There is decreased reflectivity locally in the choriocapillaris.
  - "Younger" lesions feature a conical shape of homogeneous hyperreflective material.
  - More chronic lesions feature a break in Bruch membrane with subsequent encroachment of hyperreflective material into the outer retina, causing a more "hump-shaped" appearance, resulting in disruption of the external limiting membrane, ellipsoid zone, and interdigitation zone (Figure 50.1).

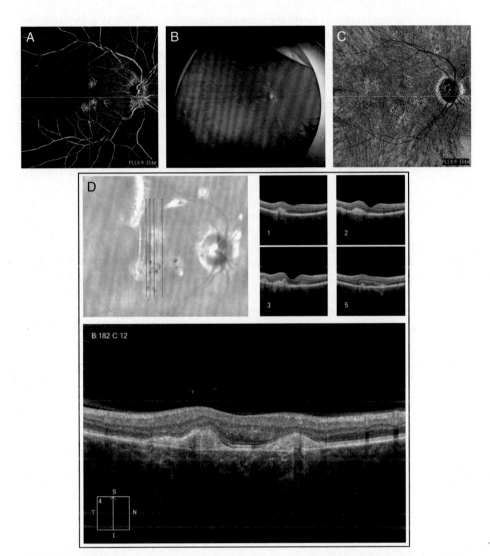

FIGURE 50.1 Multimodal imaging in punctate inner choroidopathy (PIC) (A). Optical coherence tomography angiography (OCTA) demonstrating flow abnormalities in the outer retinal slab corresponding to the pattern of spots seen in fundus photo (B) and OCT B-scan lesions (D). The choriocapillaris window demonstrates similar flow abnormalities (C). OCT B-scan reveals "hump-shaped" appearance of mature PIC lesions on OCT located over breaks in Bruch membrane.

OCTA IMAGING

- Surveillance with optical coherence tomography angiography (OCTA) for underlying choroidal neovascularization (CNV) is a key role for this emerging technology in PIC.
- OCTA patterns that have been described include "lacy wheel," "pruned large-trunk," and "dead tree aspect."[3]
- Flow voids in choroid and choriocapillaris on OCTA correspond with hypocyanescent lesions on ICG.[4]

References

1. Watzke RC, Packer AJ, Folk JC, Benson WE, Burgess D, Ober RR. Punctate inner choroidopathy. *Am J Ophthalmol.* 1984;98(5):572-584. doi:10.1016/0002-9394(84)90243-5.

2. Pichi F, Invernizzi A, Tucker WR, Munk MR. Optical coherence tomography diagnostic signs in posterior uveitis. *Prog Retin Eye Res.* 2019;75:100797. doi:10.1016/j.preteyeres.2019.100797.

3. Pohlmann D, Macedo S, Stubiger N, Pleyer U, Joussen AM, Winterhalter S. Multimodal imaging in birdshot retinochoroiditis. *Ocul Immunol Inflamm.* 2017;25(5):621-632. doi:10.1080/09273948.2017.1375532.

4. Kim EL, Thanos A, Yonekawa Y, et al. Optical coherence tomography angiography findings in punctate inner choroidopathy. *Ophthalmic Surg Lasers Imaging Retina.* 2017;48(10):786-792. doi:10.3928/23258160-20170928-02.

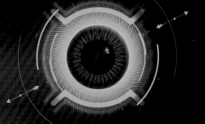

Acute Posterior Multifocal Placoid Pigment Epitheliopathy

SALIENT FEATURES

- Acute posterior multifocal placoid pigment epitheliopathy (APMPPE) is an idiopathic inflammatory condition in the differential of white dot syndromes.
- APMPPE classically presents with decreased vision, scotomas, and photopsias.
- On examination, there are typically multiple bilateral yellow-white placoid lesions at the level of the retinal pigment epithelium (RPE) and inner choroid in the posterior fundus (Figure 51.1).
- The APMPPE lesions tend to resolve within a few weeks, leaving residual pigment mottling and mild atrophy.
- Optical coherence tomography (OCT) and optical coherence tomography angiography (OCTA) are useful imaging tools that can aid in the diagnosis of APMPPE.

OCT IMAGING

- The OCT findings of APMPPE have been described in four distinct stages.[1]
  - Stage 1, acute phase—dome-shaped elevation between the ellipsoid zone (EZ) and the RPE by hyperreflective material with a variable amount of subretinal fluid, which is followed by flattening of the elevation with increased hyperreflectivity and thickening of the outer retina (Figure 51.2)

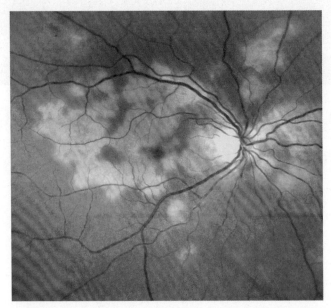

FIGURE 51.1 Fundus photo of acute-phase APMPPE lesion demonstrating characteristic yellow-white placoid lesions at the level of the RPE and inner choroid. APMPPE, acute posterior multifocal placoid pigment epitheliopathy; RPE, retinal pigment epithelium.

- Stage 2, subacute phase—separation between the EZ and the RPE with associated thinning of the outer nuclear layer (ONL)
- Stage 3, late phase—disruption and segmental loss of the EZ junction with increased hyperreflectivity of the RPE (Figure 51.3)
- Stage 4, resolution phase—reconstitution of the EZ with restoration of clear delineation from the RPE (Figure 51.4)

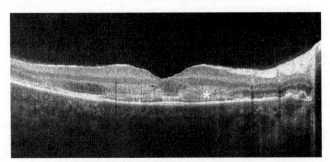

FIGURE 51.2 OCT of stage-1, late acute-phase APMPPE with segmental thickening of the ellipsoid zone and increased hyperreflectivity of the outer nuclear layers (white asterisk). APMPPE, acute posterior multifocal placoid pigment epitheliopathy; OCT, optical coherence tomography.

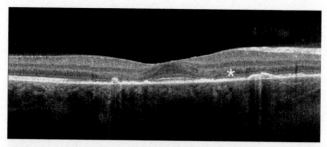

FIGURE 51.3 OCT of stage-3, late-phase APMPPE with partial disappearance of the ellipsoid zone and increased hyperreflectivity of the RPE (white asterisk). APMPPE, acute posterior multifocal placoid pigment epitheliopathy; OCT, optical coherence tomography; RPE, retinal pigment epithelium.

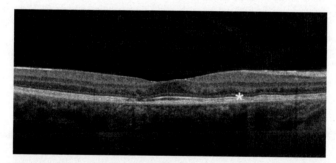

FIGURE 51.4 OCT of stage-4, resolution-phase APMPPE with return of two discrete hyperreflective bands representing the EZ and the RPE (white asterisk). APMPPE, acute posterior multifocal placoid pigment epitheliopathy; EZ, ellipsoid zone; OCT, optical coherence tomography; RPE, retinal pigment epithelium.

OCTA IMAGING

- During the acute phase of APMPPE, OCTA demonstrates flow reduction in the choriocapillaris and outer choroid suggesting that the inner choroid and choriocapillaris are the primary sites of disease pathology (Figures 51.5 and 51.6).[2]
- Furthermore, these areas of choriocapillaris flow deficits identified on OCTA correspond with and extend beyond the area of outer retina hyperreflectivity seen on OCT B-scan.[3]
- The choriocapillaris flow deficits on OCTA demonstrate improvement with plaque resolution on clinical examination and may be used to monitor disease progression and resolution.[2,3]

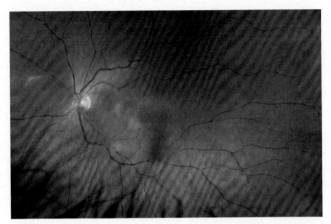

FIGURE 51.5 Fundus photo of acute-phase APMPPE lesion demonstrating characteristic yellow-white placoid lesions at the level of the RPE and inner choroid. Corresponding en-face OCTA image can be seen in Figure 51.6. APMPPE, acute posterior multifocal placoid pigment epitheliopathy; OCTA, optical coherence tomography angiography; RPE, retinal pigment epithelium.

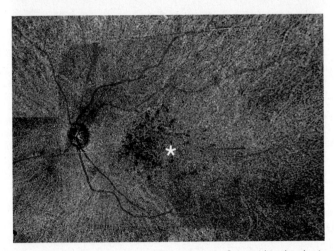

FIGURE 51.6 En-face swept-source 12 × 12 mm OCTA showing flow void in the choriocapillaris (white asterisk) corresponding to the clinical APMPPE lesions seen in Figure 51.5. APMPPE, acute posterior multifocal placoid pigment epitheliopathy; OCTA, optical coherence tomography angiography.

References

1. Goldenberg D, Habot-Wilner Z, Loewenstein A, Goldstein M. Spectral domain optical coherence tomography classification of acute posterior multifocal placoid pigment epitheliopathy. *Retina*. 2012;32(7):1403-1410.
2. Klufas MA, Phasukkijwatana N, Iafe NA, et al. Optical coherence tomography angiography reveals choriocapillaris flow reduction in placoid chorioretinitis. *Ophthalmol Retina*. 2017;1(1):77-91.
3. Burke TR, Chu CJ, Salvatore S, et al. Application of OCT-angiography to characterise the evolution of chorioretinal lesions in acute posterior multifocal placoid pigment epitheliopathy. *Eye (Lond)*. 2017;31(10):1399-1408.

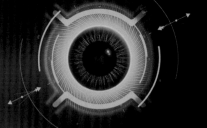

CHAPTER **52**

Multiple Evanescent White Dot Syndrome

SALIENT FEATURES

- Multiple evanescent white dot syndrome (MEWDS) was first described in 1984[1] and is considered to be a transient idiopathic outer retinal disease that affects the photoreceptors/outer retina.
- It typically presents in young healthy women as unilateral reduced visual acuity, photopsias, an enlarged blind spot, and multiple focal small white dots at the level of the outer retina in the macula (Figure 52.1). Foveal pigmentary granularity, optic disc edema, and vitreous cells may also be present.[1-3]
- Often, there is a preceding viral prodrome, which leads many to believe there is an infectious etiology to the pathogenesis of this syndrome.[1]
- MEWDS is a self-limiting process with a majority of cases demonstrating spontaneous resolution of all retinal lesions and improvement in visual acuity and photopsias within weeks of symptom onset. Treatment is typically not indicated.
- Multimodal imaging is instrumental in diagnosing MEWDS as its clinical presentation may be indistinct from other white dot syndromes.
- The hallmark imaging features of MEWDS include punctate wreathlike pattern of hyperfluorescence dots and optic disc leakage on fluorescein angiography (FA) (Figure 52.2), nummular hypocyanescent lesions on indocyanine green angiography (ICGA), and hyperautofluorescent lesions on fundus autofluorescence (FAF) (Figure 52.3).[4-7]

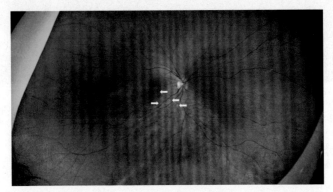

FIGURE 52.1 Wide-field fundus photograph of acute multiple evanescent white dot syndrome (MEWDS), demonstrating multiple very subtle areas of deep retinal whitening/graying (white arrows) that are better highlighted by corresponding fluorescein angiography (FA) (Figure 52.2) and fundus autofluorescence (FAF) (Figure 52.3) images.

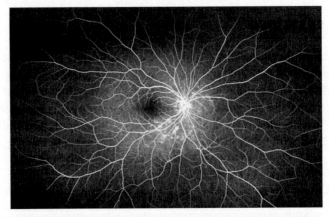

FIGURE 52.2 Corresponding wide-field fluorescein angiography (FA) of acute multiple evanescent white dot syndrome (MEWDS), demonstrating characteristic midphase wreathlike pattern of hyperfluorescence dots and mild optic disc leakage.

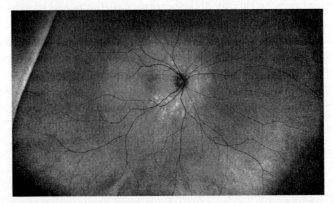

FIGURE 52.3 Corresponding wide-field fundus autofluorescence (FAF) of acute multiple evanescent white dot syndrome (MEWDS), demonstrating characteristic multifocal areas of stippled hyperautofluorescence.

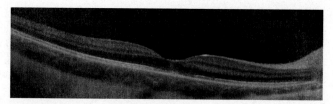

FIGURE 52.4 Optical coherence tomography (OCT) of acute multiple evanescent white dot syndrome (MEWDS), demonstrating focal area of subfoveal ellipsoid zone (EZ) disruption and punctate hyperreflective projections within the outer nuclear layer (ONL).

OCT IMAGING

- Ellipsoid zone (EZ) disruption corresponding topographically to areas of hyperautofluorescent areas on FAF (Figure 52.4)
- Punctate hyperreflective spots/projections within the outer nuclear layer (ONL)[8,9] (Figure 52.4)
- Hyperreflective dots in the inner choroid close to sites of EZ and outer retinal disruption[9,10]
- Larger hyporeflective and confluent spots colocalizing to level of EZ with smaller hyperreflective dots colocalized to level of ONL on en-face optical coherence tomography (OCT)[8,11]
- Possible transient focal choroidal thickening in areas of EZ disruption, in the acute phase
- EZ disruption, hyperreflective ONL spots, and choroidal changes appear to resolve over time[12]

OCTA IMAGING

- Remarkably normal with preserved flow in retinal and choriocapillaris vasculature[9,13]

References

1. Jampol LM, Sieving PA, Pugh D, Fishman GA, Gilbert H. Multiple evanescent white dot syndrome. *Arch Ophthalmol.* 1984;102(5):671. doi:10.1001/archopht.1984.01040030527008.
2. Olitsky SE. Multiple evanescent white-dot syndrome in a 10-year-old child. *J Pediatr Ophthalmol Strabismus.* 1998;35(5):288-289. Available at http://www.ncbi.nlm.nih.gov/pubmed/9782441. Accessed October 14, 2019.
3. Lim JI, Kokame GT, Douglas JP. Multiple evanescent white dot syndrome in older patients. *Am J Ophthalmol.* 1999;127(6):725-728. Available at http://www.ncbi.nlm.nih.gov/pubmed/10372888. Accessed October 14, 2019.
4. Marsiglia M, Gallego-Pinazo R, Cunha de Souza E, et al. Expanded clinical spectrum OF multiple evanescent white dot syndrome with multimodal imaging. *Retina.* 2016;36(1):64-74. doi:10.1097/IAE.0000000000000685.

5. Ie D, Glaser BM, Murphy RP, Gordon LW, Sjaarda RN, Thompson JT. Indocyanine green angiography in multiple evanescent white-dot syndrome. *Am J Ophthalmol.* 1994;117(1):7-12. doi:10.1016/s0002-9394(14)73008-9.

6. Furino C, Boscia F, Cardascia N, Alessio G, Sborgia C. Fundus autofluorescence and multiple evanescent white dot syndrome. *Retina.* 2009;29(1):60-63. doi:10.1097/IAE.0b013e31818c5e04.

7. Dell'Omo R, Mantovani A, Wong R, Konstantopoulou K, Kulwant S, Pavesio CE. Natural evolution of fundus autofluorescence findings IN multiple evanescent white dot syndrome. *Retina.* 2010;30(9):1479-1487. doi:10.1097/IAE.0b013e3181d50cd3.

8. Pichi F, Srvivastava SK, Chexal S, et al. En face optical coherence tomography and optical coherence tomography angiography of multiple evanescent white dot syndrome. *Retina.* 2016;36:S178-S188. doi:10.1097/IAE.0000000000001255.

9. Pereira F, Lima LH, de Azevedo AGB, et al. Swept-source OCT in patients with multiple evanescent white dot syndrome. *J Ophthalmic Inflamm Infect.* 2018;8(1):16. doi:10.1186/s12348-018-0159-2.

10. Fiore T, Iaccheri B, Cerquaglia A, et al. Outer retinal and choroidal evaluation in multiple evanescent white dot syndrome (MEWDS): an enhanced depth imaging optical coherence tomography study. *Ocul Immunol Inflamm.* 2018;26(3):428-434. doi:10.1080/09273948.2016.1231329.

11. De bats F, Wolff B, Vasseur V, et al. "En-Face" spectral-domain optical coherence tomography findings in multiple evanescent white dot syndrome. *J Ophthalmol.* 2014;2014:1-6. doi:10.1155/2014/928028.

12. Li D, Kishi S. Restored photoreceptor outer segment damage in multiple evanescent white dot syndrome. *Ophthalmology.* 2009;116(4):762-770. doi:10.1016/j.ophtha.2008.12.060.

13. Yannuzzi NA, Swaminathan SS, Zheng F, et al. Swept-Source OCT angiography shows sparing of the choriocapillaris in multiple evanescent white dot syndrome. *Ophthalmic Surg Lasers Imaging Retina.* 2017;48(1):69-74. doi:10.3928/23258160-20161219-10.

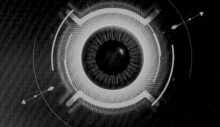

CHAPTER 53

Acute Zonal Occult Outer Retinopathy

SALIENT FEATURES

- Acute zonal occult outer retinopathy (AZOOR) is an idiopathic inflammatory disorder that classically affects young women.
- Symptoms include unilateral or bilateral photopsia and progressive visual field loss, which usually begins as enlargement of the blind spot.
- The hallmark findings in AZOOR are broad areas of concentric outer retinal abnormalities that often begin in the peripapillary zone and expand toward the periphery.
- Diagnosis is often made based on symptomology and multimodal imaging. Importantly, there needs to be evidence of progression with enlargement of the affected area over time in order for the diagnosis to be made.
- The process primarily affects the photoreceptor-RPE (retinal pigment epithelium) complex.
- The appearance on clinical examination depends on the stage at which the patient presents.[1]
  - In the early stages, the affected retina may be demarcated at the leading edge by a yellowish line. OCT through affected retina reveals outer retinal abnormalities that are correspondingly hyper-autofluorescent on fundus autofluorescence (Figure 53.1).
  - In the progressive subacute or chronic stages, the lesions become trizonal, consisting of concentric areas of normal retina (zone 1), followed by retina with evidence of photoreceptor-RPE damage (zone 2), and, finally, a zone of outer retinal and choroidal atrophy (zone 3) (Figure 53.2).

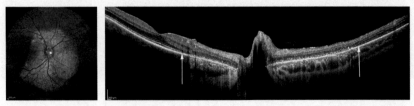

FIGURE 53.1 Early-stage acute zonal occult outer retinopathy (AZOOR). Early-stage disease may present only with disruption of the photoreceptor layer, without the classic trizonal appearance. Corresponding fundus autofluorescence demonstrates hyperautoflorescence in the regions of photoreceptor loss (white arrows).

OCT IMAGING

- Early-stage AZOOR may present only with disruption of the photoreceptor layers on optical coherence tomography (OCT), without evidence of choroidal atrophy (Figure 53.1).
- The advanced form demonstrates a trizonal pattern of outer retinal damage in AZOOR (Figure 53.2).
  - Retinal architecture in zone 1 will be normal.

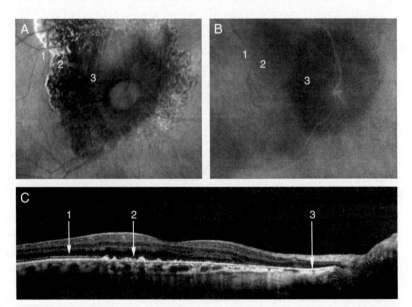

FIGURE 53.2 Trizonal nature of acute zonal occult outer retinopathy (AZOOR) on fundus autofluorescence (A), indocyanine green angiography (B), and optical coherence tomography (OCT) (C). All three zones seen in trizonal AZOOR are present in this case: zone 1 represents normal-appearing retina; zone 2 represents retina with disruption of the photoreceptor layer; and zone 3 represents areas of choroidal atrophy. The progression front occurs at the leading, hyperautofluorescent edge of zone 2.

- Zone 2 demonstrates photoreceptor-RPE disruption, including disturbances in the ellipsoid and interdigitation zones, as well as possible subretinal deposits that appear drusenoid in nature.
- Zone 3 is represented by end-stage outer retinal and choroidal atrophy.
- Choroidal neovascularization may occur as a rare complication of AZOOR and is often type 2 in nature.[2]

OCTA IMAGING

- The usefulness of optical coherence tomography angiography (OCTA) in the diagnosis of AZOOR has not been clearly established. OCTA may be useful in detecting complications of AZOOR, such as choroidal neovascularization.[3]

References

1. Mrejen S, Khan S, Gallego-Pinazo R, Jampol LM, Yannuzzi LA. Acute zonal occult outer retinopathy: a classification based on multimodal imaging. *JAMA Ophthalmol.* 2014;132(9):1089-1098.
2. Introini U, Casalino G, Dhrami-Gavazi E, et al. Clinical course of acute zonal occult outer retinopathy complicated by choroidal neovascularization. *Int J Retina Vitreous.* 2018;4:32.
3. Levison AL, Baynes K, Lowder CY, Srivastava SK. OCT angiography identification of choroidal neovascularization secondary to acute zonal occult outer retinopathy. *Ophthalmic Surg Lasers Imaging Retina.* 2016;47(1):73-75.

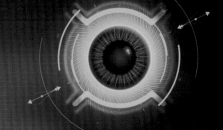

CHAPTER 54

Serpiginous and Serpiginous-like Choroiditis

SALIENT FEATURES

- Serpiginous choroiditis (SC) is a rare, bilateral, idiopathic, progressive, chronic, relapsing disease associated with geographic inflammation and scarring of the retinal pigment epithelium and inner choroid.
- SC typically presents as deep gray-yellow lesions extending outward from peripapillary area that progress to generalized retinal, retinal pigment epithelium (RPE), and inner choroidal atrophy and pigmentary degeneration (Figures 54.1 and 54.2). There is typically minimal to no vitreous inflammation. Recurrences occur at the edges of prior chorioretinal scars (Figure 54.3).
- Visual prognosis is guarded and occurs secondary to foveal atrophy and secondary choroidal neovascularization (CNV) (Figures 54.4 and 54.5).
- Autofluorescence (AF) can be an essential tool to monitor activity; active lesions or recurrences will typically demonstrate new hyper-AF signals along the edge of prior scars. Inactive scars will appear hypo-AF.
- Aggressive systemic and/or local immunosuppressive therapy is the mainstay of treatment with the addition of anti–vascular endothelial growth factor therapy should CNV be present.
- SC is part of a family of related placoid disorders:
  - In *macular serpiginous,* there is a predilection of involvement of the macular area.
  - In *ampiginous choroiditis (relentless placoid chorioretinitis),* the lesions are multifocal and resemble the more benign lesions of acute posterior multifocal placoid pigment epitheliopathy (APMPPE) but demonstrate a relentlessly progressive course that may be poorly responsive to immunomodulatory therapy.

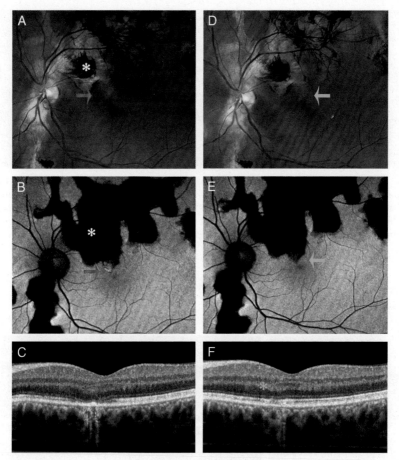

FIGURE 54.1 Fundus photograph (A) from a patient with a long-standing history of serpiginous choroiditis demonstrating a geographic, serpentine pattern of chorioretinal atrophy extending from the nerve with pigmentary degeneration. Areas of chorioretinal atrophy are hypoautofluorescent on fundus autofluorescence (FAF) (A and B, white asterisks). Red arrow over (A) highlights a small yellow-grey lesion extending from the edge of margin of chorioretinal atrophy that demonstrates a hyperautoflorescent signal (B, red arrow). Optical coherence tomography (OCT) through the involved retina demonstrates outer retinal thickening, ellipsoid zone loss, and retinal pigment epithelium (RPE) thickening confirming reactivation. After treatment with oral corticosteroids and a subsequent increase in systemic immunosuppression, the lesion is less pronounced on photography (D, green arrow) and more hypoautofluorescent (E, green arrow), and the outer retinal/RPE abnormalities appear to be improving (F, green asterisk).

- *Tuberculous serpiginous-like choroiditis* denotes a similarly behaving disease entity that carries an intraocular tuberculosis association that is more often multifocal in nature, may demonstrate vitritis, and typically affects younger individuals. Anti–tuberculosis-directed therapy is recommended in these cases, although the outcomes of these medications in modulating the disease course are not well established.

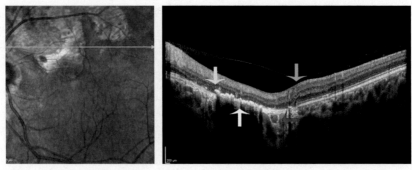

FIGURE 54.2 Optical coherence tomography (OCT) image from the same patient as Figure 55.1 through an area of prior choroiditis highlighting features of prior disease including outer retinal thinning and photoreceptor loss (yellow arrow); retinal pigment epiththelium (RPE) hypertrophy and/or atrophy (white arrow); and choriocapillaris atrophy with prominent medium to large choroidal vessels visualized under Bruch membrane (red arrow). There is a sharp demarcation between affected and unaffected retina (green arrow).

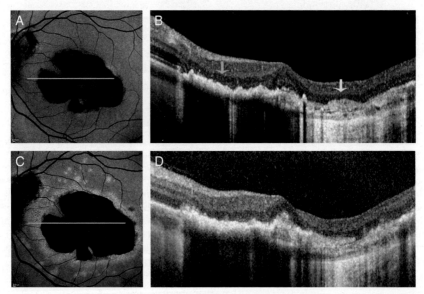

FIGURE 54.3 A and B, Fundus autofluorescence (FAF) and optical coherence tomography (OCT) images from a patient with macular serpiginous demonstrating hypoautofluorescence through the macular region. Outer retinal thinning and photoreceptor loss are present (B, green arrow) as is subretinal fibrosis (B, yellow arrow). C and D, A year later, the patient presented with blurry vision and photopsias with evidence of reactivation including a new rim of hyperautofluorescence around the main lesion and several satellite foci of hyperautofluorescence (C, red asterisks). There is ellipsoid zone (EZ) attenuation and retinal pigment epiththelium (RPE) thickening in the prior uninvolved retina at the edge of the chorioretinal scarring consistent with reactivation (red arrow).

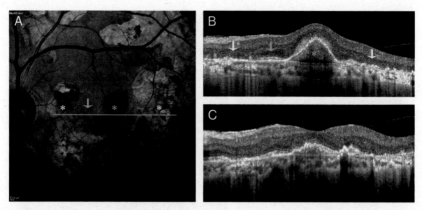

FIGURE 54.4 Multicolor photograph (A) from a patient with previously controlled serpiginous-like choroiditis who presented with new central visual loss. There is evidence of prior chorioretinal inflammation (yellow asterisks), a new foveal pigment epithelial detachment (green asterisk), and an intervening region of uninvolved retina (green arrow). Green line signifies location of optical coherence tomography (OCT) scan (B) which also demonstrates areas of chorioretinal atrophy (yellow arrows), relatively preserved retina (green arrow), and a tall pigment epithelial detachment with overlying subretinal hyperreflective material (SRHM) and moderately hyperreflective internal material (green asterisk). The patient was diagnosed with secondary choroidal neovascularization and was initiated on monthly anti–vascular endothelial growth factor therapy (C). After 1 year of therapy, vision returned to baseline, the pigment epithelial detachment has decreased in height (red asterisk), and there is some reconstitution of the subfoveal outer retinal bands (ellipsoid zone [EZ] and external limiting membrane [ELM]).

OCT IMAGING

- Active lesions demonstrate hyperreflectivity and thickening of the outer retina and RPE. Photoreceptor layer attenuation and subretinal hyperreflective material may be present (Figure 54.1C).
- Chronic, inactive lesions demonstrate RPE and retinal atrophy. Subretinal fibrosis may be present (Figure 54.2).
- The presence of new outer retinal abnormalities, pigment epithelium detachments, and subretinal hyperreflective material at the edges of atrophy may signify recurrences (Figure 54.3D).
- Inner choroidal atrophy may be present in chronic cases.
- CNV is often visualized as irregular pigment epithelial detachment with "double-layer" sign at edges of prior chorioretinal scarring (Figure 54.4B).

OCTA IMAGING

- In active lesions, optical coherence tomography angiography (OCTA) can detect choriocapillaris flow voids underlying areas of outer retinal and RPE thickening and hyperreflectivity. These may expand a larger area than is seen clinically and correspond to hypofluorescence on indocyanine green angiography.

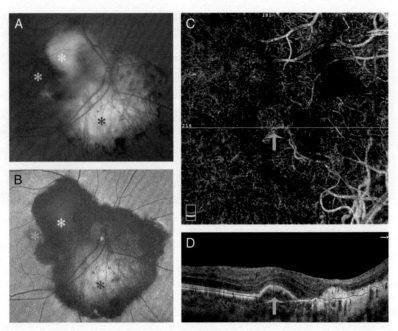

FIGURE 54.5 Fundus photograph and fundus autofluorescence (FAF) imaging (A and B) from a patient with controlled serpiginous choroiditis demonstrating peripapillary chorioretinal atrophy with areas of white fibrosis and marked hypoautofluorescence (yellow asterisks). An area of profound chorioretinal atrophy demonstrates hyperautofluorescence likely due to emergence of underlying scleral tissue (red asterisk). The patient presents with new-onset blurry vision. Optical coherence tomography (OCT) demonstrates a subtle pigment epithelial detachment that demonstrates mildly decreased autofluorescent signal (green asterisks). En-face OCT angiography image (C) demonstrates a tangle of subfoveal vessels within the pigment epithelial detachment (PED). There is segmentation artifact from retinal and large choroidal vasculature through the area of prior chorioretinal atrophy (purple asterisks). D, B-scan with flow signal overlay clearly demonstrating flow signal within the PED confirming secondary choroidal neovascularization.

- These flow voids persist in the inactive states after the development of overlying retinal and RPE atrophy, suggesting true choriocapillaris nonperfusion (vs artifactually decreased signal due to OCT signal hypotransmission).
- The superficial and deep retinal vascular plexuses may appear normal in the early disease course but ultimately demonstrate a lack of flow with progressive retinal atrophy.
- OCTA has a role in the identification and monitoring of CNV that may develop in the disease process (Figure 54.5).

References

1. Cunningham ET, Gupta A, Zierhut M. The creeping choroiditides – serpiginous and multifocal serpiginoid choroiditis. *Ocul Immunol Inflamm.* 2014;22:345-348.

2. Desai R, Nesper P, Goldstein DA, et al. OCT angiography imaging in serpiginous choroidopathy. *Ophthalmol Retina*. 2018;2:351-359.

3. Konana VK, Bhagya M, Babu K. Double-layer sign: a new OCT finding in active tubercular serpiginous-like choroiditis to monitor activity. *Ophthalmol Retina*. 2020;4(3):336-342.

4. Pakzad-Vaezi K, Khaksari K, Chu Z, et al. Swept-source OCT angiography of serpiginous choroiditis. *Ophthalmol Retina*. 2018;2:712-719.

5. Pichi F, Invernizzi A, Tucker WR, Munk MR. Optical coherence tomography diagnostic signs in posterior uveitis. *Prog Retin Eye Res*. 2019;75:100797.

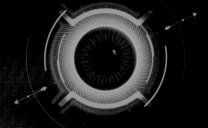

CHAPTER 55

Endogenous Endophthalmitis

SALIENT FEATURES

- Endogenous endophthalmitis (EE) is a rare but vision-threatening condition resulting from the hematogenous spread of microorganisms (bacteria, fungi, or mycobacteria) from distant foci to intraocular structures and accounts for 2% to 8% of all cases of endophthalmitis.[1]
- Risk factors include recent hospitalization, diabetes mellitus, immunosuppression, intravenous drug use, indwelling catheters, urinary tract infection, organ abscesses, and endocarditis.[2]
- A thorough systemic evaluation and a review of systems are warranted for cases of suspected EE including complete physical examination (including a full skin check), blood and urine cultures, and imaging as appropriate, often in conjunction with an internist and possibly requiring inpatient admission.[3]
- Ocular symptoms include varying degrees of decreased vision and eye pain. Systemic symptoms such as fever, chills, nausea, vomiting, and other signs may be present.
- Ocular signs include a combination of anterior chamber inflammation, hypopyon, vitreous haze, visible arteriolar septic emboli, uveal tissue abscesses, and necrotizing retinitis (Figures 55.1A and 55.2A).[4] Systemic signs will depend on the source of the infection.
- Ultrasound may reveal diffuse or compartmentalized hyperechogenicity of the vitreous cavity (Figure 55.3). Choroidal or retinal abscesses, if present, will appear as domed-shaped elevations. Chorioretinal thickening is also present.
- If the media permits, fluorescein angiography may demonstrate perivascular sheathing and leakage from diffuse vasculitis.

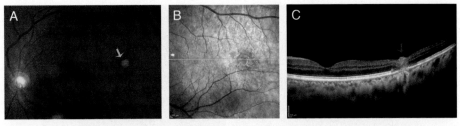

FIGURE 55.1 A, Color fundus photograph from a patient with a history of candidemia with resolved focal chorioretinitis in the temporal macula (blue arrow). The patient was previously treated with systemic and intraocular antifungals with resolution of inflammation and restoration of vision. Near-infrared image (B) demonstrates location of the cross-sectional spectral-domain optical coherence tomography (SD-OCT) image. C, SD-OCT through the fovea demonstrates a hyperreflective full-thickness retinal nodule with underlying retinal pigment epithelium (RPE) irregularity without overlying vitritis (red arrow) signifying chronicity and inactivity.

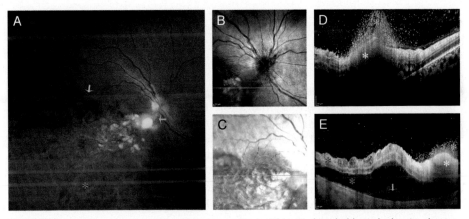

FIGURE 55.2 A, Color photograph from a young patient with acute lymphoblastic leukemia who presented to the emergency room with fevers and blurry vision. The patient was found to have methicillin-sensitive *Staphylococcus aureus* (MSSA) bacteremia secondary to an infected indwelling catheter. The catheter was replaced, and the patient was placed on systemic antibiotics. Fundus examination revealed a single, creamy-white septic embolus extending from a retinal arteriole (green arrow) with secondary branch retinal vein occlusion and hemorrhagic vasculitis (red asterisk) with diffuse preretinal and intraretinal hemorrhages (blue arrow). B and C, Near-infrared images demonstrating locations of the adjacent spectral-domain optical coherence tomography (SD-OCT) photos through the embolus (D) and the macula (E). D, SD-OCT through the lesion demonstrates extensive vitreous hyperreflectivity over the lesion (green asterisk) and a hyperreflective mass in the retina (yellow asterisk). E, SD-OCT through the fovea catches the nasal focus of vitreous hyperreflectivity (green asterisk) and the embolus (yellow asterisk). Retinal layers are hyperreflective and disorganized (red asterisk). There are outer retinal cystoid spaces (pink asterisk) and a difficult-to-appreciate focus of subretinal fluid (green arrow). The patient received vitreous aspiration which also yielded MSSA. A single injection of intravitreal vancomycin and ceftazidime along with prolonged systemic antibiotic course resulted in resolution of the systemic and intraocular infection. The patient received several rounds of intravitreal anti–vascular endothelial growth factor to treat secondary macular edema with ultimate quiescence and some restoration of vision.

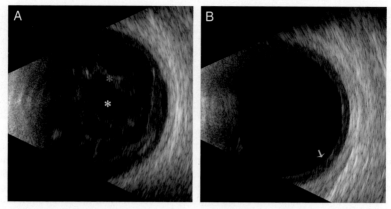

FIGURE 55.3 A, Ocular B-scan ultrasound image from a patient with endogenous endophthalmitis with significant vitritis. There are hyperechogenic vitreous septae (red asterisk) with intervening hypoechogenic spaces (yellow asterisk). There is no retinal or choroidal detachment. B, Ocular B-scan ultrasound of the same patient 1 month after pars plana vitrectomy, vitreous culture, and injection of intravitreal antibiotics. The central vitreous cavity is hypoechogenic, and there is a thin rim of remaining vitreous.

- Prompt diagnosis with vitreous aspiration or pars plana vitrectomy and initiation of intravitreal and/or systemic antimicrobials are critical in preserving visual acuity in this ocular emergency.[5]
- Pars plana vitrectomy has a role in reducing microbial load, increasing diagnostic yield, and delivering intravitreal therapy and may be employed per the treating clinician's judgment. Systemic treatment for the underlying etiology is indicated and should be performed in concert with an internist.
- Visual prognosis is guarded, even with prompt and aggressive treatment. Presenting visual acuity is the greatest predictor of outcome.[6]

OCT FEATURES

- If there is a view of the posterior segment, vitreous inflammation on optical coherence tomography (OCT) can present as multiple discrete hyperreflective foci in the vitreous cavity that may aggregate on the posterior hyaloid or retinal surface (Figure 55.2D).[7]
- Retinal (Figures 55.1C and 55.2D), subretinal, and/or choroidal abscesses appear as discrete hyperreflective masses that are accompanied by hyperreflective foci in the vitreous (vitritis) and varying degrees of choroidal thickening.[8]
- Varying degrees of retinal hyperreflectivity and layer obscuration may be present depending on location and severity of the retinitis (Figure 55.2D).

OCTA FEATURES

- There is currently no role for optical coherence tomography angiography (OCTA) in endophthalmitis.

References

1. Sadiq MA, Hassan M, Agarwal A, et al. Endogenous endophthalmitis: diagnosis, management, and prognosis. *J Ophthalmic Inflamm Infect.* 2015;5(1):32. doi:10.1186/s12348-015-0063-y.

2. Vaziri K, Schwartz SG, Kishor K, Flynn HW Jr. Endophthalmitis: state of the art. *Clin Ophthalmol.* 2015;9:95-108. doi:10.2147/OPTH.S76406.

3. Cho H, Shin YU, Siegel NH, et al. Endogenous endophthalmitis in the American and Korean population: an 8-year retrospective study. *Ocul Immunol Inflamm.* 2018;26(4):496-503. doi:10.1080/09273948.2016.1195000.

4. Fortun J, Modi YS, Bessette A, et al. Clinical features and management of subretinal abscesses secondary to methicillin-resistant *Staphylococcus aureus* endogenous endophthalmitis. *Ophthalmic Surg Lasers Imaging Retina.* 2017;48(2):134-142. doi:10.3928/23258160-20170130-07.

5. Shenoy SB, Thotakura M, Kamath Y, Bekur R. Endogenous endophthalmitis in patients with MRSA septicemia: a case series and review of literature. *Ocul Immunol Inflamm.* 2016;24(5):515-520. doi:10.3109/09273948.2015.1020173.

6. Bjerrum SS, la Cour M. 59 eyes with endogenous endophthalmitis- causes, outcomes and mortality in a Danish population between 2000 and 2016. *Graefes Arch Clin Exp Ophthalmol.* 2017;255(10):2023-2027. doi:10.1007/s00417-017-3760-4.

7. Lavine JA, Mititelu M. Multimodal imaging of refractory Candida chorioretinitis progressing to endogenous endophthalmitis. *J Ophthalmic Inflamm Infect.* 2015;5(1):54. doi:10.1186/s12348-015-0054-z.

8. Invernizzi A, Symes R, Miserocchi E, et al. Spectral domain optical coherence tomography findings in endogenous Candida endophthalmitis and their clinical relevance. *Retina.* 2018;38(5):1011-1018. doi:10.1097/IAE.0000000000001630.

Part 6
Inherited Retinal Degenerations

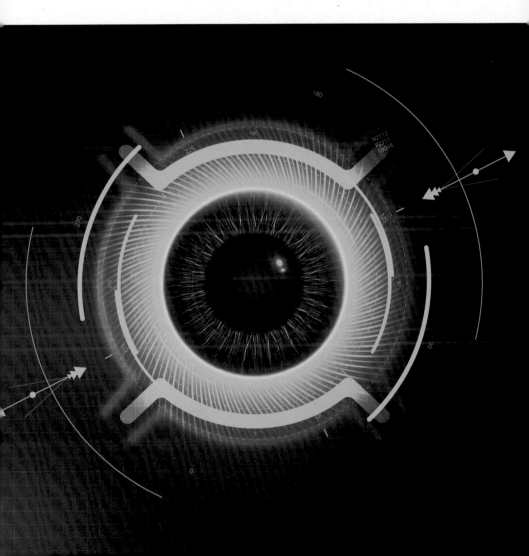

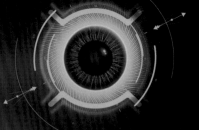

CHAPTER 56

Retinitis Pigmentosa

SALIENT FEATURES

- Retinitis pigmentosa (RP) is the most common hereditary retinal degeneration (approximately 1 in 4000) which results in bilateral progressive vision loss secondary to photoreceptor loss.
- Symptoms of RP include progressive nyctalopia and visual field loss; typically, central vision is maintained until late in the disease.
- Ocular examination findings consistent with RP include pale/waxy optic nerve, severe arteriolar attenuation, and pigmentary deposits within the peripheral retina, classically referred to as "bone spicules." Additional examination findings include posterior subcapsular cataract, vitreous cell, and cystoid macular edema.
- RP can be diagnosed by clinical examination but is also supported through multimodal diagnostics.
- Goldmann visual fields—which classically demonstrate ring scotoma— and electroretinography (ERG)—which reveal reduced amplitude of A- and B-waves in earlier stages but can progress to nondetectible amplitudes in advanced disease. Visual fields and ERG are also helpful in identifying disease severity and tracking disease progression.
- Genetics evaluation is also now frequently utilized to identify the underlying gene defect.
- Optical coherence tomography (OCT) is routinely used in RP to assess retinal thickness, photoreceptor integrity, and for macular edema.
- Optical coherence tomography angiography (OCTA) is an emerging modality for RP but may play a role in the future to evaluate severity and disease progression based on retinal vascular plexus changes.

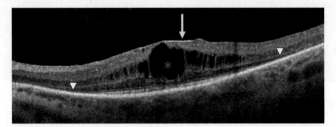

FIGURE 56.1 Optical coherence tomography (OCT) in retinitis pigmentosa (RP) and confirmed RP-1 mutation. Cystoid macular edema is present causing loss of normal foveal pit (red asterisk). Concomitant epiretinal membrane is also noted (yellow arrow). Loss of the ellipsoid zone can be seen just outside of the fovea with extension of loss both nasal and temporal (white arrowheads).

OCT IMAGING

- OCT imaging abnormalities can be seen in both the inner and outer retina in RP patients (Figures 56.1-56.4).
- RP patients frequently demonstrate generalized retinal atrophy with macular thinning (Figure 56.5).[2]
- As photoreceptor loss extends more posteriorly, ellipsoid zone (EZ) loss is to be visualized on the macular OCT often with foveal sparing (Figure 56.2).
- Irregularity, shortening, or absence of the macular EZ line in RP patients has been correlated with decreased best corrected visual acuity (BCVA) and decreased retinal sensitivity.[3]

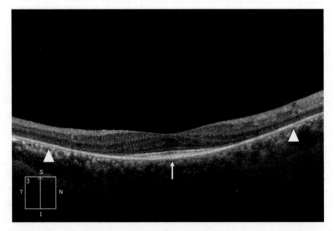

FIGURE 56.2 Optical coherence tomography (OCT) in retinitis pigmentosa with loss of ellipsoid zone nasally and temporally (white arrowheads) with foveal sparing (white arrow).

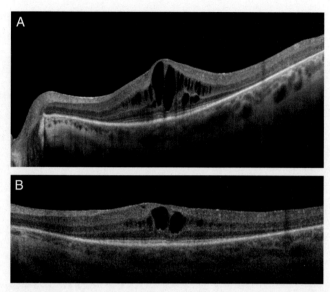

FIGURE 56.3 Optical coherence tomography (OCT) in retinitis pigmentosa complicated by cystoid macular edema (A). Following treatment with topical carbonic anhydrase inhibitor drops, the macular edema improved over 4 months (B).

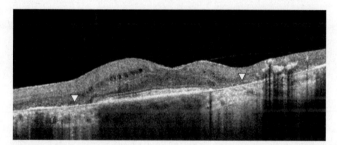

FIGURE 56.4 Advanced retinal atrophy secondary to retinitis pigmentosa. Optical coherence tomography (OCT) demonstrates minimal epiretinal membrane with mild intraretinal fluid (red asterisk). Diffuse thinning of the retina is noted along with parafoveal complete ellipsoid zone loss and retinal pigment epithelium (RPE) atrophy (white arrowhead).

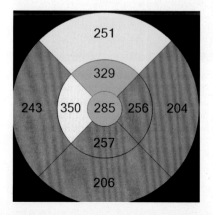

FIGURE 56.5 Retinal thickness map in retinitis pigmentosa with significant retinal thinning and relative sparing of the central subfield.

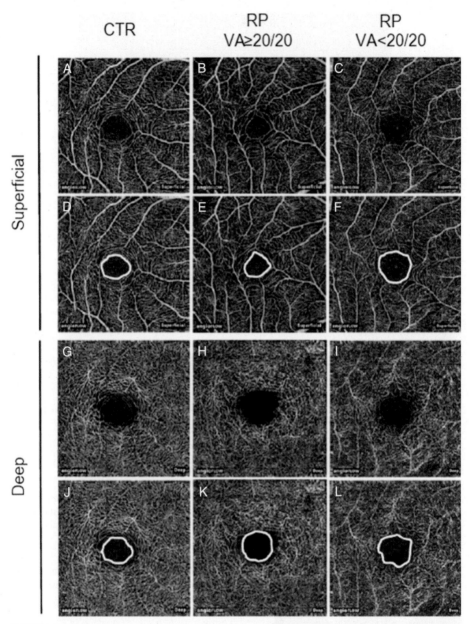

FIGURE 56.6 Comparative imaging of superficial and deep plexus optical coherence tomography angiography (OCTA) in a control patient (left) versus two retinitis pigmentosa patients (RPs) with (middle) and without central vision loss (right). Images show the superficial foveal avascular zone (FAZ) seemingly enlarged in RP with vision loss. (Reprinted with permission from Koyanagi Y, Murakami Y, Funatsu J, et al. Optical coherence tomography angiography of the macular microvasculature changes in retinitis pigmentosa. *Acta Ophthalmol.* 2018;96:e58-e67.)

- Epiretinal membrane and cystoid macular edema are common complications associated with RP (Figures 56.1, 56.3, and 56.4); OCT is used to track progression as well as response to intervention.[4]
- Emerging treatments, such as the retinal prosthesis and gene therapy, will also utilize OCT for screening candidates, assessing the device/therapeutic placement during surgery with intraoperative OCT, and evaluating postoperative factors such as array placement or retinal alterations following gene therapy.[5]

OCTA IMAGING

- Decreased retinal vascular density in both the superficial capillary plexus (SCP) and deep capillary plexus (DCP) along with larger foveal avascular zone at the SCP and DCP level has been reported in RP (Figure 56.6).[6,7]
- Reduced vascular density of the level of the optic nerve may explain the development of nerve pallor seen on examination.[3]

References

1. Harong DT, Berson EL, Dryja TP. Retinitis pigmentosa. *Lancet.* 2006;368(9549):1795-1809.
2. Arrigo A, Romano F, Albertini G, et al. Vascular patterns in Retinitis Pigmentosa on swept-source optical coherence tomography angiography. *J Clin Med.* 2019;8(9):1425.
3. Mitamura Y, Aizawa S, Baba T, et al. Correlation between retinal sensitivity and photoreceptor inner/outer segment junction in patients with retinitis pigmentosa. *Br J Ophthalmol.* 2009;93:125-126.
4. Liew G, Srong S, Bradley P, et al. Prevalence of cystoid macular edema, epiretinal membrane and cataract in retinitis pigmentosa. *Br J Ophthalmol.* 2019;103(8):1163-1166.
5. Parmeggini F, De Nadai K, Piovan A, et al. Optical coherence tomography imaging in the management of the Argus II retinal prosthesis system. *Eur J Ophthalmol.* 2017;27(1):e16-e21.
6. Battaglia Parodi M, Cicinelli MV, Rabiolo A, et al. Vessel density analysis in patients with retinitis pigmentosa by means of optical coherence tomography angiography. *Br J Ophthalmol.* 2017;101:428-432.
7. Koyanagi Y, Murakami Y, Funatsu J, et al. Optical coherence tomography angiography of the macular microvasculature changes in retinitis pigmentosa. *Acta Ophthalmol.* 2018;96:e58-e67.

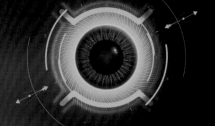

CHAPTER 57

Choroideremia

SALIENT FEATURES

- Choroideremia is an X-linked recessive disease, due to a mutation in CHM gene. CHM gene encodes for Rab escort protein-1, a protein that regulates intracellular trafficking in photoreceptors and the retinal pigment epithelium (RPE).[1]
- Prevalence is estimated to be 1/50,000 to 100,000.[1,2]
- Nyctalopia and peripheral visual field loss (most often a ring scotoma) are early symptoms, followed by central vision loss later in life (approximately age 50-70 years).[3]
- Fundus appearance is notable for "salt and pepper" mottling, most prominent in the midperiphery that later involves the center.
- Electroretinography (ERG) is abnormal even in early stage of the disease.[4]
- Female carriers can have mild presentations, although there are some case reports of severe phenotype that matches phenotype of male patients. The pigmentary changes in the carrier are thought to be secondary to X-chromosome lyonization.[5]
- Choroideremia can be complicated by choroidal neovascularization (CNV).[6]

OCT IMAGING

- Optical coherence tomography (OCT) shows sharp transitional zone between the areas of outer retinal atrophy and normal outer retina (Figure 57.1).[6]

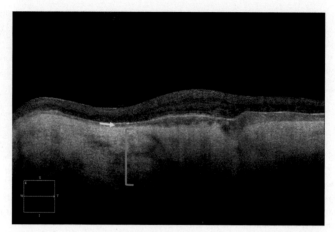

FIGURE 57.1 Choroideremia optical coherence tomography (OCT) with central preservation. Transition zone between choroidal loss and partial preservation noted (yellow arrow). Increased retinal layer integrity, including ellipsoid zone preservation, overlying the area of partially preserve choroid. Increased visualization of the sclera related to overlying atrophy (blue bracket).

- Outer retinal tubulation (ORT) may be present near the margin of the sharp transition zone. These appear as hyperreflective ring surrounding hyporeflective center (Figure 57.2).[6]
- Interlaminar bridge, a wedged-shaped hypo- or hyperreflective structure that "bridges" inner and outer retina may be present as well (Figures 57.1 and 57.3).[7,8]
- OCT may also identify CNV and associated sequelae (eg, intraretinal fluid, subretinal fluid) (Figure 57.3).[6]

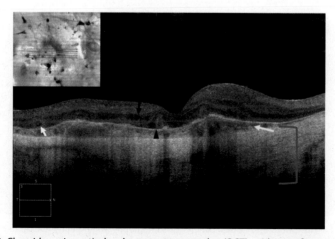

FIGURE 57.2 Choroideremia optical coherence tomography (OCT) with significant atrophy. Near-infrared image on the top left corner shows generalized atrophy partial sparing of the central island. OCT B-scan demonstrating outer retinal atrophy, possible outer retinal tubulation (white arrow), interlaminar bridge (black arrowhead) as well as intraretinal fluid (black arrow) and choroidal thinning (yellow arrow). Increased visibility of the sclera is noted due to overlying atrophy (blue bracket).

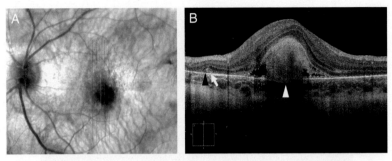

FIGURE 57.3 Choroideremia with choroidal neovascularization (CNV). (a) Near-infrared image shows generalized atrophy sparing the central island. (B) Optical coherence tomography (OCT) B-scan shows marked outer retinal atrophy in the periphery with possible outer retinal tubulation (white arrow) and extensive attenuation of the ellipsoid zone (black arrowhead) at the margin. Centrally, a large CNV is present with surrounding subretinal fluid (white arrowhead).

OCTA IMAGING

- Optical coherence tomography angiography (OCTA) shows significant choriocapillaris loss that correlates with loss of ellipsoid zone on OCT (Figure 57.4). RPE loss is more extensive than choriocapillaris loss.[6,9]
- There is loss of significant superficial retinal vessel network compared to normal population.[9]
- OCTA may also be diagnostic of CNV presence (Figure 57.4).[6]

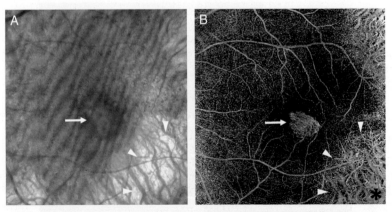

FIGURE 57.4 Fundus photo and optical coherence tomography angiography (OCTA) of choroideremia with choroidal neovascularization (CNV) from Figure 57.3. Central CNV (arrow) is visualized in both fundus photo and OCTA. Note that choroidal vessels are visible in the temporal periphery in OCTA (black asterisk) given retinal/retinal pigment epithelium (RPE) atrophy and choriocapillaris loss. RPE loss as noted on the fundus photo (arrowhead) while underlying choriocapillaris remodeling and early loss is noted in same area on the OCTA (arrowhead).

References

1. van den Hurk JA, Schwartz M, van Bokhoven H, et al. Molecular basis of choroideremia (CHM): mutations involving the Rab escort protein-1 (REP-1) gene. *Hum Mutat.* 1997;9:110-117.

2. MacDonald IM, Hume S, Chan S, Seabra MC. Choroideremia. In: Pagon RA, Adam MP, Ardinger HH et al, eds. *GeneReviews(R).*Seattle, WA: University of Washington; 1993-2017.

3. Roberts MF, Fishman GA, Roberts DK, et al. Retrospective, longitudinal, and cross sectional study of visual acuity impairment in choroideraemia. *Br J Ophthalmol.* 2002;86:658-662.

4. Grover S, Fishman GA. Hereditary choroidal diseases. In: Schachat A, Sadda SR, Hinton DR, et al, eds. *Ryan's Retina.* Philadelphia, PA: Elsevier; 2018:997-1005.

5. Lorda-Sanchez IJ, Ibañez AJ, Sanz RJ, et al. Choroideremia, sensorineural deafness, and primary ovarian failure in a woman with a balanced X-4 translocation. *Ophthalmic Genet.* 2000;21:185-189.

6. Jain N, Jia Y, Gao SS, et al. Optical coherence tomography angiography in choroideremia: correlating choriocapillaris loss with overlying degeneration. *JAMA Ophthalmol.* 2016;134(6):697-702.

7. Syed R, Sundquist SM, Ratnam K, et al. High-resolution images of retinal structure in patients with choroideremia. *Invest Ophthalmol Vis Sci.* 2013;54:950-961.

8. Sun LW, Johnson RD, Williams V, et al. Multimodal imaging of photoreceptor structure in choroideremia. *PLoS One.* 2016;11:e0167526.

9. Abbouda A, Dubis AM, Webster AR, et al. Identifying characteristic features of the retinal and choroidal vasculature in choroideremia using optical coherence tomography angiography. *Eye.* 2017;32:563-571.

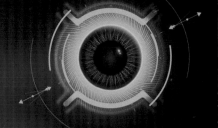

CHAPTER 58

Stargardt Disease

SALIENT FEATURES

- Stargardt disease (SD) is a predominantly autosomal recessive condition most commonly due to a mutation in the ABCA4 gene, which leads to the accumulation of bisretinoid diretinoid-phosphatidylethanolamine (A2PE) and diretinoid-pyridinium-ethanolamine (A2E) in photoreceptor outer segments and retinal pigment epitheium (RPE) cells, respectively, leading to cell death.[1]
- SD is the most common juvenile macular dystrophy, occurring in approximately 1 out of 10,000, and characterized by macular atrophy, pisciform flecks, and visual decline.[2]
- Optical coherence tomography (OCT) shows progressive loss of the ellipsoid zone (EZ) as well as deeper structures, including the RPE and choroid, which has been correlated with visual decline.[1-3]
- Optical coherence tomography angiography (OCTA) has shown a decline in both the retinal superficial capillary plexus (SCP) and deep capillary plexus (DCP).[4]
- Additionally, OCTA has shown a loss in choriocapillaris vascular density associated with overlying areas of ellipsoid zone and RPE atrophy.[1]

OCT IMAGING

- OCT demonstrates EZ loss, RPE atrophy, and choriocapillaris loss, as well as the presence of both retinal and choroidal flecks (Figure 58.1 and 58.2).[1,3]
- EZ loss likely precedes the presence of RPE atrophy.[1,5]

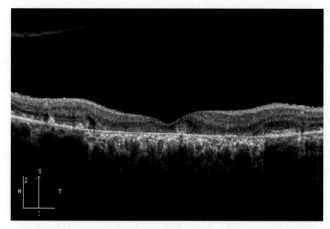

FIGURE 58.1 Optical coherence tomography in a patient with Stargardt disease displaying an abnormal foveal contour and outer retinal atrophy with marked disruption of the ellipsoid zone. Retinal pigment epithelium (RPE) atrophy is present centrally with surrounding focal areas of RPE hypertrophy.

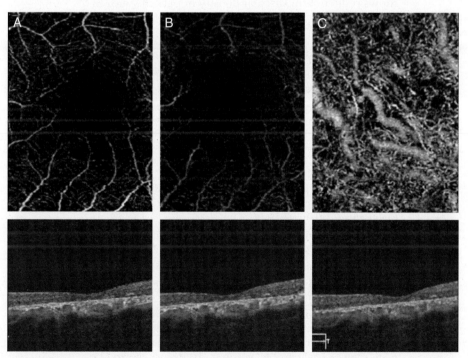

FIGURE 58.2 Optical coherence tomography angiography demonstrating reduction in the vascular density and enlargement of the foveal avascular zone in both the superficial (A) and deep capillary plexus with associated projection artifact (B). Choriocapillaris atrophy is also noted with visualization of the remaining larger choroidal vessels (C).

- RPE hypertrophy areas may be seen between the RPE atrophy areas in the OCT images (Figure 58.1).
- EZ loss has been correlated with visual acuity decline in SD patients.[2]
- In terms of choroidal changes, loss of the Sattler and Haller layers is associated with worsening visual outcomes, severity of retinal architectural decline, and disease progression.[3]
- Retinal flecks can span from the outer nuclear layer to the RPE/Bruch membrane complex.[6]
- Choroidal flecks have been associated with SD and found to correlate with declining visual function and retinal atrophy.[7]

OCTA IMAGING

- OCTA imaging is instrumental in documenting the decreased vascular presence in SD.
- Both the vascular complexes of the retina and the choriocapillaris show loss in SD.[1,4]
- In terms of retinal vasculature, analysis of both the SCP and DCP shows reduction in vascular density in patients with SD.[4]
- When analyzing choroidal changes, both the EZ and RPE loss are associated with declining choriocapillaris vascular density, alone or in combination with each other when compared to normal controls.[1,3,8]
- Furthermore, focal choriocapillaris defects have also been linked to overlying, corresponding pisciform flecks.[4]
- Declining choriocapillaris vascular density has been correlated with visual decline.[9]

References

1. Alabduljalil T, Patel RC, Alqahtani AA, et al. Correlation of outer retinal degeneration and choriocapillaris loss in stargardt disease using en face optical coherence tomography and optical coherence tomography angiography. *Am J Ophthalmol*. 2019;202:79-90.
2. Arepalli S, Traboulsi EI, Ehlers JP. Ellipsoid zone mapping and outer retinal assesment in stargardt disease. *Retina*. 2018;38(7):1427-1431.
3. Arrigo A, Grazioli A, Romano F, et al. Choroidal patterns in stargardt disease: correlations with visual acuity and disease progression. *J Clin Med*. 2019;8(9):1388.
4. Battaglia Parodi M, Cicinelli MV, Rabiolo A, Pierro L, Bolognesi G, Bandello F. Vascular abnormalities in patients with Stargardt disease assessed with optical coherence tomography angiography. *Br J Ophthalmol*. 2017;101(6):780-785.
5. Sodi A, Mucciolo DP, Cipollini F, et al. En face OCT in Stargardt disease. *Graefes Arch Clin Exp Ophthalmol*. 2016;254(9):1669-1679.
6. Voigt M, Querques G, Atmani K, et al. Analysis of retinal flecks in fundus flavimaculatus using high-definition spectral-domain optical coherence tomography. *Am J Ophthalmol*. 2010;150(3):330-337.

7. Piri N, Nesmith BL, Schaal S. Choroidal hyperreflective foci in Stargardt disease shown by spectral-domain optical coherence tomography imaging: correlation with disease severity. *JAMA Ophthalmol.* 2015;133(4):398-405.

8. Pellegrini M, Acquistapace A, Oldani M, et al. Dark atrophy: an optical coherence tomography angiography study. *Ophthalmology.* 2016;123(9):1879-1886.

9. Ratra D, Tan R, Jaishankar D, et al. Choroidal structural changes and vascularity index in stargardt disease on swept source optical coherence tomography. *Retina.* 2018;38(12):2395-2400.

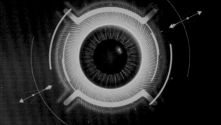

CHAPTER **59**

Sorsby Fundus Dystrophy

SALIENT FEATURES

- Sorsby fundus dystrophy (SFD) is an autosomal-dominant, fully pene-trant, fundus dystrophy caused by mutations in the tissue inhibitor of metalloproteinase-3 (TIMP3) gene.
- Sudden and progressive bilateral central vision loss begins in the fourth or fifth decade of life.
- Multiple yellowish drusenlike deposits are a hallmark of SFD.
- Progression to geographic atrophy and fibrotic lesions occurs over the course of the disease (Figure 59.1).
- Choroidal neovascularization may be present in the late stages of disease.

OCT IMAGING

- Optical coherence tomography (OCT) reveals drusenoid pigment epithelial detachments, reticular pseudodrusen, peripheral psuedod-rusen, and soft drusen.
- Central and peripheral chorioretinal atrophy are observed on OCT in late stages of the disease (Figure 59.2).
- OCT can be used to detect pockets of subretinal and intraretinal fluid secondary to exudative choroidal neovascularization (Figure 59.3), which may progress to areas of fibrosis and disciform scarring.

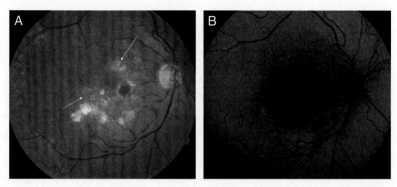

FIGURE 59.1 Color fundus and fundus autofluorescence (FAF) imaging of patient with Sorsby fundus dystrophy (SFD). A, Fundus photography shows fine, yellowish flecks around the macula (arrows). B, Generalized macular hypoautofluorescence signifying retinal pigment epithelium dysfunction is visible on FAF.

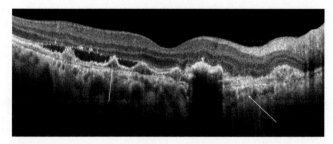

FIGURE 59.2 Optical coherence tomography (OCT) of a patient with Sorsby fundus dystrophy (SFD) highlighting common features of the disease including drusenoid pigment epithelial detachments (yellow arrow), intraretinal hyperreflective foci, and chorioretinal atrophy (white arrow).

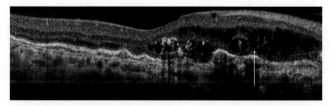

FIGURE 59.3 Optical coherence tomography (OCT) image from a patient with Sorsby fundus dystrophy (SFD) demonstrates broad-based, shallow fibrovascular pigment epithelium detachment, intraretinal fluid, and hyperreflective foci secondary to active choroidal neovascularization.

OCTA IMAGING

- OCT angiography can detect choroidal neovascularization and monitor response to treatment in SFD patients.

References

1. Gliem M, Muller PL, Mangold E, et al. Sorsby fundus dystrophy: novel mutations, novel phenotypic characteristics, and treatment outcomes. *Invest Ophthalmol Vis Sci.* 2015;56(4):2664-2676.

2. Gliem M, Muller PL, Mangold E, et al. Reticular pseudodrusen in sorsby fundus dystrophy. *Ophthalmology.* 2015;122(8):1555-1562.

3. Mohla A, Khan K, Kasilian M, Michaelides M. OCT angiography in the management of choroidal neovascular membrane secondary to Sorsby fundus dystrophy. *BMJ Case Rep.* 2016;2016:bcr2016216453.

4. Sivaprasad S, Webster AR, Egan CA, Bird AC, Tufail A. Clinical course and treatment outcomes of Sorsby fundus dystrophy. *Am J Ophthalmol.* 2008;146(2):228-234.

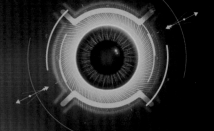

CHAPTER 60

North Carolina Macular Dystrophy

SALIENT FEATURES

- North Carolina macular dystrophy (NCMD) is an autosomal-dominant developmental abnormality of the macula caused by overexpression of PRDM13, a retinal transcription factor.
- NCMD demonstrates complete penetrance with congenital or infantile onset, and patients exhibit bilateral visual loss and symmetrical macular abnormalities.
- NCMD is generally nonprogressive with phenotypic variability categorized into grades instead of stages.
  - Grade 1 is characterized by good visual acuity and yellow drusenlike lesions in the macula.
  - Grade 2 is characterized by good to moderate visual acuity with confluent bilateral macular yellow specks, retinal pigment epithelial (RPE) atrophy, and a disciform scar.
  - Grade 3 is characterized by moderate to poor visual acuity with severe central chorioretinal atrophy, referred to as a macular caldera (Figure 60.1).

OCT IMAGING

- Optical coherence tomography (OCT) characteristics are respective to the NCMD grade.[1]
  - Grade 1—The retinal layers are mostly intact with mild hyperreflective deposits noted at the level of the RPE.

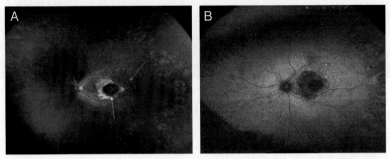

FIGURE 60.1 Ultra-wide-field (UWF) color fundus and fundus autofluoresence (FAF) imaging of patient with grade-3 North Carolina macular dystrophy (NCMD). A, Color imaging reveals an excavated coloboma-like lesion on fundus photography (white arrow) with yellow specks around the macula (green arrow). B, FAF demonstrates central hypoautofluorescence.

- Grade 2—OCT across the macular lesion demonstrates intact inner retinal layers and outer retinal/RPE atrophy.
- Grade 3—Within the caldera, OCT shows complete atrophy of the retina and choroid with hyporeflective cystic spaces (Figure 60.2). The caldera may be surrounded by subretinal fibrosis.

OCTA IMAGING

- Retinal vasculature on optical coherence tomography angiography (OCTA) is relatively intact regardless of NCMD grade.[2]

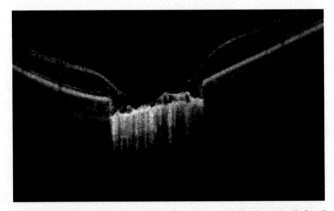

FIGURE 60.2 Optical coherence tomography (OCT) of a patient with grade-3 North Carolina macular dystrophy (NCMD). An excavated atrophic chorioretinal lesion known as a caldera is observed. There is well-circumscribed full-thickness disruption of the central retina with loss of the retinal pigment epithelium (RPE) and choroid. The location of normal-appearing retinal layers is considered the caldera edge.

References

1. Khurana RN, Sun X, Pearson E, et al. A reappraisal of the clinical spectrum of North Carolina macular dystrophy. *Ophthalmology*. 2009;116(10):1976-1983.

2. Small KW, Tran EM, Small L, Rao RC, Shaya F. Multimodal imaging and functional testing in a North Carolina macular disease family: toxoplasmosis, fovea plana, and Torpedo maculopathy are phenocopies. *Ophthalmol Retina*. 2019;3(7):607-614.

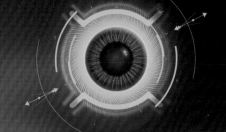

CHAPTER 61

Best Disease

SALIENT FEATURES

- Best disease is an autosomal-dominant macular dystrophy with variable phenotypic expression associated with the BEST1 gene.
- It is the second most common macular dystrophy, affecting approximately 1 in 10,000.[1]
- Best disease typically presents in childhood to early adulthood with good prognosis.
- Visual acuity is minimally affected in early stages; as the disease slowly progresses, patients may have declining visual acuity, a central scotoma, or metamorphopsia.
- The classic appearance of Best disease is a bilateral, single yellow "egg-yolk" deposit at the macula, but up to 30% of patients can present with multiple lesions (multifocal Best).[1]
- Best disease has six clinical stages based on the phenotype of the vitelliform lesions (Figure 61.1A-E and Figure 61.2)
  - Stage 1: Previtelliform with normal or subtle retinal pigment epithelium (RPE) changes
  - Stage 2: Vitelliform with classic "egg-yolk" lesion
  - Stage 3: Pseudohypopyon with disruption of vitelliform lesion due to layering of lipofuscin
  - Stage 4: Vitelleruptive with "scrambled egg" appearance with further disruption of vitelliform lesion and irregular distribution
  - Stage 5: Atrophic with central RPE and retinal atrophy
  - Stage 6: Lesion with choroidal neovascularization (Figure 61.2)

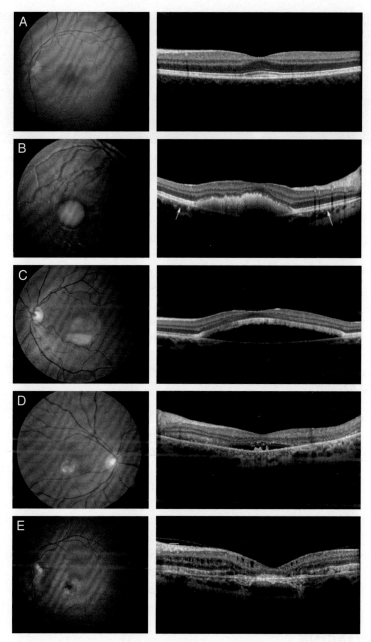

FIGURE 61.1 Fundus photography and optical coherence tomography (OCT) of Best disease throughout stages: A, Previtelliform lesion with subtle RPE change. B, Vitelliform lesion affecting outer retinal integrity with overlying ellipsoid zone loss. Peripheral to the lesion, the ellipsoid zone remains intact with possible increased prominence of the interdigitation zone (arrows). C, Pseudohypopyon lesion with lesion liquefaction. D, Vitelleruptive lesion with further liquefication and outer retinal layer deterioration. E, Atrophic lesion with complete loss of the outer retina, fibrotic changes, and intraretinal cysts. (Reprinted with permission from Qian CX, Charran D, Strong CR, Steffens TJ, Jayasundera T, Heckenlively JR. Optical coherence tomography examination of the retinal pigment epithelium in Best vitelliform macular dystrophy. *Ophthalmology.* 2017;124(4):456-463.)

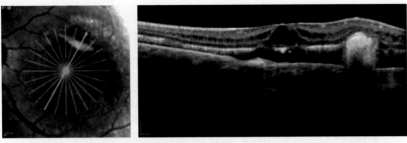

FIGURE 61.2 Late-stage Best disease with resulting choroidal neovascularization causing intraretinal and subretinal fluid. (Reprinted with permission from Fineman M, Ho A. *Retina*. 3rd ed. Philadelphia, PA: Wolters Kluwer; 2018.)

- Electrooculography (EOG) shows Arden ratio of <1.5. Electroretinography (ERG) is normal. Diagnosis is most reliably confirmed with genetic testing.[2]
- FA shows hypofluorescence of early vitelliform lesions, progressing to mixed hyper- and hypofluorescence, and finally hyperfluorescence of the atrophic stage.
- Hyperautofluorescence (FAF) shows hyperautofluorescence of early vitelliform lesions and hypoautofluorescence when lesions become fibrotic or atrophic.

OCT IMAGING

- Optical coherence tomography (OCT) can be used to localize the vitelliform lesion to the subretinal space, evaluate features of the vitelliform lesion, and evaluate for associated subretinal fluid.
- Classic vitelliform lesions appear homogenous and hyperreflective; over time, some of the material is replaced by fluid which is hyporeflective[3] (Figure 61.1).
- In advanced disease, a fibrotic pillar from the sub-RPE space can be visualized elevating the retina like a "circus tent"[1] (Figure 61.1).
- Subretinal vitelliform material accumulation leads to a clear separation of the outer retinal layers[4] (Figure 61.1).
- OCT may also be utilized to evaluate for associated choroidal neovascularization (CNV).

OCTA IMAGING

- Optical coherence tomography angiography (OCTA) shows foveal avascular zone (FAZ) abnormalities and patchy loss of vascularity in the superficial and deep retinal layers.[5,6]
- OCTA may be particularly helpful for identifying CNV[5] (Figure 61.3).

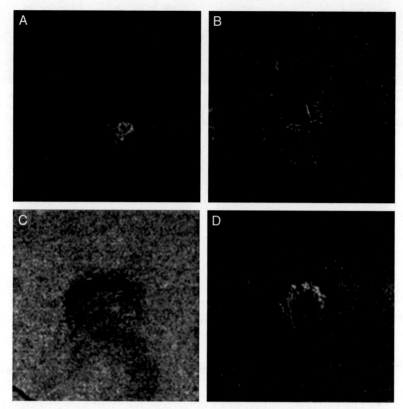

FIGURE 61.3 Optical coherence tomography (OCT) angiography for choroidal neovascularization patterns in Best disease (A) dense net, (B) loose net, (C) unidentifiable, and (D) ring shaped. (Reprinted with permission from Guduru A, Gupta A, Tyagi M, et al. Optical coherence tomography angiography characterisation of Best disease and associated choroidal neovascularization. *Br J Ophthalmol.* 2018;102:444-447.)

References

1. Schachat AP, Wilisoson CP, Hinton DR, Sadda SR, Wiedemann P. *Ryan's Retina.* 6th ed. Amsterdam, Netherlands: Elsevier; 2018.
2. MacDonald IM, Lee T. Best vitelliform macular dystrophy. In: Adam MP, Ardinger HH, Pagon RA, et al, eds. *GeneReviews® [Internet].* Seattle, WA: University of Washington; 2003;1993-2019. [Updated 2013 Dec 12].
3. Denniston A, Murray P, eds. *Oxford Handbook of Ophthalmology.* Oxford: Oxford University Press; 2014
4. Qian CX, Charran D, Strong CR, Steffens TJ, Jayasundera T, Heckenlively JR. Optical coherence tomography examination of the retinal pigment epithelium in Best vitelliform macular dystrophy. *Ophthalmology.* 2017;124(4):456-463.
5. Guduru A, Gupta A, Tyagi M, et al. Optical coherence tomography angiography characterisation of Best disease and associated choroidal neovascularization. *Br J Ophthalmol.* 2018;102:444-447.
6. Wang XN, You QS, Li Q, et al. Findings of optical coherence tomography angiography in Best vitelliform macular dystrophy. *Ophthalmic Res.* 2018;60(4):214-220.

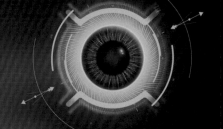

CHAPTER 62

Cone Dystrophy

SALIENT FEATURES

- Cone dystrophy defines a heterogeneous group of heritable retinal dystrophies with a broad presenting phenotype that can impair swift diagnosis.
- These disorders are characterized by isolated degeneration of the cone photoreceptors.
- The two major subtypes are congenital stationary cone dystrophy and the progressive variant.
- Several gene mutations in different inheritance patterns can cause cone dystrophy including *CNGB3* (autosomal recessive), *OPN1LW* (X-linked), and *GUCA1A* (autosomal dominant).
- A bulls-eye pattern of retinal pigment epithelium (RPE) atrophy is a common but nonspecific feature of cone dystrophies.

OCT IMAGING

- Early stages demonstrate minimal to no macular changes.
- The hallmark findings are focal loss of the outer nuclear layer, the ellipsoid zone, and the retinal pigment epithelium (Figure 62.1).
- Notably the central macula is usually affected with sparing of the peripheral macula and remainder of the retina. More severe disease is characterized by macular atrophy (Figure 62.2).
- In progressive cone dystrophy, the fovea thins before the macula eventually becomes atrophic.
- Visual acuity is associated with ellipsoid zone integrity.

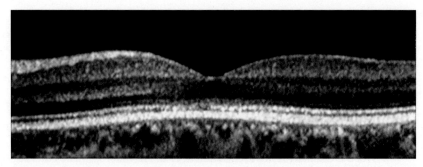

FIGURE 62.1 Optical coherence tomography (OCT) B-scan through the fovea demonstrates central ellipsoid zone and ELM signal attenuation with thinning of the outer nuclear layer.

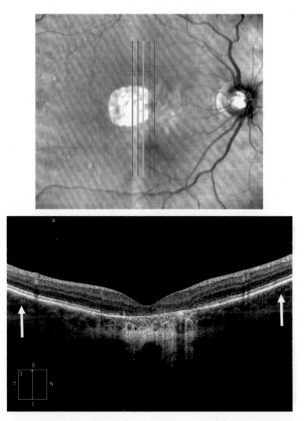

FIGURE 62.2 *En-face* near-infrared and optical coherence tomography showing complete outer retinal loss localized to the foveal region of the macula sparing the peripheral macula and remainder of the retina (arrows).

References

1. Gill JS, Georgiou M, Kalitzeos A, Moore AT, Michaelides M. Progressive cone and cone-rod dystrophies: clinical features, molecular genetics and prospects for therapy. *Br J Ophthalmol.* 2019;103(5):711-720.

2. Zahlava J, Lestak J, Karel I. Optical coherence tomography in progressive cone dystrophy. *Biomed Pap Med Fac Palacky Univ Olomouc.* 2014;158(4).

3. Cho SC, Woo SJ, Park KH, Hwang JM. Morphologic characteristics of the outer retina in cone dystrophy on spectral-domain optical coherence tomography. *Korean J Ophthalmol.* 2013;27(1):19-27.

4. Hood DC, Zhang X, Ramachandran R, et al. The inner segment/outer segment border seen on optical coherence tomography is less intense in patients with diminished cone function. *Invest Ophthalmol Vis Sci.* 2011;52(13):9703-9709.

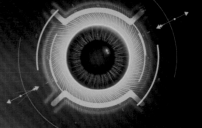

CHAPTER 63

Adult Vitelliform Dystropy

SALIENT FEATURES

- Pattern dystrophies are a group of autosomal-dominant retinal disorders characterized by pigment deposition in the macula.
- Adult vitelliform dystrophy (also known as adult-onset foveomacular vitelliform dystrophy [AOFVD]) is the most common pattern dystrophy and is characterized by bilateral, symmetric yellow or grayish round lesions in the macular area.
- Adult vitelliform dystrophy typically presents in middle age with mild metamorphopsia or reduced central vision.
- Progression is typically slow.
- Vision loss is typically mild-moderate.
- Choroidal neovascularization (CNV) is a rare complication.[1]
- Fluorescein angiography demonstrates hypofluorescence at the vitelliform lesion with a ring of hyperfluorescence.
- Fundus autofluorescence reveals significant hyperautofluorescence of the vitelliform material.[2]
- Electro-oculogram (EOG) is normal; however, multifocal electro-retinogram(ERG) may be reduced.

OCT IMAGING

- OCT in the early stage demonstrates a well-defined, hyperreflective central subretinal thickening in the vitelliform stage that progresses to hyporeflective areas in the pseudohypopyon or vitelliruptive stages (Figures 63.1 and 63.2).[3]
- The vitelliform stage may appear to be simultaneously continuous with the RPE and the ellipsoid zone.
- OCT may also show subretinal fluid which may be related to alterations in the vitelliform stage. It is important to distinguish exudative subretinal fluid related to an associated CNV compared to degenerative fluid related to the vitelliform process.[3]

OCTA IMAGING

- Optical coherence tomography angiography (OCTA) demonstrates vascular rarefaction with fewer blood vessels at the superficial and deep capillary plexuses, and the choriocapillaris layer, likely secondary to anatomic distortion (Figure 63.3).[2]
- OCTA also serves as an important modality for identifying CNV (Figure 63.4).[5,6]

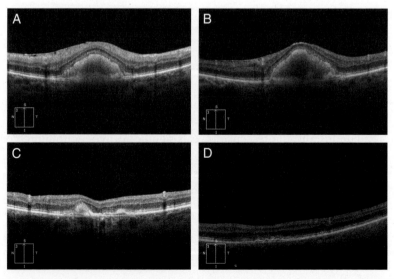

FIGURE 63.1 Optical coherence tomography (OCT) demonstrating longitudinal macular changes in adult vitelliform macular dystrophy. Significant hyperreflective central subretinal material is followed by progressive atrophy over the course of 4 years, from (A) to (D).

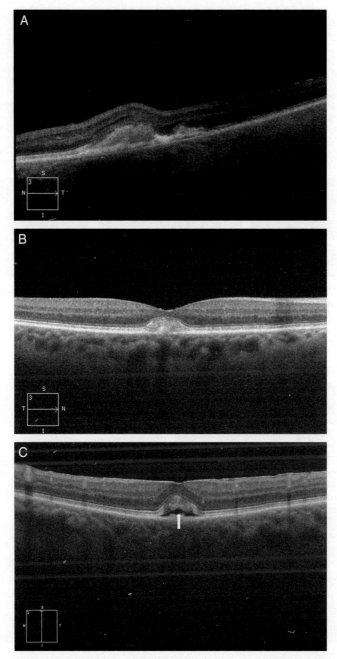

FIGURE 63.2 Optical coherence tomography (OCT) findings in vitelliform macular dystrophy. A, Multilobular vitelliform material with central collapse and overlying retinal atrophy. B, Central hyperreflective vitelliform lesion with overlying ellipsoid zone attenuation. C, Mixed reflectivity of the central vitelliform lesion, consistent with the pseudohypopyon stage. Hyporeflective subretinal fluid is noted secondary to the vitelliform lesion evolution (arrow). No evidence of choroidal neovascularization (CNV) was noted.

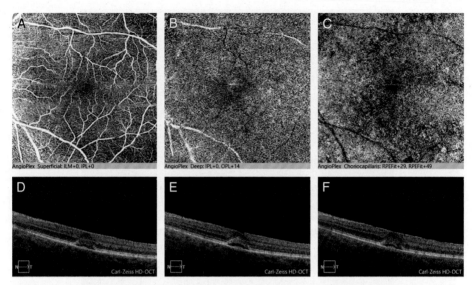

FIGURE 63.3 Optical coherence tomography angiography (OCTA) in vitelliform macular dystrophy. A-C, A 3 × 3 mm macular cube OCTA with *en-face* projection capturing the superficial, deep, and choriocapillaris layers of the left eye from a patient with adult vitelliform pattern dystrophy with associated subretinal fluid. D-F, B-scans with decorrelation overlay centered on the fovea show the segmentation of the superficial, deep, and choriocapillaris layers. No evidence of choroidal neovascularization (CNV) is identified.

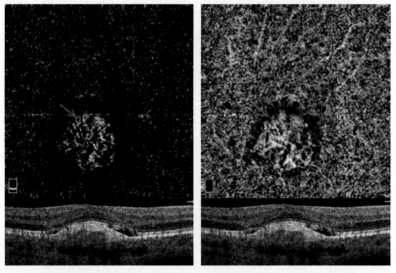

FIGURE 63.4 Optical coherence tomography angiography (OCTA) in vitelliform macular dystrophy with associated choroidal neovascularization (CNV). (Top row) OCTA with *en-face* visualization of well-defined CNV (red arrows) within the vitelliform lesion. (Bottom row) B-scans centered on the fovea demonstrate decorrelation overlay with signal within the vitelliform lesion and associated subretinal fluid. (Reprinted with permission from Joshi KM, Nesper PL, Fawzi AA, Mirza RG. Optical coherence tomography angiography in adult-onset foveomacular vitelliform dystrophy. *Retina.* 2018;38(3):600-605.)

References

1. Da Pozzo S, Parodi MB, Toto L, et al. Occult choroidal neovascularization in adult-onset foveomacular vitelliform dystrophy. *Ophthalmologica*. 2001;215:412-414.

2. Querques G, Zambrowski O, Corvi F, et al. Optical coherence tomography angiography in adult-onset foveomacular vitelliform dystrophy. *Br J Ophthalmol*. 2016;100:1724-1730.

3. Pierro L, Tremolada G, Introini U, Calori G, Brancato R. Optical coherence tomography findings in adult-onset foveomacular vitelliform dystrophy. *Am J Ophthalmol*. 2002;134(5):675-680.

4. Treder M, Lauermann JL, Alnawaiseh M, Heiduschka P, Eter N. Quantitative changes in flow density in patients with adult-onset foveomacular vitelliform dystrophy: an OCT angiography study. *Graefes Arch Clin Exp Ophthalmol*. 2018;256(1):23-28.

5. Joshi KM, Nesper PL, Fawzi AA, Mirza RG. Optical coherence tomography angiography in adult-onset foveomacular vitelliform dystrophy. *Retina*. 2018;38(3):600-605.

6. Lupidi M, Coscas G, Cagini C, Coscas F. Optical coherence tomography angiography of choroidal neovascularization in adult onset foveomacular vitelliform dystrophy: pearls and pitfalls. *Invest Ophthalmol Vis Sci*. 2015;56:7638-7645.

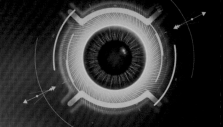

CHAPTER 64

Achromatopsia

SALIENT FEATURES

- Achromatopsia is an autosomal-recessive cone-photoreceptor disorder with an estimated prevalence of 1 in 300,000.[1]
- It is characterized by abnormal color discrimination, poor visual acuity, photophobia, central scotoma with eccentric fixation, and nystagmus. These clinical findings are present at birth.[2]
- Achromatopsia and blue cone monochromatism are difficult to distinguish clinically without ERG. Optical coherence tomography (OCT) has detected subtle morphological differences between these two cone diseases.[2]
- Causative mutations in CNGA3, CNGB3, GNAT2, and PDE6C genes are involved in the cone photoreceptor dysfunction. These are gene-encoding proteins involved in the retinal phototransduction pathway.[3]
- Full-field electroretinography (ff-ERG) reveals significantly reduced cone response with normal rod response (Figure 64.1).[1]
- Fundus autofluorescence (FAF) imaging typically reveals areas of reduced autofluorescence in the fovea (Figure 64.2).[2]

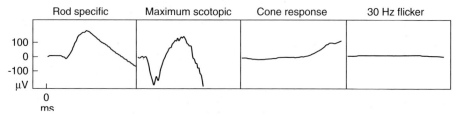

FIGURE 64.1 Full-field electroretinogram (ff-ERG) in achromatopsia demonstrates attenuated cone response with normal rod function.

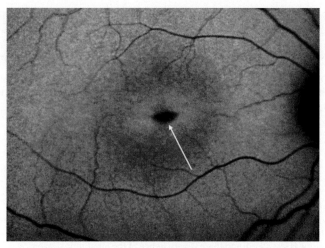

FIGURE 64.2 Fundus autofluorescence imaging of an achromatopsia patient highlights central hypoaut-ofluorescence (arrow) signifying central retinal pigment epithelium (RPE) disruption.

OCT IMAGING

- Focal disruption or complete loss of the ellipsoid zone (EZ) with a remaining hyporeflective space is a hallmark of achromatopsia on OCT (Figures 64.3 and 64.4).[1]
- Late stages of achromatopsia typically demonstrate retinal pigment epithelium (RPE) layer disruption.[1]
- Foveal hypoplasia, evident as a poorly defined foveal contour and persistence of inner retinal layers, is occasionally observed (Figure 64.5).[1]
- The distinct foveal reflectiveness patterns and normal macular thickness on OCT differentiates achromatopsia from blue cone monochromatism, which typically demonstrates less prominent EZ disruption and overt macular thinning.

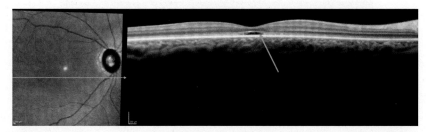

FIGURE 64.3 Optical coherence tomography (OCT) scan through the fovea demonstrates ellipsoid zone (EZ) disruption with a hyporeflective space remaining in its place (green arrow).

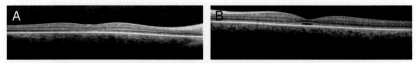

FIGURE 64.4 Optical coherence tomography (OCT) images of an achromatopsia patient 6 years apart. A, In 2012, intermittent attenuation of the ellipsoid zone (EZ) is present. B, By 2018, focal loss of the EZ is evident with a hyporeflective space.

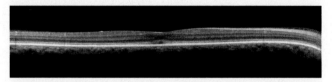

FIGURE 64.5 Optical coherence tomography (OCT) image showing partial loss of the foveal dip (fovea plana or foveal hypoplasia) in a patient with achromatopsia. There is also attenuation of the ellipsoid zone (EZ). The foveal slope is less steep, and there is persistence of the inner retinal layers.

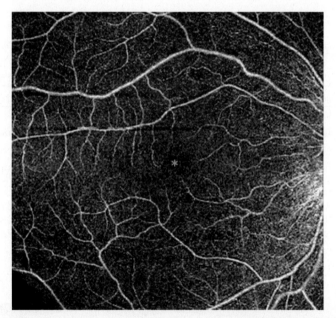

FIGURE 64.6 Optical coherence tomography angiography (OCTA) demonstrating a small foveal avascular zone consistent with foveal hypoplasia (green asterisk) in a patient with achromatopsia.

OCTA IMAGING

- Nystagmus and poor fixation make image acquisition difficult.
- Decreased size of the foveal avascular zone can be visualized on optical coherence tomography angiography (OCTA) (Figure 64.6).

References

1. Greenberg JP, Sherman J, Zweifel SA, et al. Spectral-domain optical coherence tomography staging and autofluorescence imaging in achromatopsia. *JAMA Ophthal.* 2014;132(4):437-445.

2. Barthelmes D, Sutter FK, Kurz-Levin MM, et al. Quantitative analysis of OCT characteristics in patients with achromatopsia and blue-cone monochromatism. *Invest Ophthalmol Vis Sci.* 2006;47(3):1161-1166.

3. Khan NW, Wissinger B, Kohl S, Sieving PA. CNGB3 achromatopsia with progressive loss of residual cone function and impaired rod-mediated function. *Invest Ophthalmol Vis Sci.* 2007;48(8):3864-3871.

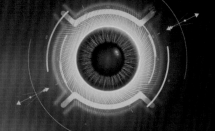

CHAPTER 65

Oculocutaneous and Ocular Albinism

SALIENT FEATURES

- Oculocutaneous albinism (OCA) is an autosomal-recessive condition of reduced melanin synthesis visibly involving the eyes, skin, and hair.[1]
- Cases of ocular involvement without associated changes in skin and hair, termed ocular albinism (OA), are typically X-linked.[2]
- In OA, there is a reduction in the total number of melanosomes although each melanosome has a normal level of melanin.[3]
- Classic retinal findings include hypopigmented fundi and foveal hypoplasia. Foveal hypoplasia is thought to be related to arrested foveal development resulting in the absence or reduction of the foveal avascular zone and subsequent impaired development of the foveal pit.[4]
- OA is also associated with an increased number of chiasmal decussations of nerve fibers from the temporal retina.[5]

OCT IMAGING

- While there are variable presentations, patients with OCA or OA often display fovea plana (Figure 65.1).
- In fovea plana, there is an absence of a central foveal depression and preservation of the retinal nerve fiber layer, inner plexiform layer, and inner nuclear layers.
- Outer retinal abnormalities such as thinning of the outer nuclear layer and lack of central thickening of the ellipsoid zone (EZ) are also seen in fovea plana.

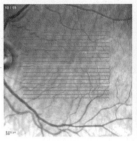 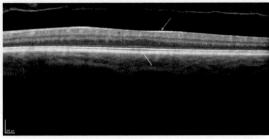

FIGURE 65.1 Spectral-domain optical coherence tomography (SD-OCT) image of a patient with oculocutaneous albinism demonstrates foveal plana with absence of a foveal pit. The hyperreflectivity along the surface of the retina (blue arrow) is consistent with aberrant preservation of the nerve fiber layer. There is also persistence of the inner retinal layers (red asterisk). There is also absence of elevation of the ellipsoid zone (EZ) at the fovea (yellow arrow) which is seen in normal patients. There is increased reflectivity of choroidal anatomy in a patient with oculocutaneous albinism (OCA), perhaps secondary to decreased signal attenuation from altered pigmentation of the retinal pigment epithelium.

- Other findings of OCA or OA on OCT include increased choroid reflectivity likely secondary to decreased OCT signal attenuation from a melanin-poor retinal pigment epithelium (Figure 65.1).

OCTA IMAGING

- There is paucity of optical coherence tomography angiography (OCTA) imaging in OCA and OA due to inability of patients to fixate due to nystagmus.
- As there is often foveal hypoplasia in patients with OCA and OA, OCTA may demonstrate a reduced or absent foveal avascular zone (FAZ).[6]

References

1. Harvey PS, King RA, Summers CG. Spectrum of foveal development in albinism detected with optical coherence tomography. *J Am Assoc Pediatr Ophthalmol Strabismus*. 2006;10(3):237-242.

2. Shen B, Samaraweera P, Rosenberg B, Orlow SJ. Ocular albinism type 1: more than meets the eye. *Pigment Cell Res*. 2001;14(4):243-248.

3. Cortese K, Giordano F, Surace EM, et al. The ocular albinism type 1 (OA1) gene controls melanosome maturation and size. *Invest Ophthalmol Vis Sci*. 2005;46(12):4358-4364.

4. Wilk MA, McAllister JT, Cooper RF, et al. Relationship between foveal cone specialization and pit morphology in albinism. *Invest Ophthalmol Vis Sci*. 2014;55(7):4186-4198.

5. Ather S, Proudlock FA, Welton T, et al. Aberrant visual pathway development in albinism: from retina to cortex. *Hum Brain Mapp*. 2019;40(3):777-788.

6. Pakzad-Vaezi K, Keane PA, Cardoso JN, Egan C, Tufail A. Optical coherence tomography angiography of foveal hypoplasia. *Br J Ophthalmol*. 2017;101(7):985-988. doi:10.1136/bjophthalmol-2016-309200.

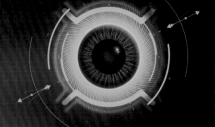

CHAPTER 66

X-Linked Retinoschisis

SALIENT FEATURES

- X-linked retinoschisis (XLRS) is an early-onset retinal dystrophy secondary to mutations in the RS1 gene that encodes the retinoschisin protein.
- XLRS is clinically characterized by a spoke-wheel pattern of schisis in the macula, with peripheral retinoschisis commonly observed as well (Figure 66.1).
- Symptoms include amblyopia, nystagmus, strabismus, and vision loss.

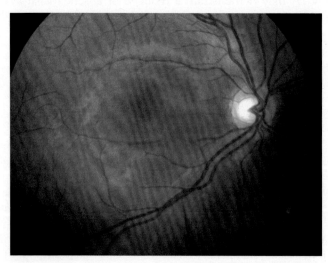

FIGURE 66.1 Color fundus photograph of eye with genetically confirmed X-linked retinoschisis (XLRS). Note the characteristic spoke-wheel pattern of schisis in the macula.

- There is currently no treatment indicated for the foveal and peripheral retinal splitting in XLRS, although secondary complications such as development of a retinal detachment or vitreous hemorrhage may require treatment.
- Gene therapy is currently being evaluated as a potential future therapy.

OCT IMAGING

- Optical coherence tomography (OCT) is the gold standard for visualizing the macular alterations in XLRS.
- Foveomacular splitting is most frequently observed in the inner nuclear layer (INL), outer plexiform layer (OPL), and outer nuclear layer (ONL).
- Schisis is often most prominent in the INL, with the largest spaces occurring in the central macula and sometimes extending out beyond the major temporal arcades. These spaces can extend into the underlying OPL (Figure 66.2).
- Schisis is variably present in the ONL.
- Small, slitlike spaces are sometimes seen perifoveally in the ganglion cell layer (GCL) (Figure 66.2).
- In some cases, in advanced stage, the traditional schisis appearance disappears and retinal atrophy is observed.

OCTA IMAGING

- Literature on vascular abnormalities in XLRS patients is limited.
- Microvascular changes in the superficial capillary plexus (SCP) and flow loss in the deep capillary plexus (DCP) in eyes with XLRS have been described (Figure 66.3). Microvascular changes usually present as abnormal protrusions of the microvascular walls and/or tortuosity of the vessels.

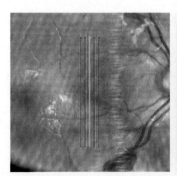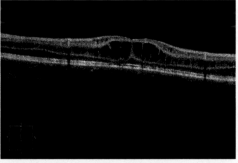

FIGURE 66.2 Optical coherence tomography (OCT) in X-linked retinoschisis (XLRS). B-scan OCT of eye from Figure 66.1 demonstrating schisis predominantly in the inner nuclear layer (INL) and minimally in the outer nuclear layer (ONL) nasally. Several small cysts can also be observed in the ganglion cell layer (GCL).

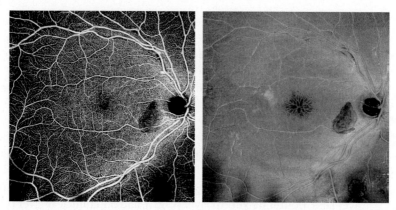

FIGURE 66.3 A, Superficial optical coherence tomography angiography (OCTA) of the same eye from Figure 66.1. B, Structural image reveals the characteristic spoke-wheel pattern in the macula.

References

1. Han IC, Whitmore SS, Critser DB, et al. Wide-field swept-source OCT and angiography in X-linked retinoschisis. *Ophthalmol Retina*. 2018;3(2):178-185.
2. Gregori NZ, Lam BL, Gregori G, et al. Wide-field spectral-domain optical coherence tomography in patients and carriers of X-linked retinoschisis. *Ophthalmology*. 2013;120(1):169-174.
3. Sikkink SK, Biswas S, Parry NR, Stanga PE, Trump D. X-linked retinoschisis: an update. *J Med Genet*. 2007;44(4):225-232.
4. Stringa F, Tsamis E, Papayannis A, et al. Segmented swept source optical coherence tomography angiography assessment of the perifoveal vasculature in patients with X-linked juvenile retinoschisis: a serial case report. *Int Med Case Rep J*. 2017;10:329-335. doi:10.2147/IMCRJ.S136310.
5. Yu J, Ni Y, Keane PA, Jiang C, Wang W, Xu G. Foveomacular schisis in juvenile X-linked retinoschisis: an optical coherence tomography study. *Am J Ophthalmol*. 2010;149(6):973-978.e2.

Part 7

Retinal, Choroidal, and Scleral Lesions

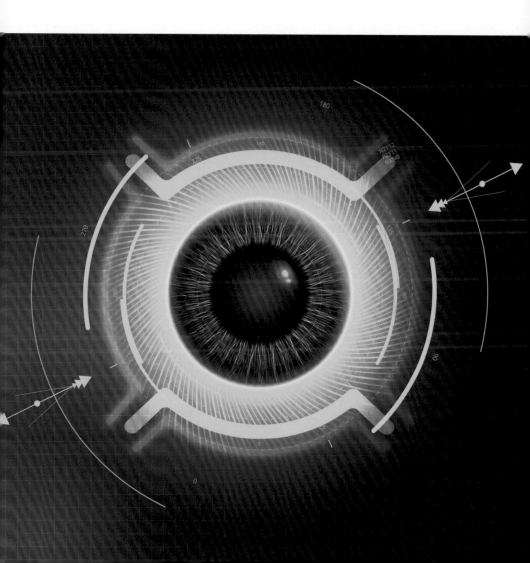

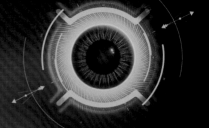

CHAPTER 67

Choroidal Nevus

SALIENT FEATURES

- Histologically, a choroidal nevus is composed entirely of spindle A cells that occupy the choroid space but spare the choriocapillaris.[1]
- Defined by the Collaborative Ocular Melanoma Study (COMS) criteria, choroidal nevus is a choroidal melanocytic lesion less than 5 mm in diameter or less than 1 mm thick.[2] However, others have expanded these parameters to less than 3 mm in thickness.[3]

OCT IMAGING

- Optical coherence tomography (OCT) can facilitate the diagnosis of nevus by determining the presence of drusen (Figure 67.1C, green arrows), irregularly thickened Bruch membrane (Figure 67.1C, yellow arrows), and occasionally outer retinal atrophy/photoreceptor loss (Figure 67.4C).[3]
- OCT also aids in evaluation of subretinal fluid versus overlying schisis (Figures 67.2C and 67.3, green arrows).
- Some clinicians have used OCT to monitor choroidal nevus height to evaluate growth[4]; however, this is technically challenging given that it is difficult to measure the exact same location, even with image registration at follow-up visits.
- Melanocytic nevi tend to have high anterior choroidal tumor reflectivity (Figure 67.1C, white asterisks); however, amelanotic nevi often demonstrate only medium reflectivity.[5]

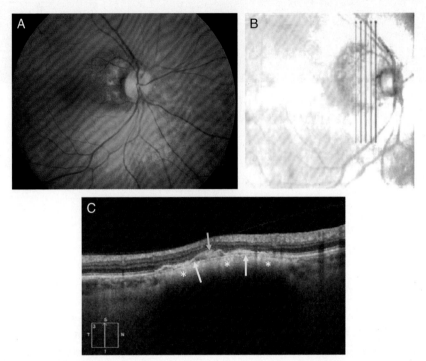

FIGURE 67.1 A, Color fundus photograph of a melanocytic circumpapillary choroidal nevus with overlying drusen of the right eye. B, Near-infrared reflectance with vertical lines through nevus. C, Optical coherence tomography (OCT) illustrating hyperreflectivity of the anterior choroidal lesion compressing the choriocapillaris (white asterisks). Irregularity in Bruch membrane (yellow arrows) with drusen deposits (green arrow) suggesting chronicity.

OCTA IMAGING

- Optical coherence tomography angiography (OCTA) has been proposed to distinguish between a benign nevus and a small malignant melanoma in the following ways:
  - The choriocapillaris flow density over a nevus has been reported to be the same as the corresponding location in the contralateral eye. Conversely, the choriocapillaris flow density over choroidal melanoma has been reduced. A limitation to this study is the lack of explanation for the criteria definition for melanoma cases.[6] It is possible that a thicker nevi may result in greater compression of the choriocapillaris compared to a flat nevus, limiting the flow.

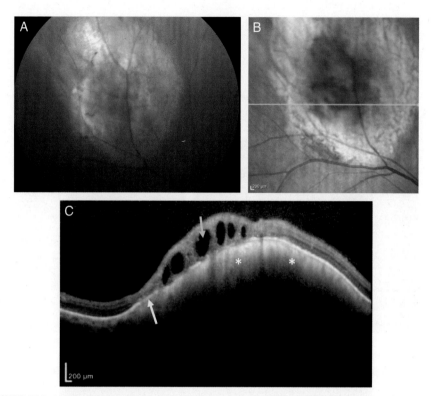

FIGURE 67.2 A, Color fundus photograph of a halo nevus. B, Near-infrared shows hyperreflective ring around nevus illustrating atrophy with horizontal line. C, Optical coherence tomography (OCT) over nevus shows outer retina atrophy (yellow arrow), schisis overlying nevus (green arrow), and hyperreflectivity (white asterisks) highlighting the anterior choroidal nevus with posterior shadowing.

- One group has suggested that increased central macular thickness and enlarged deep foveal avascular zones were associated with patients with small melanomas compared to nevi.[7]
- Nevi have been described on OCTA as hyperreflective in 82% of the cases (Figure 67.5F and G, and Figure 67.6), while 17% were either isoreflective or hyporeflective at the choriocapillaris layer. This was in contrast to choroidal melanoma which were described as isoreflective or hyporeflective in 63% of the cases.[8]

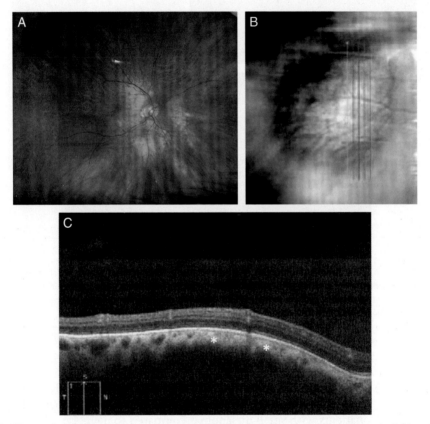

FIGURE 67.3 A, Color fundus photograph of a small flat choroidal nevus without drusen in right eye. B, Near-infrared reflectance of nevus with vertical lines. C, Mild choroidal elevation and compression with isoreflectivity and posterior shadowing of choroidal nevus without drusen, retinal atrophy, retinal pigment epithelium (RPE) abnormality, nor changes in Bruch membrane.

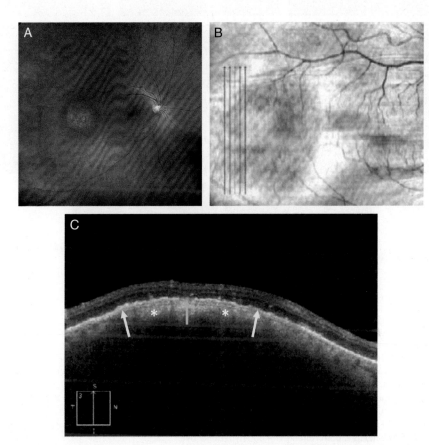

FIGURE 67.4 A, Color fundus photography of a choroidal nevus with chronic drusen in the right eye. B, Near-infrared reflectance of nevus with vertical lines. C, Choroidal elevation with isoreflectance (white asterisks), drusen and ellipsoid layer irregularity (yellow arrows) with outer retina atrophy (green arrow) indicating chronicity.

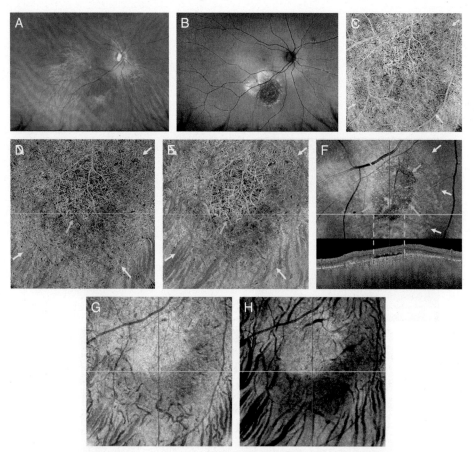

FIGURE 67.5 A, Color fundus photograph and (B) fundus autofluorescence of a choroidal nevus. C, Swept-source optical coherence tomography angiography (OCTA) 6 × 6 mm layers shows choroidal nevus (outlined by yellow arrows) with mild hyperreflectivity in center (green arrow) with minor reduction of vascular density at level of outer retina to choriocapillaris (ORCC). Similar vascular reduction (voids) seen at choriocapillaris (D) and deeper choroid (E). En-face OCTA (F) at the structural ORCC illustrates a hyperreflective lesion (nevus outlined by yellow arrows) with a central hyporeflective region (green arrows) suggestive of subretinal fluid when compared to OCTA B-scan below. However, at the choriocapillaris (G) and deeper choroid (H), the nevus is both isoreflective and hyperreflective.

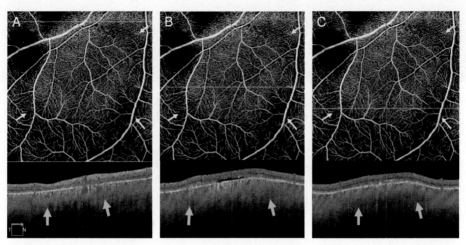

FIGURE 67.6 Swept-source optical coherence tomography angiography (OCTA) 6 × 6 mm layer with choroidal nevus. A-C, Margins of the choroidal nevus (yellow arrows). Horizontal lines correspond to the OCTA B-scan below. The decorrelation signal of the nevus indicates that the nevus maintains good choroidal vascular flow with some reduction as the nevus thickens (green arrows).

References

1. Naumann G, Yanoff M, Zimmerman LE. Histogenesis of malignant melanomas of the uvea. I: Histopathologic characteristics of nevi of the choroid and ciliary body. *Arch Ophthalmol.* 1966;76(6):784-796.

2. Factors predictive of growth and treatment of small choroidal melanoma: COMS Report No. 5. The collaborative ocular melanoma study group. *Arch Ophthalmol.* 1997;115(12):1537-1544.

3. Say EA, Shah SU, Ferenczy S, Shields CL. Optical coherence tomography of retinal and choroidal tumors. *J Ophthalmol.* 2012;2012:385058.

4. Jonna G, Daniels AB. Enhanced depth imaging OCT of ultrasonographically flat choroidal nevi demonstrates 5 distinct patterns. *Ophthalmol Retina.* 2019;3(3):270-277.

5. Torres VL, Brugnoni N, Kaiser PK, Singh AD. Optical coherence tomography enhanced depth imaging of choroidal tumors. *Am J Ophthalmol* 2011;151(4):586-593.e2.

6. Ghassemi F, Mirshahi R, Fadakar K, Sabour S. Optical coherence tomography angiography in choroidal melanoma and nevus. *Clin Ophthalmol.* 2018;12:207-214.

7. Valverde-Megias A, Say EA, Ferenczy SR, Shields CL. Differential macular features on optical coherence tomography angiography in eyes with choroidal nevus and melanoma. *Retina.* 2017;37(4):731-740.

8. Toledo JJ, Asencio M, Garcia JR, et al. OCT angiography: imaging of choroidal and retinal tumors. *Ophthalmol Retina.* 2018;2(6):613-622.

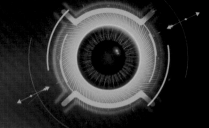

CHAPTER 68

Congenital Hypertrophy of the Retinal Pigment Epithelium

SALIENT FEATURES

- Congenital hypertrophy of the retinal pigment epithelium (CHRPE) is a unilateral, asymptomatic, hyperpigmented smooth or scalloped congenital hamartoma that can either be solitary or grouped. Color variation may be present from gray to black. Larger lesions often have inner "punched out" lacunae with hypopigmentation.
- Multiple diffuse CHRPE-like lesions are associated with Gardner and Turcot syndromes.

OCT IMAGING

- The typical findings of CHRPE on optical coherence tomography (OCT) include thinning of the overlying retina and photoreceptor loss (Figure 68.1). In one study, the neurosensory retina was measured at 68% thickness of adjacent normal retina, which likely accounts for the visual field deficit that may be associated with these lesions.
- For pigmented CHRPE, the retinal pigment epithelium (RPE) has been reported to be 52% thicker than adjacent RPE in normal tissue. However, amelanotic CHRPE have lacunae with thinner RPE allowing visualization of the choroid.[1]
- Lacunae are common within CHRPE and present on OCT as an absence of RPE, resulting in increased optical transmission.[2]

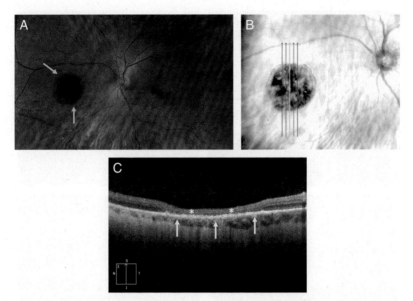

FIGURE 68.1 Congenital hypertrophy of the retinal pigment epithelium (CHRPE). A, Color fundus photograph depicts a circular CHRPE (green arrows) in a 44-year-old patient. B, Near-infrared image with vertical line through lesion. C, Hyperreflective thickening of the retinal pigment epithelium (yellow arrows) with thinning of overlying retina and photoreceptor loss (white asterisks).

OCTA IMAGING

- CHRPE presentation on optical coherence tomography angiography (OCTA) will vary from normal retinal and choroidal vascularity to disorganized plexus with vascular tortuosity (Figure 68.2).[3,4]

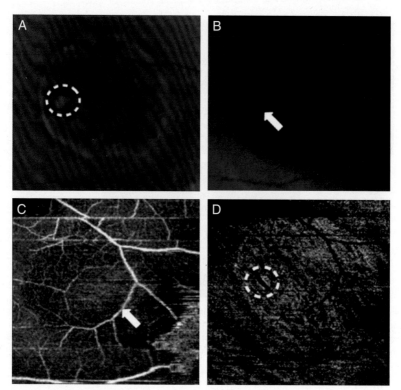

FIGURE 68.2 Optical coherence tomography angiography (OCTA) in congenital hypertrophy of the retinal pigment epithelium (CHRPE). A, Fundus image demonstrating CHRPE with lacunae (dotted circle). B, Fundus autofluorescence demonstrating hypoautofluorescence in area of CHRPE and relative hyperautofluorescence at lacunae (white arrow). C, Superficial slab from OCTA demonstrating normal retinal vasculature with inferior branching of retinal vessel over the CHRPE lesion (white arrow). Motion artifacts are present. D, OCTA with choroidal slab demonstrating projection artifact removal of retinal vessels and slight increased reflectivity adjacent to lacunae (dotted line). Minimal choroidal flow is noted. (Reprinted with permission from Shanmugam PM, Konana VK, Ramanjulu R, et al. Ocular coherence tomography angiography features of congenital hypertrophy of retinal pigment epithelium. *Indian J Ophthalmol.* 2019;67(4):563-566.)

References

1. Say EA, Shah SU, Ferenczy S, Shields CL. Optical coherence tomography of retinal and choroidal tumors. *J Ophthalmol.* 2012;2012:385058.
2. Fung AT, Pellegrini M, Shields CL. Congenital hypertrophy of the retinal pigment epithelium: enhanced-depth imaging optical coherence tomography in 18 cases. *Ophthalmology.* 2014;121(1):251-256.
3. Shanmugam PM, Konana VK, Ramanjulu R, et al. Ocular coherence tomography angiography features of congenital hypertrophy of retinal pigment epithelium. *Indian J Ophthalmol.* 2019;67(4):563-566.
4. Toledo JJ, Asencio M, Garcia JR, et al. OCT angiography: imaging of choroidal and retinal tumors. *Ophthalmol Retina.* 2018;2(6):613-622.

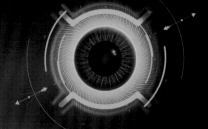

CHAPTER 69

Choroidal Melanoma

SALIENT FEATURES

- Choroidal melanoma is the most common primary choroidal tumor of the eye with an incidence of 5.2 per 1,000,000 per year in the United States.[1]
- Malignant melanoma transformation from choroidal nevus occurs at a rate of approximately 1 in 8000.[2]

OCT IMAGING

- Optical coherence tomography (OCT) of melanoma demonstrates choroidal shadowing, thinning/loss of overlying choriocapillaris, subretinal fluid, subretinal lipofuscin deposits, and "shaggy" or absent photoreceptors (Figure 69.1C).[3]
- OCT is not diagnostic for melanoma but can aid in identifying risk factors of melanoma, such as subretinal fluid and lipofusin, which is clinically observed as orange pigment (Figure 69.2C).

OCTA IMAGING

- Optical coherence tomography angiography (OCTA) may become a useful tool in differentiating malignant melanoma from benign nevi. Choroidal melanoma have been described as predominately isoreflective or hyporeflective (Figure 69.3A) with or without a hyperreflective halo (Figure 69.3E) in 63% of cases ($N = 11$) seen at the choriocapillaris layer. Conversely, nevi were mostly

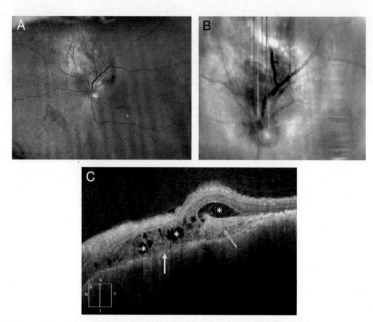

FIGURE 69.1 A, Color fundus photograph of a peripapillary choroidal melanoma with subretinal hemorrhage and subretinal fluid. B, Near-infrared. C, Thinning/loss of overlying choriocapillaris with shaggy photoreceptors and retinal pigment epithelium (RPE) cells (yellow arrow). Subretinal and intraretinal fluid (white asterisks), partially due to RPE cells malfunction and suggestive of possible CNV (green arrow). Although fluid can be seen secondary to the tumor alone without CNV.

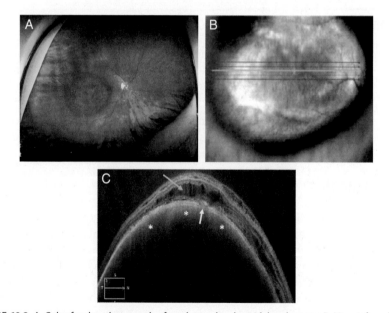

FIGURE 69.2 A, Color fundus photograph of a submacular choroidal melanoma. B, Near-infrared image over tumor. C, Compressive thinning of overlying choroid and choriocapillaris (white asterisks) with posterior choroidal shadowing. Retinal schisis overlying tumor (green arrow). Shaggy photoreceptors with subretinal lipofuscin deposit (yellow arrow).

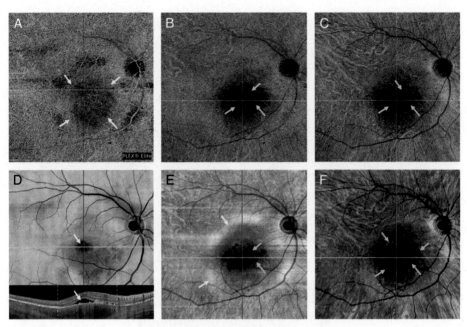

FIGURE 69.3 Swept-source optical coherence tomography angiography (OCTA) 12 × 12 mm image focused on a submacular choroidal melanoma. A, Hyporeflectivity with mild reduction of vascular density at level of outer retina to choriocapillaris (ORCC). Hyporeflective vascular voids (green arrows) seen at choriocapillaris (B) and deeper choroid (C). D, *En-face* OCTA at the structural ORCC shows a patchy hyporeflective region over the melanoma (green arrows with lines corresponding to OCTA B-scan) with a darker hyporeflective area which corresponds with the subretinal fluid seen on the OCTA B-scan below (yellow arrows). E, A hyporeflective region with multiple nonflow "void area" signals (green arrows) surrounded by a hyperreflective halo (yellow arrows) at the structural choriocapillaris layer. F, The en-face OCTA deeper choroid demonstrates hyporeflectivity with multiple nonflow "void area" signals (green arrows).

hyperreflective (82%; $N = 55$).[4] Consequently, a hyporreflective plexus or hyperreflective ring at the layer of the choriocapillaris has been associated with increased risk for malignancy (Figure 69.3E) in contrast to the hyperreflective plexus seen in nevi (Chapter 67) (Figure 69.4).

- One study proposed increased central macular thickness, enlarged deep foveal avascular zone, and reduced capillary vascular density in eye with choroidal melanoma compared to normal contralateral eye.[5] However, further large size trials will be needed to validate this proposal.

- Following plaque brachytherapy or proton beam therapy for uveal melanoma treatment, reduction in vascular density with capillary dropout, and microaneurysms can be visualized by OCTA indicating the development of radiation retinopathy.[6]

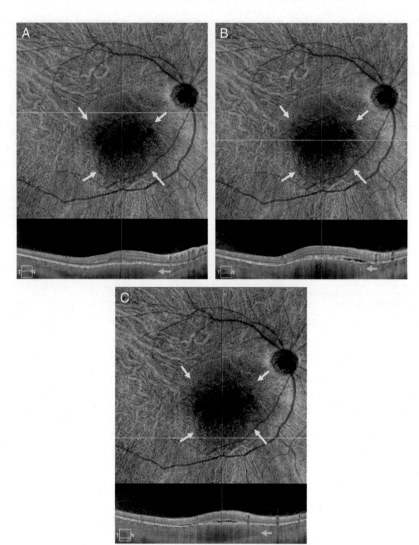

FIGURE 69.4 Swept-source optical coherence tomography angiography (OCTA) 12 × 12 mm choroidal layer. A-C, Hyporeflective region depicting the choroidal melanoma (yellow arrows). Below shows corresponding vascular flow at different segments of the melanoma. Melanoma appears to have reduced vascular flow (green arrow) compared to nevi (Chapter 67).

References

1. Aronow ME, Topham AK, Singh AD. Uveal melanoma: 5-year update on incidence, treatment, and survival (SEER 1973-2013). *Ocul Oncol Pathol.* 2018;4(3):145-151.
2. Singh AD, Kalyani P, Topham A. Estimating the risk of malignant transformation of a choroidal nevus. *Ophthalmology.* 2005;112(10):1784-1789.

3. Shields CL, Kaliki S, Rojanaporn D, et al. Enhanced depth imaging optical coherence tomography of small choroidal melanoma: comparison with choroidal nevus. *Arch Ophthalmol.* 2012;130(7):850-856.

4. Toledo JJ, Asencio M, Garcia JR, et al. OCT angiography: imaging of choroidal and retinal tumors. *Ophthalmol Retina.* 2018;2(6):613-622.

5. Valverde-Megias A, Say EA, Ferenczy SR, Shields CL. Differential macular features on optical coherence tomography angiography in eyes with choroidal nevus and melanoma. *Retina.* 2017;37(4):731-740.

6. Sellam A, Coscas F, Lumbroso-Le Rouic L, et al. Optical coherence tomography angiography of macular features after proton beam radiotherapy for small choroidal melanoma. *Am J Ophthalmol.* 2017;181:12-19.

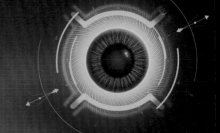

CHAPTER 70

Choroidal Hemangioma

SALIENT FEATURES

- Choroidal hemangiomas display a pattern of circumscribed or diffuse choroidal involvement. Circumscribed hemangioma presents as an orange-colored raised choroidal lesion located most commonly in the posterior pole with overlying retinal edema, subretinal fluid, and retinal pigment epithelium (RPE) fibrosis.[1]
- Indocyanine green shows early bright hypercyanescence with choroidal filling and late "wash out" hypocyanescence compared to surrounding choroid.
- Exudative fluid that is visually significant warrants treatment to preserve vision or prevent intractable neovascularization.

OCT IMAGING

- Both circumscribed and diffuse hemangiomas will often manifest with subretinal fluid (Figure 70.1C, green arrow), retinal edema, and photoreceptor loss (Figure 70.1C, yellow arrows).[2]
- The presentation of photoreceptor loss, retinoschisis, and intraretinal edema is a sign of chronicity of repeated episodes of subretinal fluid.[3]
- Optical coherence tomography (OCT) shows medium to low reflectivity of uniform intensity on the anterior surface of the tumor with large vascular choroidal vessels (Figure 70.1C, asterisks).[4]

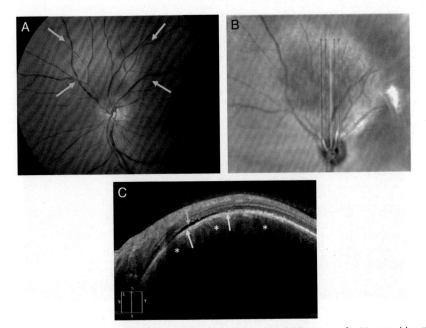

FIGURE 70.1 Spectral-domain optical coherence tomography (SD-OCT) image of a 51-year-old patient with a circumscribed choroidal hemangioma. A, Note the orange hue superior to the optic nerve with evidence of elevation (green arrows). B, Near-infrared. C, Evidence of chronic subretinal fluid overlying tumor with the loss and irregularity of photoreceptors (yellow arrows). Active subretinal fluid present with abnormal retinal pigment epithelium–appearing cells (green arrow). The choroidal hemangioma has medium to low reflectivity, in contrast to melanocytic nevi or melanoma which typically has high anterior choroidal reflectivity.[8] Large intrinsic choroidal vessels of the choroidal mass (asterisks).

OCTA IMAGING

- The outer borders of choroidal hemangiomas demonstrate a hyper-reflective margin at the level of the outer retina to choriocapillaris (ORCC) (Figure 70.2A). Inward branching vessels from the outer margins of the hemangioma in a spoke-wheel manner have been described.[5]

- Swept-source optical coherence tomography angiography (OCTA) details the multiple dilated interconnected, irregularly arranged, superficial and deep choroidal vessels which are larger in diameter compared to normal adjacent vessels (Figures 70.2C and 70.3).[6]

- Wide-field OCTA may provide information regarding the response to treatment based on reduction in vascular density on OCTA maps.[7]

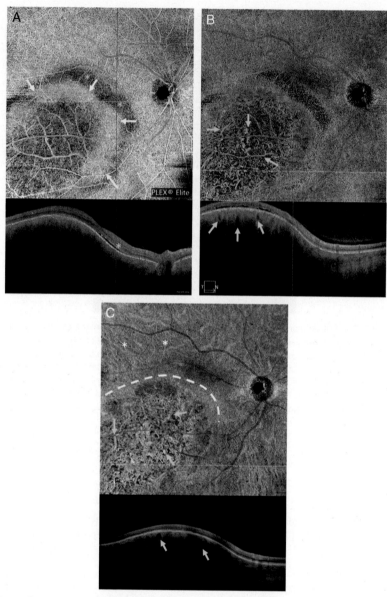

FIGURE 70.2 Swept-source optical coherence tomography angiography (SS-OCTA) of the right eye in a 55-year-old female with choroidal hemangioma on a 12 × 12 mm scan. A, The border of the choroidal hemangioma is outlined by a hyperreflective margin (yellow arrows) at the level of the outer retina to choriocapillaris (ORCC). Hyporeflective surrounding "halo" at ORCC illustrates subretinal fluid (green asterisks). B, The choroid demonstrates multiple dilated interconnected irregular vessels (green arrows) which are larger in diameter compared to normal choriocapillaris which is correlated with the OCTA B-scan below. C, The yellow line delineates the larger vascular choroidal vessels (green arrows) compared to normal vessels (white asterisks). Below, corresponding high-definition OCT shows larger choroidal vessels (green arrows).

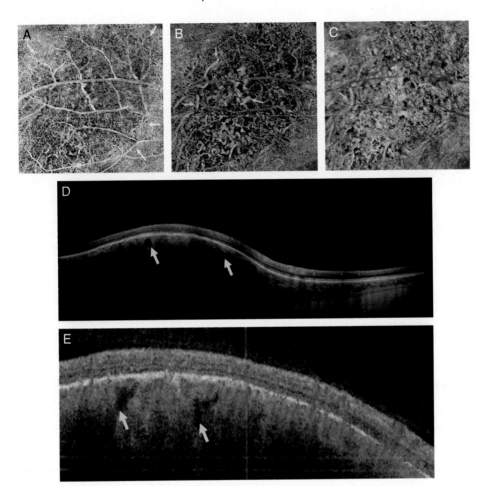

FIGURE 70.3 Swept-source optical coherence tomography angiography (OCTA) of right eye in a 55-year-old female with choroidal hemangioma on a 6 × 6 mm image scale (A-C). A, The borders of the choroidal hemangioma are outlined by a hyperreflective margin (yellow arrows) at the level of the outer retina to choriocapillaris (ORCC). B and C, The choroidal demonstrates multiple dilated interconnected irregular vessels (green arrows) which are larger in diameter compared to choriocapillaris (B) and choroid (C). D, A 16-mm high-definition (HD) OCT line exemplifies the large choroidal vessels (black voids, green arrows). E, Decorrelation OCTA B-scan demonstrating low flow.

References

1. Krohn J, Rishi P, Froystein T, Singh AD. Circumscribed choroidal haemangioma: clinical and topographical features. *Br J Ophthalmol.* 2019;103(10):1448-1452.

2. Ramasubramanian A, Shields CL, Harmon SA, Shields JA. Autofluorescence of choroidal hemangioma in 34 consecutive eyes. *Retina.* 2010;30(1):16-22.

3. Shields CL, Materin MA, Shields JA. Review of optical coherence tomography for intraocular tumors. *Curr Opin Ophthalmol.* 2005;16(3):141-154.

4. Sayanagi K, Pelayes DE, Kaiser PK, Singh AD. 3D Spectral domain optical coherence tomography findings in choroidal tumors. *Eur J Ophthalmol.* 2011;21(3):271-275.

5. Takkar B, Azad S, Shakrawal J, et al. Blood flow pattern in a choroidal hemangioma imaged on swept-source-optical coherence tomography angiography. *Indian J Ophthalmol.* 2017;65(11):1240-1242.

6. Rojanaporn D, Kaliki S, Ferenczy SR, Shields CL. Enhanced depth imaging optical coherence tomography of circumscribed choroidal hemangioma in 10 consecutive cases. *Middle East Afr J Ophthalmol.* 2015;22(2):192-197.

7. Sagar P, Shanmugam PM, Konana VK, et al. Optical coherence tomography angiography in assessment of response to therapy in retinal capillary hemangioblastoma and diffuse choroidal hemangioma. *Indian J Ophthalmol.* 2019;67(5):701-703.

8. Torres VL, Brugnoni N, Kaiser PK, Singh AD. Optical coherence tomography enhanced depth imaging of choroidal tumors. *Am J Ophthalmol.* 2011;151(4):586-593.e2.

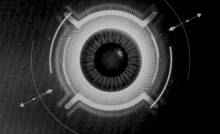

CHAPTER 71

Retinal Capillary Hemangioblastoma

SALIENT FEATURES

- Retinal hemangioblastoma is a cluster of retinal capillary endothelial cells with engorged retinal arteriole feeding into the lesion with an enlarged venule exiting the lesion. Although the lesion itself is benign, the risk of significant subretinal and intraretinal exudation can be vision threatening.

OCT IMAGING

- Identification of an isoreflective to hyperreflective vascular mass throughout all layers of the retina with posterior shadowing. Adjacent subretinal or intraretinal exudation may be present if lesion is actively leaking (Figure 71.1).[1]
- Outer retinal atrophy/photoreceptor loss may develop following fluid resolution and may also be associated with the actual lesion.
- Following laser therapy, optical coherence tomography (OCT) may be used for documenting tumor shrinkage.

OCTA IMAGING

- Optical coherence tomography angiography (OCTA) may demonstrate retinal vascular abnormalities which may then be evaluated for treatment response following laser. These acute changes include vasoconstriction of vessels and discontinuation of blood flow. Additionally, OCTA provides follow-up evaluation on vessel attenuation and straightening as well as shrinkage of the endothelial tumor mass following laser therapy.[1]
- OCTA imaging currently has limited peripheral retina visualization abilities which restrict evaluation to posteriorly located tumors.[2]

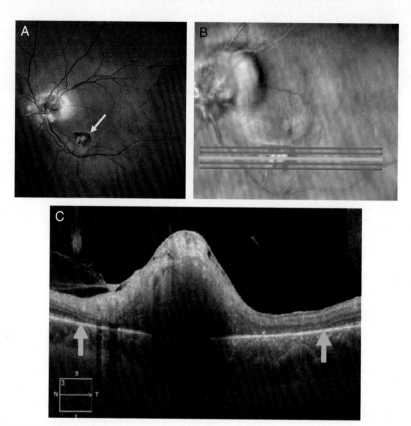

FIGURE 71.1 Retinal capillary hemangioblastoma (RCH) in a patient with von Hippel-Lindau disease. A, RCH noted adjacent to the optic nerve as well as along the inferior arcade. B, Near red-free with horizontal line over RCH. C, Vascular mass throughout all layers of the retina (arrows) with posterior shadowing. Disruption and loss of outer segment/photoreceptors beneath the tumor mass.

References

1. Chou BW, Nesper PL, Jampol LM, Mirza RG. Solitary retinal hemangioblastoma findings in OCTA pre- and post-laser therapy. *Am J Ophthalmol Case Rep.* 2018;10:59-61.

2. Sagar P, Rajesh R, Shanmugam M, et al. Comparison of optical coherence tomography angiography and fundus fluorescein angiography features of retinal capillary hemangioblastoma. *Indian J Ophthalmol.* 2018;66;872-876.

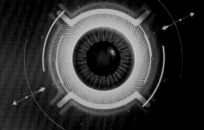

CHAPTER 72

Retinal Cavernous Hemangioma

SALIENT FEATURES

- Retinal cavernous hemangioma presents as multiple dark red–purple saccular vascular lesions that drain into a single venule (Figure 72.2A). The lack of retinal exudate and absence of a feeding artery help separate this lesion from a hemangioblastoma. Fibroglial tissue is commonly seen overlying the lesion.
- Fluorescein angiography (FA) is a useful adjunct imaging modality that can identify early hypoflourescence due to slow filling of the saccular lesions with late nonleaking filling (staining) of the cavernous saccules (Figure 72.2E). A "caplike fluorescence" is often seen due to the blood cells settling inferiorly from gravity, while the plasma separates and rises superiorly.[1]
- Given the potential central nervous system (CNS) association, magnetic resonance imaging (MRI) to evaluate for cerebral and spinal cavernous hemangiomas is recommended.

OCT IMAGING

- The typical findings are numerous cavernous spaces within the inner and outer retina layers that protrude superficially into the vitreous cavity (Figure 72.1).
- Due to blood cell settling, on optical coherence tomography (OCT), the lower region is hyporeflective with hyperreflective "cap" superiorly of plasma that separates out.[1]

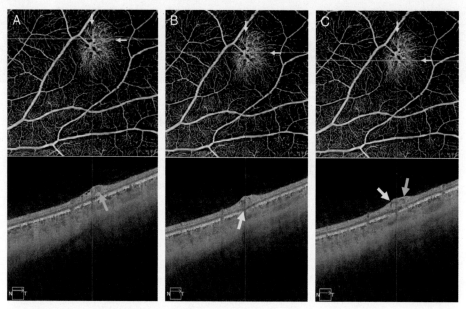

FIGURE 72.1 A-C, Swept-source optical coherence tomography angiography (OCTA) 6 × 6 mm superficial retinal layer shows the retinal cavernous hemangioma at different cross sections (yellow arrows, horizontal lines). With decorrelation overlay of the retinal cavernous compartments note areas of reduced flow (hyporeflective, green arrows) and increased flow (yellow arrows).

OCTA IMAGING

- The irregular multilobulated saccular dilation of the venous system is readily seen on optical coherence tomography angiography (OCTA) (Figures 72.1 and 72.2B and C).
- OCTA provides clear visualization of the retinal cavernous hemangioma with a single vein that drains the lesion (Figures 72.1 and 72.2B, yellow arrow).[2]

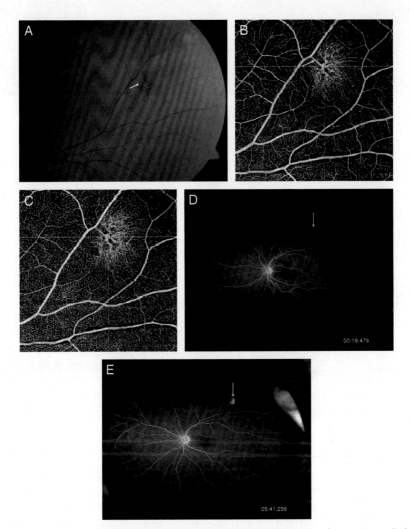

FIGURE 72.2 A, Color fundus photography of patient with retinal cavernous hemangioma. B, Swept-source optical coherence tomography angiography (OCTA) of the superficial retina illustrates the branched venule (yellow arrow) leading to multiple hyperreflective lobular "grapelike" cavernous lesions. C, Deep retina highlights the hyperreflective cavernous lesions and capillary junctions adjacent to arterioles (green arrow). D, Optos fundus fluorescein angiography at 19 seconds does not show a lesion, however, at (E) late phase (5:41 minutes), hyperflourescence is seen at the site of retinal cavernous hemangioma.

References

1. Lyu S, Zhang M, Wang RK, et al. Analysis of the characteristics of optical coherence tomography angiography for retinal cavernous hemangioma: a case report. *Medicine (Baltimore)*. 2018;97(7):e9940.

2. Kalevar A, Patel KH, McDonald HR. Optical coherence tomography angiography of retinal cavernous hemangioma. *Retina*. 2017;37(5):e50-e51.

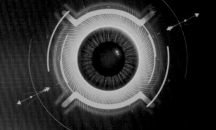

CHAPTER 73

Choroidal Metastasis

SALIENT FEATURES

- Two-thirds of patients with choroidal metastases have a known history of cancer, with lung cancer the most common in men and breast cancer in women. Of the 34% without a known cancer history, lung cancer is the most common discovered primary source.[1]
- Most commonly presents as an amelanotic elevated choroidal lesion with overlying retinal pigment epithelium (RPE) changes.

OCT IMAGING

- Choroidal metastases frequently demonstrate a hyporeflective band in the deeper choroid with enlargement of the suprachoroidal space (Figure 73.1C, yellow arrows).[2] Often the mass height is larger than the depth of the optical coherence tomography (OCT) which only allows visualization of the anterior hyporeflective portion of the metastasis (Figure 73.2B).
- The RPE often demonstrates thickening and detachment (Figure 73.1C, Figure 73.2B, Figure 73.3C). Subretinal fluid with highly reflective subretinal deposits have been reported (Figure 73.1C, white arrow).[3]
- OCT allows for monitoring of tumor size in treated metastases (Figure 73.2B and C).
- The L51 line provides enhanced depth to characterize the depth of tumor which is helpful in assessing response to systemic treatment (Figure 73.4A).

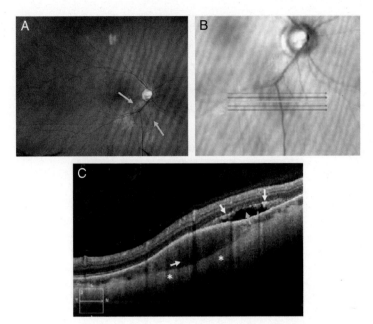

FIGURE 73.1 A, Color fundus photography of a patient with a pulmonary neuroendocrine cancer with choroidal metastasis. B, Near-infrared with horizontal lines over tumor. C, Optical coherence tomography (OCT) demonstrates a hyporeflective band along posterior choroidal mass (yellow arrow) with visible anterior edge of sclera (asterisks). Adjacent subretinal fluid (green arrow) with irregular ellipsoid zone (EZ) layer and hyperreflective subretinal deposits (white arrow).

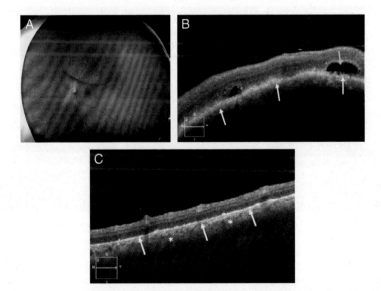

FIGURE 73.2 A, Color fundus photography of a patient with an adenoid cystic carcinoma choroidal metastasis. B, Optical coherence tomography (OCT) preplaque radiation therapy illustrates choroidal mass with thickening of the retinal pigment epithelium (RPE) (yellow arrows) and associated fluid (green arrow). C, OCT over peripheral retina postplaque radiation therapy demonstrates resolution of the choroidal mass with return of visible choriocapillaris (asterisks) and improvement in RPE thickening and detachments (yellow arrow).

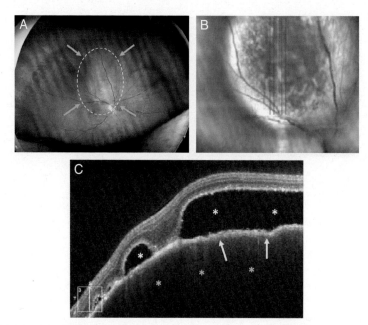

FIGURE 73.3 A, Color fundus photography of a patient with a non–small-cell lung cancer choroidal metastasis (outlined by dotted circles and green arrows). B, Near-infrared. C, Optical coherence tomography OCT image shows choroidal mass (green asterisks) with thickened retinal pigment epithelium (RPE) (yellow arrows) and subretinal fluid (white asterisks).

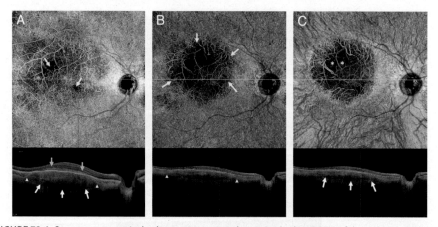

FIGURE 73.4 Swept-source optical coherence tomography angiography (OCTA) of the right eye with choroidal metastasis from breast cancer on a 12 × 12 mm image scale. A, At the layer of the outer retina to choriocapillaris (ORCC), flow voids (green asterisks) are seen with thinning of the choriocapillaris (dark voids with yellow arrows). OCT image demonstrates the metastasis compressing the choroid and choriocapillaris anteriorly (yellow arrowheads). Posterior edge of tumor appreciated with enhanced-depth analysis (white arrows). Irregular outer retina and photoreceptors anterior to metastasis (green arrows). B, The compressed choriocapillaris from the metastatic mass is prominently demonstrated by the hyporeflective void (yellow arrows). The corresponding OCTA B-scan (image below) emphasizes the compressed choroidal vasculature by the mass (yellow arrows). C, Minimal choroidal vessels with associated flow void at location of tumor (white asterisks). Below: OCT B-scan with decorrelation overlay shows hyporeflective tumor base against an isoreflective anterior margin of the sclera.

OCTA IMAGING

- A choroidal metastasis is readily seen on the optical coherence tomography angiography (OCTA) as a dark void of the choriocapillaris and choroid (Figure 73.4B and C).
- Wide-field OCTA B-scan provides visualization of the anteriorly compressed choriocapillary vasculature by the tumor (Figure 73.4B).

References

1. Shields CL, Materin MA, Shields JA. Review of optical coherence tomography for intraocular tumors. *Curr Opin Ophthalmol.* 2005;16(3):141-154.
2. Torres VL, Brugnoni N, Kaiser PK, Singh AD. Optical coherence tomography enhanced depth imaging of choroidal tumors. *Am J Ophthalmol.* 2011;151(4):586-593.e2.
3. Natesh S, Chin KJ, Finger PT. Choroidal metastases fundus autofluorescence imaging: correlation to clinical, OCT, and fluorescein angiographic findings. *Ophthalmic Surg Lasers Imaging.* 2010;41(4):406-412.

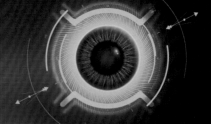

74

Vitreoretinal Lymphoma

SALIENT FEATURES

- Vitreoretinal lymphoma (VRL) is a rare lymphocytic neoplasm, most commonly an extranodal, high-grade, diffuse large B-cell lymphoma, affecting the retina, vitreous, or optic nerve.
- VRL is often on a continuum with primary central nervous system lymphoma (PCNSL), which itself represents an estimated 1% to 2% of all extranodal lymphomas.
- Greater than 80% of patients who present with intraocular disease develop intracranial involvement.[1] In this scenario, the VRL is termed "primary."
- While most common among elderly and immunocompromised patients, the incidence of primary vitreoretinal lymphoma (PVRL) and PCNSL in immunocompetent patients is on the rise.
- VRL can also arise from outside of the central nervous system. VRL should be distinguished from primary choroidal lymphoma as well as metastatic uveal or VRL associated with systemic lymphoma as they have different prognoses.
- Often masquerading as bilateral intraocular inflammation, VRL presents physicians with a unique challenge and is commonly misdiagnosed as an idiopathic uveitis and treated with corticosteroids, which can delay diagnosis and treatment of concurrent central nervous system (CNS) or systemic disease. Moreover, there are high false-negative rates of vitreoretinal biopsies.
- Classic findings include fine vitreous cellular clumping often in sheets and multifocal yellow subretinal pigment epithelial (RPE) deposits with overlying solid pigment epithelial detachments.

OCT IMAGING

- Optical coherence tomography (OCT) can differentiate VRL, which occurs anterior to Bruch membrane, from choroidal lymphoma, found posterior to Bruch membrane.
- OCT can highlight VRL lesions across multiple retinal layers, either in the form of discrete nodules or confluent hyperreflective bands (Figures 74.1 and 74.2).

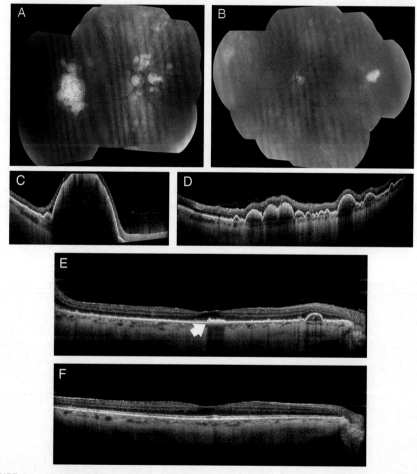

FIGURE 74.1 Fundus photos and optical coherence tomographies (OCTs) in a 76-year-old patient with bilateral keratic precipitates and multiple creamy yellow-white subretinal pigment epithelium (RPE) lesions with overlying pigmentary changes in both eyes (A and B). OCT confirms that all lesions are anterior to Bruch membrane, most appear as mounded lesions in the sub-RPE space (C and D). Subsequent brain imaging demonstrated a frontal lobe mass and biopsy revealed diffuse large B-cell lymphoma. The patient developed a focal, hyperreflective subfoveal lesion in the RPE layer with shadowing (E, white arrow), which subsequently resolved (F) with intravitreal methotrexate and rituximab. Best corrected visual acuity (BCVA) improved from 20/100 OD and 20/40 OS to 20/25 OD and 20/20 OS following therapy.

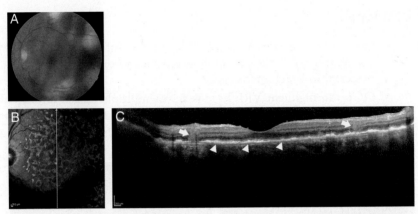

FIGURE 74.2 Fundus photo and optical coherence tomography (OCT) of a 71-year-old patient with vitreous biopsy confirmed vitreoretinal lymphoma. The elevated creamy white lesions (A) are shown to be in the subretinal pigment epithelium (RPE) space, but above Bruch membrane, on OCT. There are focal areas of full-thickness hyperreflectivity disrupting the laminations of the retina (white arrow). There are also multifocal clumps of hyperreflective lesions in the RPE layer (white arrowhead) throughout the macula, correlating with the reticular pattern seen on infrared reflectance imaging (B and C).

- Other common morphologic features of PVRL include sub-RPE hyperreflective infiltration between the RPE and Bruch membrane, hyperreflective foci in the subretinal space, irregularity of the RPE, inner retina hyperreflective infiltration, and undulation of the RPE (Figure 74.3).

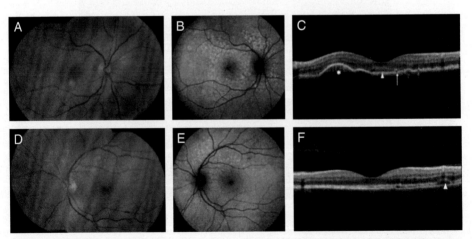

FIGURE 74.3 Multimodal imaging of a patient with bilateral primary vitreoretinal lymphoma (PVRL). A and D, Fundus photos showing diffuse, multifocal, yellowish subretinal infiltrates. B and E, Fundus autofluorescence demonstrating diffuse areas of hyperautofluorescence. C and F, Optical coherence tomography (OCT) highlighting subretinal (arrowheads) and subretinal pigment epithelium (RPE) (asterisk) infiltration, with outer retinal hyperreflective foci (arrow). (Photo courtesy of Shields and Shields MD PC.)

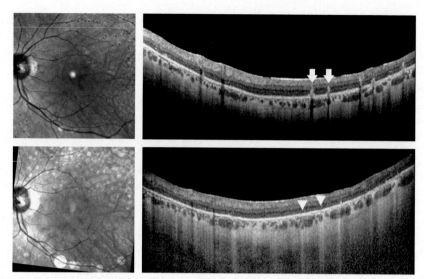

FIGURE 74.4 Optical coherence tomography (OCT) of a 59-year-old immunocompetent patient with mild vitritis and numerous punctate outer retinal lesions (A, white arrows). Brain imaging revealed central nervous system (CNS) lymphoma involving the corpus callosum and midbrain. Following systemic and intravitreal chemotherapy, the outer retinal lesions resolved with residual focal retinal pigment epithelium (RPE) atrophy, highlighted on infrared reflectance imaging and OCT as foci of hypertransmission (B, white arrowheads).

- Vertical hyperreflective lesions located between the inner retinal layers of the retina and the RPE may also be seen.
- Intraretinal and subretinal fluid may also be seen on occasion.
- Diffuse hyperreflective foci in the posterior vitreous are commonly seen on OCT and represent lymphoma cell aggregates in the vitreous, which often form cellular sheets visible when examining the anterior vitreous.
- Focal RPE atrophy with hypertransmission can be seen on OCT after resolution of outer retinal or subretinal lesions (Figure 74.4). VRL lesions can spontaneously involute and then appear elsewhere or involute with treatment.
- Some authors have reported that recurrent VRL is more likely to demonstrate atypical OCT findings, including focal, round intraretinal lesions, and villous-shaped projections from the retinal surface into the vitreous cavity.[6]

OCTA IMAGING

- Diagnostic features of VRL on optical coherence tomography angiography (OCTA) are still being studied and can vary widely between patients.

- Shadowing artifacts may be seen on OCTA due to VRL related vitritis and retinal lesions.
- Unlike some retinal or choroidal malignancies, OCTA will not typically demonstrate prominent feeder vessels or inherent vasculature associated with VRL lesions.

References

1. Chan CC, Sen HN. Current concepts in diagnosing and managing primary vitreoretinal (intraocular) lymphoma. *Discov Med.* 2013;15(81):93-100.
2. Shiels MS, Pfeiffer RM, Besson C, et al. Trends in primary central nervous system lymphoma incidence and survival in the US. *Br J Haematol.* 2016;174(3):417-424.
3. Enblad G, Martinsson G, Baecklund E, et al. Population-based experience on primary central nervous system lymphoma 2000-2012: the incidence is increasing. *Acta Oncol.* 2017;56(4):599-607.
4. Barry RJ, Tasiopoulou A, Murray PI, et al. Characteristic optical coherence tomography findings in patients with primary vitreoretinal lymphoma: a novel aid to early diagnosis. *Br J Ophthalmol.* 2018;102(10):1362-1366.
5. Liu TY, Ibrahim M, Bittencourt M, Sepah YJ, Do DV, Nguyen QD. Retinal optical coherence tomography manifestations of intraocular lymphoma. *J Ophthalmic Inflamm Infect.* 2012;2(4):215-218.
6. Saito T, Ohguro N, Iwahashi C, Hashida N. Optical coherence tomography manifestations of primary vitreoretinal lymphoma. *Graefes archive Clin Exp Ophthalmol.* 2016;254(12):2319-2326.
7. Davis JL. Intraocular lymphoma: a clinical perspective. *Eye (Lond).* 2013;27(2):153-162.
8. Deák GG, Goldstein DA, Zhou M, Fawzi AA, Jampol LM. Vertical hyperreflective lesions on optical coherence tomography in vitreoretinal lymphoma. *JAMA Ophthalmol.* 2019;137(2):194-198.
9. Lavine JA, Singh AD, Sharma S, Baynes K, Lowder CY, Srivastava SK. Ultra-widefield multimodal imaging of primary vitreoretinal lymphoma. *Retina.* 2019;39(10):1861-1871.

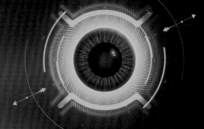

CHAPTER 75

Retinoblastoma

SALIENT FEATURES

- Retinoblastoma is the most common primary intraocular malignancy of childhood, with 95% of the cases occurring in children older than 5 years.
- Diagnosis is established by fundus examination using indirect ophthalmoscopy. Classically, the tumor appears as single or multiple dome-shaped cream white lesions with dilated retinal blood vessels feeding into and draining from the tumor. Areas of calcification within the tumor appear as white specks.
- Tumor growth pattern can be divided into endophytic and exophytic. Endophytic is described as a white hazy mass that seeds into the vitreous cavity. Exophytic tumor grows subretinally and is often accompanied by exudative retinal detachment and subretinal seeds.
- B-scan ultrasonography typically shows a dome-shaped lesion with medium to high internal echogenicity and acoustic shadowing from calcification.
- As this is predominantly a disease of children, examinations are performed under anesthesia.
- Handheld optical coherence tomography (OCT) (HH-OCT) has obviated for the patient to focus on target. HH-OCT overcomes the issues arising from lack of patient cooperation and positioning difficulties and, hence, can be conveniently used to examine children under anesthesia.
- In recent times, it has become a valuable tool in detecting "clinically invisible" lesions, subtle recurrences, monitoring treatment response, and evaluating the macular anatomy, thereby predicting the visual potential.

OCT IMAGING

- The characteristic features of retinoblastoma on OCT are divided into tumor and seeding pattern.
- The tumor shows a relatively homogenous hyperreflective dome-shaped lesion arising from inner, middle, or outer retinal layers with disorganized retinal layers and occasional cavities (Figure 75.1).
- At times, the tumor is localized in the outer retina with a normal-appearing inner retina, termed "retinal draping."
- The heterogeneity is related to the percentage of calcification within the tumor. Highly calcific tumors (like those with type 1 and type III regression) show areas of intralesional hyperreflectivity with corresponding back-shadowing.
- A cavitary variant of retinoblastoma shows a hyporeflective cavity within the intraretinal tumor.
- Tumor seeds appear as hyperreflective structures with posterior back-shadowing. While diagnosis of a prehyaloid (Figure 75.2) seed is easy, distinguishing a retrohyaloid from subretinal seed can be tricky.
- OCT helps to clearly demonstrate the location of seeds as prehyaloid, retrohyaloid, or subretinal (Figure 75.3). This allows appropriate monitoring and treatment when required.

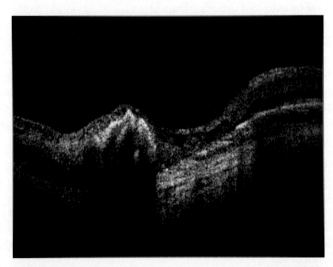

FIGURE 75.1 Handheld spectral-domain optical coherence tomography (HH-SD-OCT) of a retinoblastoma lesion. HH-SD-OCT demonstrates a heterogenous hyperreflective dome-shaped lesion (marked as red star) involving the inner and middle retina with back-shadowing suggestive of intralesional calcification. Retinal layers appear disorganized.

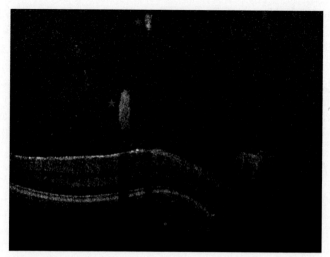

FIGURE 75.2 Handheld spectral-domain optical coherence tomography (HH-SD-OCT) showing preretinal seeds in a child with retinoblastoma. HH-SD-OCT shows two hyperreflective structures (marked as red star) in the vitreous cavity with posterior back-shadowing suggestive of partially calcified vitreous seeds.

- Small tumors (submillimeter or clinically invisible) are at times not observed on fundus examination.
- Tumor recurrences generally occur at the edge of preexisting regressed tumors. In the setting of scarring, seeding, and calcification, it can be difficult to recognize subtle recurrences. OCT helps in identifying and measuring slow growing recurrences.

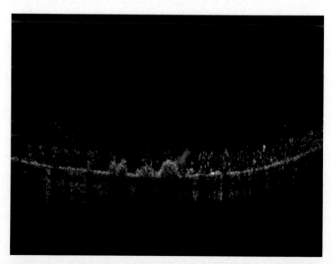

FIGURE 75.3 Handheld spectral-domain optical coherence tomography (HH-SD-OCT) showing subretinal seeds in a child with retinoblastoma. HH-SD-OCT shows multiple hyperreflective deposits (marked in red arrow) of subretinal tumor seeding.

- In macular tumors, identification of integrity of fovea can be difficult clinically as the fovea is often draped over the tumor. OCT helps in identifying an intact foveal contour thus predicting visual potential.
- OCT can visualize reduction in the size and more homogeneity of the lesion post treatment.
- In the era of intra-arterial chemotherapy, enhanced-depth imaging of the choroid is valuable in measuring choroidal thickness as choroidal thinning is known to occur with intra-arterial chemotherapy.

OCTA IMAGING

- At present, there is no clinical use of optical coherence tomography angiography (OCTA) for retinoblastoma diagnosis or management.
- However, with advent in studies, it may be pertinent to understand how retinal perfusion affects the tumor dynamics.

References

1. Broaddus E, Topham A, Singh AD. Incidence of retinoblastoma in the USA:1975-2004. *Br J Ophthalmol.* 2009;93(1):21-23.
2. Shields CL, Shields JA..Basic understanding of current classification and management of retinoblastoma. *Curr Opin Ophthalmol.* 2006;17(3):228-234.
3. Maldonado RS, Izatt JA, Sarin N, et al. Optimizing hand-held spectral domain optical coherence tomography imaging for neonates, infants, and children. *Invest Ophthalmol Vis Sci.* 2010;51:2678-2685.
4. Shields CL, Manalac J, Das C, Saktanasate J, Shields JA. Review of spectral domain-enhanced depth imaging optical coherence tomography of tumors of the retina and retinal pigment epithelium in children and adults. *Indian J Ophthalmol.* 2015;63(2):128-132.
5. Shields CL, Pellegrini M, Ferenczy SR, et al. Enhanced depth imaging optical coherence tomography of intraocular tumors: from placid to seasick to rock and rolling topography--the 2013 Francesco Orzalesi Lecture. *Retina.* 2014;34(8):1495-1512.
6. Ellsworth RM. The practical management of retinoblastoma. *Trans Am Ophthalmol Soc* 1969;67:462-534.
7. Munier FL. Classification and management of seeds in retinoblastoma. Ellsworth lecture ghent August 24th 2013. *Ophthalmic Genet.* 2014;35(4):193-207.
8. Seider MI, Grewal DS, Mruthyunjaya P. Portable optical coherence tomography detection or confirmation of ophthalmoscopically invisible or indeterminate active retinoblastoma. *Ophthalmic Surg Lasers Imaging Retina.* 2016;47(10):965-968.
9. Berry JL, Cobrinik D, Kim JW. Detection and intraretinal localization of an "invisible" retinoblastoma using optical coherence tomography. *Ocul Oncol Pathol.* 2015;2(3):148-152.

10. Park K, Sioufi K, Shields CL. Clinically invisible retinoblastoma recurrence in an infant. *Retina Cases Brief Rep.* 2019;13(2):108-110.

11. Samara WA, Pointdujour-Lim R, Say EA, Shields CL. Foveal microanatomy documented by SD-OCT following treatment of advanced retinoblastoma. *J AAPOS.* 2015;19(4):368-372.

12. Maidana DE, Pellegrini M, Shields JA, Shields CL. Choroidal thickness after intraarterial chemotherapy for retinoblastoma. *Retina.* 2014;34:2103-2109.

13. Sioufi K, Say EAT, Ferenczy SC, Leahey AM, Shields CL. Optical coherence tomography angiography findings of deep capillary plexus microischemia after intravenous chemotherapy for retinoblastoma. *Retina.* 2019;39(2):371-378.

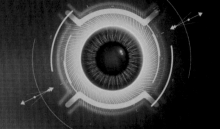
Choroidal Osteoma

SALIENT FEATURES

- Choroidal osteoma (CO) is a benign, rare, ossifying tumor of the choroid.
- It usually occurs in otherwise healthy young adults and is unilateral in approximately 75% of cases.[1]
- It can be asymptomatic or present with symptoms of blurry vision, metamorphopsia, or scotoma.
- The pathogenesis of choroidal osteoma is not well understood.
- Poor visual prognosis is associated with tumor growth, tumor decalcification (deossification), and associated choroidal neovascularization (CNV).[2] Regular long-term follow-up imaging is important to detect these changes.
- On funduscopic examination, CO appears as a deep, yellow-white to orange-white lesion typically in the juxtapapillary or peripapillary area and sometimes with overlying retinal pigment epithelium (RPE) alterations (Figures 76.1A and 76.2A).
- On funduscopic examination, decalcification may appear as a thin, atrophic, gray region.
- Ultrasonography, which is highly diagnostic for CO, exhibits high echogenicity and acoustic shadowing posterior to the lesion, often creating the appearance of a pseudonerve (Figure 76.1C).
- Fluorescein angiography demonstrates hyperfluorescence (with leakage in the presence of CNV), while indocyanine green angiography shows hypocyanescence (Figures 76.2B and 76.1B).

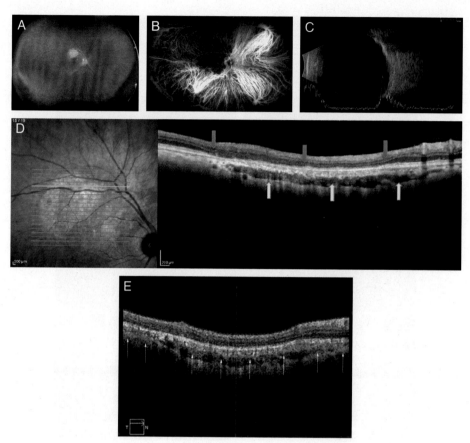

FIGURE 76.1 A, Fundus photo of a 56-year-old asymptomatic male showing a well-circumscribed white/yellow mass along the superior arcade with associated retinal pigment epithelium (RPE) alterations along the temporal edge. B, Indocyanine green angiography (ICG) demonstrating hypocyanescence in the region of choroidal osteoma (CO). C, B-scan ultrasound shows high echogenicity with acoustic shadowing, confirming the diagnosis of choroidal osteoma. D, Spectral-domain optical coherence tomography (SD-OCT) showing thinning of the outer retina with collapse of the outer nuclear layer and loss of the ellipsoid zone (EZ) and external limiting membrane (ELM) (blue arrows) overlying the choroidal osteoma (yellow arrows). The inner retinal layers are relatively well preserved. E, Optical coherence tomography angiography (OCTA) showing normal choriocapillaris (yellow arrows) and compression of the choriocapillaris (white arrows) by the CO which is most evident on the cross-sectional B-scan with flow overlay.

OCT IMAGING

- Spectral-domain optical coherence tomography (SD-OCT) imaging shows an intact overlying retina in calcified areas of choroidal osteomas. Decalcified regions show an intact inner retina with thin to absent outer retina and photoreceptor loss corresponding to poor visual acuity[3] (Figure 76.1D).

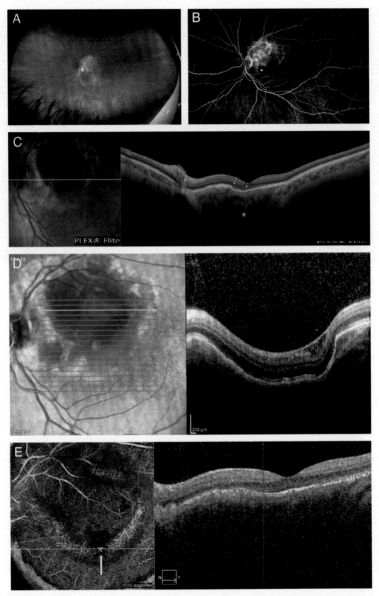

FIGURE 76.2 A, Fundus photo of a 26-year-old male who presented with blurry vision and metamorphopsia, showing an orange round juxtapapillary lesion with a focal area of subretinal hemorrhage along the inferior edge. B, Fluorescein angiography (FA) shows hyperfluorescence corresponding to a classic choroidal neovascularization. C, Swept-source optical coherence tomography (OCT) through the fovea showing a thick choroidal osteoma (asterisk), compression of the overlying choriocapillaris, retinal pigment epithelium (RPE) undulations in the region of choroidal neovascularization (CNV) (white arrow), and disruption of photoreceptor layer overlying the CO (yellow arrow) (Courtesy of K. Bailey Freund, MD). D, SD-OCT demonstrating choroidal excavation. E, OCT angiography (OCTA) of this choroidal osteoma with choroidal excavation is limited by segmentation artifact given the multiple vertical planes with the majority of the osteoma out of the vertical axis. A manual evaluation of the OCTA is helpful which localizes increased vessel density (with corresponding increased flow on the cross-sectional image) at and above the level of the RPE consistent with choroidal neovascularization (arrow).

- In eyes with both calcified and decalcified components, a sharp transition in the retinal architecture overlying the CO can be seen.
- SD-OCT is limited in posterior visualization when the osteoma extends to the sclerochoroidal junction.[4]
- Enhanced-depth OCT (EDI-OCT) and swept-source OCT (SS-OCT) can help reveal a dome or undulating surface with horizontal lamellar lines and horizontal or vertical tubules within the tumor, presumably representing bone lamellae and intralesional vessels.[5]
- Other features found on EDI-OCT and SS-OCT include compression of the choriocapillaris, a spongelike appearance with multiple hyperreflective dots and layers, and transparency to the sclerochoroidal junction[6] (Figure 76.2C).
- Focal choroidal excavation may be present (Figure 76.2D).
- Outer retinal tubulations (ORT) are branching tubular structures seen on OCT as oval-shaped hyporeflective lumens with hyperreflective borders. ORTs have been found to overlay areas of CNV and over the decalcified portions of CO.[7]

OCTA IMAGING

- Optical coherence tomography angiography (OCTA) imaging may demonstrate increased capillary density in the choroid and deep retinal vascular plexus.[8]
- OCTA may aid in the diagnosis of CNV particularly when the fluorescein angiography is limited by the inherent hyperfluorescence of the lesion[9] (Figure 76.2D).

References

1. Shields CL, Shields JA, Augsburger JJ. Choroidal osteoma. *Surv Ophthalmol.* 1988;33:17-27.
2. Shields CL, Sun H, Demirci H, Shields JA. Factors predictive of tumor growth, tumor decalcification, choroidal neovascularization, and visual outcome in 74 eyes with choroidal osteoma. *Arch Ophthalmol.* 2005;123:1658-1666.
3. Shields CL, Perez B, Materin MA, Mehta S, Shields JA. Optical coherence tomography of choroidal osteoma in 22 cases: evidence for photoreceptor atrophy over the decalcified portion of the tumor. *Ophthalmology.* 2007;114:e53-e58.
4. Freton A, Finger PT. Spectral domain-optical coherence tomography analysis of choroidal osteoma. *Br J Ophthalmol.* 2012;96:224-228.
5. Shields CL, Arepalli S, Atalay HT, Ferenczy SR, Fulco E, Shields JA. Choroidal osteoma shows bone lamella and vascular channels on enhanced depth imaging optical coherence tomography in 15 eyes. *Retina.* 2015;35:750-757.
6. Pellegrini M, Invernizzi A, Giani A, Staurenghi G. Enhanced depth imaging optical coherence tomography features of choroidal osteoma. *Retina.* 2014;34:958-963.

7. Xuan Y, Zhang Y, Wang M, et al. Multimodal fundus imaging of outer retinal tubulations in choroidal osteoma patients. *Retina.* 2018;38:49-59.

8. Cennamo G, Romano MR, Breve MA, et al. Evaluation of choroidal tumors with optical coherence tomography: enhanced depth imaging and OCT-angiography features. *Eye (Lond).* 2017;31:906-915.

9. Szelog JT, Filho MAB, Lally DR, de Carlo TE, Duker JS. Optical coherence tomography angiography for detecting choroidal neovascularization secondary to choroidal osteoma. *Ophthalmic Surg Lasers Imaging Retina.* 2016;47:69-72.

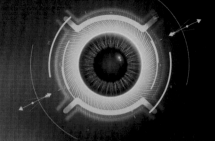

CHAPTER 77

Sclerochoroidal Calcification

SALIENT FEATURES

- Usually asymptomatic; detected on routine eye examination.
- Sclerochoroidal calcifications are bilateral benign amorphous acellular calcium accumulations within the sclera.
- On fundus examination, sclerochoroidal calcifications present as yellow-white lesions with ill-defined margins, most commonly found in regions of the retinal vascular arcades (Figure 77.1).
- The protrusion from the scleral calcification compresses the choroid and can cause atrophy of the retinal pigment epithelium atrophy and overlying retina.[1,2] Rarely are choroidal neovascular membranes (CNVMs) associated with sclerochoroidal calcifications.
- On fluorescence angiography, the lesions show late staining.
- B-scan shows hyperechogencity with dense shadowing (Figure 77.1).
- Most commonly associated with increased age.
- Also been associated with hyperparathyroidism and pseudohyperparathyroidism.[3]
- These are distinguished from osteomas due to bilaterality (85%), onset later in life (mean age: 78 years), commonly found in temporal arcades (not juxtapapillary), occurrence same in men and women and multifocal locality.[4]
- Patients with sclerochoroidal calcifications should obtain serum vitamin D, calcium, and magnesium levels to assess calcium metabolism.
- Treatment includes management of calcium metabolism disorders as well as visually significant CNVM (rare).
- Reports have shown calcification erosions through the choroid and retina into the vitreous resulting in "secondary asteroid hyalosis."[5]

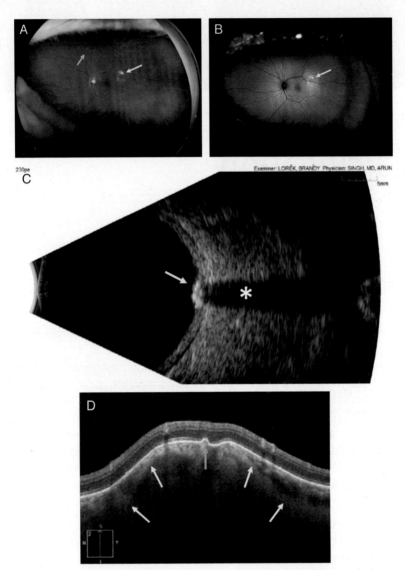

FIGURE 77.1 Optical coherence tomography (OCT) images from a 69-year-old patient with bilateral sclerochoroidal calcifications. A, Fundus photo with larger sclerochoroidal calcification along superior temporal arcade (yellow arrow) and smaller sclerochoroidal calcification at 12 o'clock in midperiphery (green arrow). B, Fundus autofluorescence with hyperautofluorescense at site of calcification (yellow arrow). C, B-scan demonstrating hyperreflectivity (yellow arrow) at the site of calcific lesion with shadowing (asterisks). D, Scleral-based calcium lesions causing compressive choroidal thinning (yellow arrows). Abnormal retinal pigment epithelium with disrupted ellipsoid zone at apex (blue arrow).

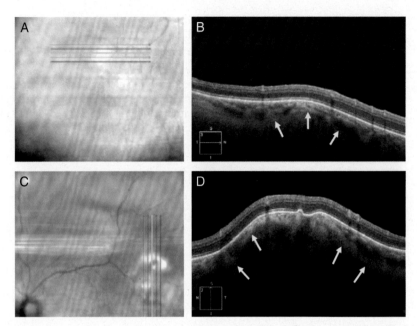

FIGURE 77.2 Comparison of a small versus a large sclerochoroidal calcification imaged by optical coherence tomography (OCT) seen within the same person. A and C, On infrared, the lesion has hyperreflectance. B, Mild choroidal thinning (yellow arrows) appreciated with reduced shadowing and normal retinal pigment epithelium and ellipsoid in the smaller scleral calcification compared to (D) significant compressive choroidal thinning (yellow arrows) and abnormal retinal pigment epithelium (RPE) and outer retina in the larger scleral calcification.

OCT IMAGING

- Optical coherence tomography (OCT) demonstrates the scleral-based calcium lesion resulting in compressive choroidal thinning (Figures 77.1 and 77.2, yellow arrows).
- Size of the calcification can result in apical or lateral disruption and thinning of the retinal pigment epithelium and ellipsoid zone with posterior shadowing.[6]

References

1. Wong S, Zakov ZN, Albert DM. Scleral and choroidal calcifications in a patient with pseudohypoparathyroidism. *Br J Ophthalmol.* 1979;63(3):177-180.
2. Jensen OA. Ouclar calcifications in primary hyper-parathyroidism. Histochemical and ultrastructural study of a case: Comparison with ocular calcifications in idiopathic hypercalcaemia of infancy and in renal failure. *Acta Ophthalmol.* 1975;53(2):173-186.
3. Goldstein BG, Miller J. Metastatic calcification of the choroid in a patient with primary hyperparathyroidism. *Retina.* 1982;2(2):76-79.

4. Choudhary MM, Singh AD. Asteroid opactities in sclerochoroidal calcification. *Lat Am J Ophthalmol.* 2019;1(1):5-7.

5. Schachat AP, Robertson DM, Mieler WF, et al. Sclerochoroidal calcification. *Arch Ophthalmol.* 1992;110(2):196-199.

6. Hasanreisoglu M, Saktanasate J, Shields PW, Shields CL. Classification of sclerochoroidal calcification based on enhanced depth imaging opitcal coherence tomography "mountain-like" featuers. *Retina.* 2015;35(7):1407-1414.

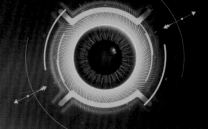

Combined Hamartoma of the Retina and Retinal Pigment Epithelium

SALIENT FEATURES

- Combined hamartoma of the retina and retinal pigment epithelium (CHRRPE) is a rare, benign intraocular tumor with variable clinical features first described by Gass in 1973.

- This lesion is comprised of vascular, glial, and melanocytic tissue. It is generally believed to be congenital and nonhereditary.

- The etiology of CHRRPE remains uncertain. It is often seen as an isolated condition but can be associated with neurofibromatosis type 1 and type 2.

- CHRRPE characteristically presents as an ill-defined, grayish retinal mass with tortuous or straightened vessels and a variable amount of retinal gliosis and vitreous traction (Figure 78.1A).

- Assessing the degree of retinal involvement (epiretinal only, partial retinal involvement, or complete retinal and RPE involvement); the proximity to the foveal center; and presence of traction-induced retinoschisis and/or neurosensory detachment can help guide follow-up intervals and the necessity of surgical intervention.

- Pars plana vitrectomy with membrane delamination may be employed in cases with visual loss and/or distortion, macular involvement, and neurosensory detachment with variable visual and anatomic outcome.

OCT IMAGING

- Optical coherence tomography (OCT) can help ascertain the depth of retinal involvement in CHRRPE.
- Commonly described OCT features include retinal thickening, retinal disorganization, epiretinal membrane, retinal folding and striae, vitreoretinal adhesion or traction, and intraretinal hyporeflective spaces corresponding to schisis or cystoid spaces (Figures 78.1 and 78.2).
- Traction from epiretinal CHRRPE may cause inner retinal folding in a "saw-tooth" pattern. Deeper involvement may distort the inner retina into an "omega" shape, lined posteriorly by the outer plexiform layer (Figures 78.1 and 78.2).

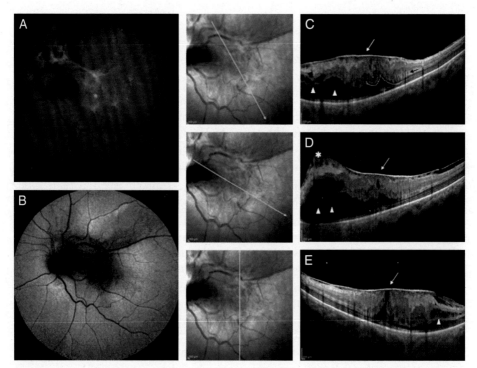

FIGURE 78.1 Multimodal imaging of a patient with combined hamartoma of the retina and retinal pigment epithelium (CHRRPE). A, Multicolor image showing a grayish-white lesion involving the macula and the peripapillary area superiorly with extensive epiretinal membrane. B, Fundus autofluorescence demonstrating hypoautofluorescence in the area corresponding to the lesion. C-E, Spectral-domain optical coherence tomography (SD-OCT) highlighting many common features of this condition including retinal thickening and folds, epiretinal membrane (arrow), vitreoretinal traction (asterisk), and hyporeflective areas corresponding to intraretinal schisis and cystoid spaces (arrowheads). The ellipsoid zone is attenuated and there is an "omega" sign at the fovea consistent with traction.

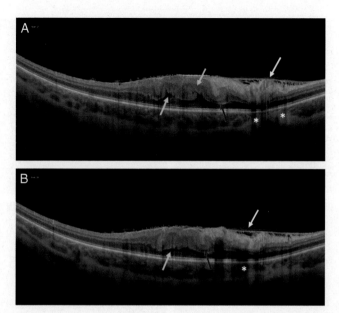

FIGURE 78.2 Enhanced-depth imaging optical coherence tomography (OCT) of a 21-year-old patient with a combined hamartoma of the retina and retinal pigment epithelium (CHRRPE). A and B are two adjacent OCT slices in the foveal region. CHRRPE characterized by the thickened inner retina with secondary retinal traction caused by excessive glial tissue (yellow arrows) on the surface of the lesion primarily involving the inner retinal layers which extend to outer plexiform layer (OPL) creating a "saw-tooth" appearance (green arrow) and extending deeper resulting in retinal folded in an "omega" pattern (purple arrow). The retinal pigment epithelium is intact, and there is no choroidal mass (white asterisks).

- In the majority of cases, the retina adjacent to the lesion appears flat and displays normal architecture with progressive thickening toward the lesion. Triangular hyperreflective alterations located at the edges of the lesion in the outer retina with no posterior shadowing have been described ("shark-teeth sign").
- Resolution of traction-induced changes on OCT can be seen post surgical repair.
- A higher frequency of full-thickness retinal involvement with ellipsoid and RPE disruption, intraretinal cystoid spaces, and choroidal neovascularization has been seen on OCT imaging of peripapillary lesions compared to macular lesions.

OCTA IMAGING

- Increased vascular tortuosity and disorganization of the superficial and deep capillary plexus can readily be seen on optical coherence tomography angiography (OCTA). Reduced or absent foveal avascular zone is a common finding that is highlighted by OCTA (Figures 78.3 and 78.4).

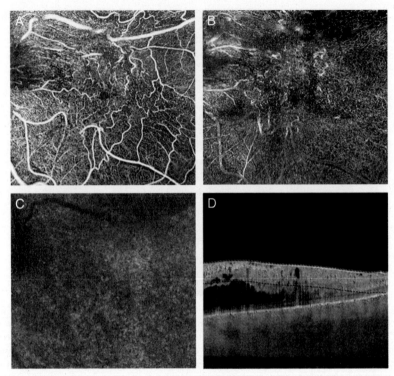

FIGURE 78.3 Spectral-domain optical coherence tomography angiography (OCTA) of the case shown in Figure 82.1. A and B, Vascular alteration with increased tortuosity and traction is visible at the level of both the superficial and deep capillary plexus. Note the almost complete loss of the foveal avascular zone (FAZ). C, The choriocapillaris does not show any appreciable alteration. D, B-scan demonstrating vascular flow overlay.

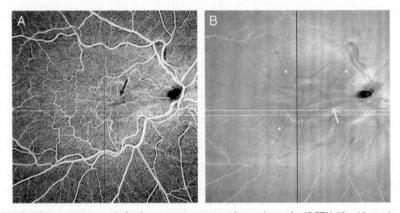

FIGURE 78.4 Swept-source optical coherence tomogrography angiography (OCTA) 12 × 12 mm image of combined hamartoma of the retina and retinal pigment epithelium (CHRRPE). A, The OCTA image of the inner retina demonstrates increased vascular tortuosity temporal to fovea with straightened vessels from optic nerve to the lesion (green arrow) secondary to traction. Absence of the foveal avascular zone (purple arrow). B, En-face OCT of inner retina shows excessive hyperreflective tissue on the surface of the lesion (yellow arrow) extending from optic nerve temporally resulting in significant retinal traction as seen by the 360 degrees of tractional lines (white asterisks).

- Quantitatively, decreased vascular density of the superficial capillary plexus (SCP), deep capillary plexus (DCP), and choriocapillaris has been noted.
- OCTA can be used to monitor the normalization of vascular anatomy that may occur after surgical repair.

References

1. Gass JD. An unusual hamartoma of the pigment epithelium and retina simulating choroidal melanoma and retinoblastoma. *Trans Am Ophthalmol Soc.* 1973;71:171-183; discussions 184-175.
2. Schachat AP, Shields JA, Fine SL, et al. Combined hamartomas of the retina and retinal pigment epithelium. *Ophthalmology.* 1984;91(12):1609-1615.
3. Shields CL, Mashayekhi A, Dai VV, Materin MA, Shields JA. Optical coherence tomographic findings of combined hamartoma of the retina and retinal pigment epithelium in 11 patients. *Arch Ophthalmol.* 2005;123(12):1746-1750.
4. Arepalli S, Pellegrini M, Ferenczy SR, Shields CL. Combined hamartoma of the retina and retinal pigment epithelium: findings on enhanced depth imaging optical coherence tomography in eight eyes. *Retina.* 2014;34(11):2202-2207.
5. Kumar V, Chawla R, Tripathy K. Omega sign: a distinct optical coherence tomography finding in macular combined hamartoma of retina and retinal pigment epithelium. *Ophthalmic Surg Lasers Imaging Retina.* 2017;48(2):122-125.
6. Arrigo A, Corbelli E, Aragona E, et al. Optical coherence tomography and optical coherence tomography angiography evaluation of combined hamartoma of the retina and retinal pigment epithelium. *Retina.* 2019;39(5):1009-1015.
7. Gupta R, Fung AT, Lupidi M, et al. Peripapillary versus macular combined hamartoma of the retina and retinal pigment epithelium: imaging characteristics. *Am J Ophthalmol.* 2019;200:263-269.
8. Scupola A, Grimaldi G, Sammarco MG, Sasso P, Marullo M, Blasi MA. Multimodal imaging evaluation of combined hamartoma of the retina and retinal pigment epithelium. *Eur J Ophthalmol.* 2020;30(3):555-599. doi:10.1177/1120672119831223.
9. Sridhar J, Shahlaee A, Rahimy E, Hong B, Shields CL. Optical coherence tomography angiography of combined hamartoma of the retina and retinal pigment epithelium. *Retina.* 2016;36(7):e60-e62.
10. Dedania VS, Ozgonul C, Zacks DN, Besirli CG. Novel classification system for combined hamartoma OF the retina and retinal pigment epithelium. *Retina.* 2018;38(1):12-19.
11. Chawla R, Temkar S, Sagar P, Venkatesh P. An unusual case of congenital hypertrophy of retinal pigment epithelium with overlying hemorrhages. *Indian J Ophthalmol.* 2016;64(9):672-673.

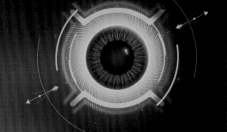

CHAPTER 79

Retinal Astrocytic Hamartoma and Presumed Solitary Circumscribed Retinal Astrocytic Proliferation

SALIENT FEATURES

- Retinal astrocytic hamartoma (RAH) and presumed solitary circum-scribed retinal astrocytic proliferation (PSCRAP) are intraocular tumors presumed to derive from retinal glial cells.
- RAH is a benign intraocular tumor composed of retinal astrocytes with minimally dilated vessels. Ophthalmoscopically, it appears as a superficial gray-yellow mass, with possible fine vitreoretinal traction and a variable amount of calcification (Figure 79.1A). If calcified, glistening yellow spherules are seen.[1,2]
- RAH is believed to be congenital in most cases but can also be acquired. It is frequently associated with tuberous sclerosis complex (TSC).[1]
- PSCRAP appears ophthalmoscopically as a well-defined, round, elevated, white-yellow retinal mass, obscuring retinal vessels (Figure 79.4A). This lesion is most commonly located in the postequatorial region.[3]
- PSCRAP generally presents in eyes with no previous ocular insult, and it is not associated with TSC. Its pathogenesis remains unknown.[3]

OCT IMAGING

- Common optical coherence tomography (OCT) findings in RAH include localized hyperreflective thickening of the retinal nerve fiber layer (RNFL) with gradual transition to adjacent normal retina, variable degree of retinal disorganization, inward and outward bowing with variable compression of the middle and outer retinal layers, and possible vitreoretinal adhesion/traction (Figure 79.1C and D, Figure 79.2C, and Figure 79.3). Based on OCT appearance, this tumor is thought to originate from the RNFL.[2,4-6]
- Calcified spherules within the tumor appear as optically empty spaces with a typical "moth-eaten" appearance. They usually occur one-third of the depth into the tumor and can be associated with posterior optical shadowing (Figure 79.2C).[5-7]
- A classification of RAH based on spectral-domain optical coherence tomography (SD-OCT) has been proposed. It correlates each type of RAH with systemic manifestations of TSC.[7]

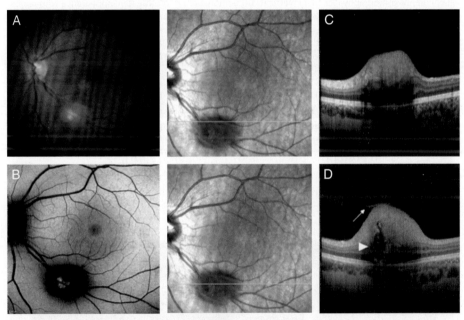

FIGURE 79.1 Multimodal imaging of a patient with retinal astrocytic hamartoma. A, Fundus photograph showing a yellow translucent lesion along the inferotemporal arcade. B, Fundus autofluorescence demonstrating hypoautofluorescence of the tumor with a central area of hyperautofluorescence corresponding to calcification within the lesion. C and D, Spectral-domain optical coherence tomography (SD-OCT) highlighting many common features of this condition including hyperreflective thickening at the level of the nerve fiber layer, with some inward and outward bowing, compression of the middle and outer retina, minimal posterior shadowing and subtle vitreoretinal adhesion (arrow). A cut through the calcified portion of the lesion demonstrates a round optically empty space (arrowhead).

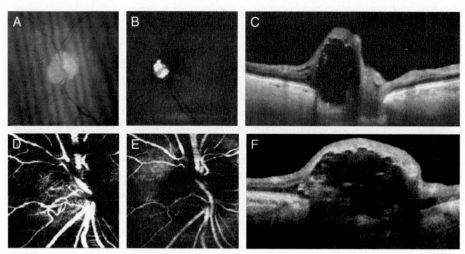

FIGURE 79.2 Multimodal imaging of a patient with retinal astrocytic hamartoma. A, Fundus photograph showing a small yellow papillary lesion with prominent calcified glistening spherules. B, Fundus autofluorescence demonstrating hyperautofluorescence of the tumor due to calcification. C, Spectral-domain optical coherence tomography (SD-OCT) (vertical cut) demonstrating "moth-eaten" appearance with almost complete hyporeflectivity of the lesion due to extensive calcification. D and E, Optical coherence tomography angiography (OCTA) at the level of the superficial capillary plexus shows a dense irregular vascular network with deep posterior shadowing at the level of the deep capillary plexus. F, Corresponding B-scan (horizontal cut) demonstrates intrinsic vascular flow within the superficial portion of the lesion.

- OCT imaging of PSCRAP typically demonstrates an abruptly elevated lesion ("snowball configuration") with smooth or slightly irregular surface, compression of the overlying retina, and visible interface between the mass and the retinal nerve fiber layer. The mass frequently shows deep posterior optical shadowing (Figure 79.4B).[4,8]
- Based on OCT appearance, recent reports have indicated that PSCRAP might originate from the deep retina or the RPE as opposed to retinal astrocytes.[4,8,9]

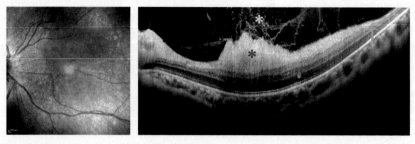

FIGURE 79.3 Spectral-domain optical coherence tomography (SD-OCT) imaging of a patient with retinal astrocytic hamartoma. There is localized hyperreflective thickening of the retinal nerve fiber layer (blue asterisk) with gradual transition to adjacent normal retina (green arrow) and vitreoretinal adhesion/traction (yellow asterisk).

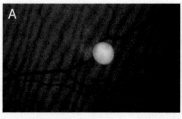
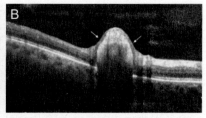

FIGURE 79.4 Presumed solitary circumscribed retinal astrocytic proliferation. A, Fundus photograph showing a "pearly" white retinal mass, obscuring retinal vessels. B, Spectral-domain optical coherence tomography (SD-OCT) demonstrates typical findings of this condition including abrupt elevation, smooth surface, posterior optical shadowing, and compression of the overlying retina, with a visible interface (arrows). (Photo courtesy of Shields and Shields, MD, PC.)

OCTA IMAGING

- Optical coherence tomography angiography (OCTA) findings in RAH suggest intrinsic tumor vascularity versus disorganized superficial and deep capillary plexi. The lesion might appear dark at the level of deeper layers (outer retina, choriocapillaris) due to shadowing effect (Figure 79.2D and E).[10,11]
- OCTA of PSCRAP has demonstrated lack of intrinsic vascularity of the lesion, with intact overlying SCP, intact vasculature of the retina surrounding the lesion, and lack of vascular flow entering into the tumor.[9]

References

1. Nyboer JH, Robertson DM, Gomez MR. Retinal lesions in tuberous sclerosis. *Arch Ophthalmol.* 1976;94(8):1277-1280.
2. Say EA, Shah SU, Ferenczy S, Shields CL. Optical coherence tomography of retinal and choroidal tumors. *J Ophthalmology.* 2011;2011:385058.
3. Shields JA, Bianciotto CG, Kivela T, Shields CL. Presumed solitary circumscribed retinal astrocytic proliferation: the 2010 Jonathan W. Wirtschafter Lecture. *Arch Ophthalmol.* 2011;129(9):1189-1194.
4. Schwartz SG, Harbour JW. Spectral-domain optical coherence tomography of presumed solitary circumscribed retinal astrocytic proliferation versus astrocytic hamartoma. *Ophthalmic Surg Lasers Imaging Retina.* 2015;46(5):586-588.
5. Shields CL, Benevides R, Materin MA, Shields JA. Optical coherence tomography of retinal astrocytic hamartoma in 15 cases. *Ophthalmology.* 2006;113(9):1553-1557.
6. Shields CL, Say EAT, Fuller T, Arora S, Samara WA, Shields JA. Retinal astrocytic hamartoma arises in nerve fiber layer and shows "Moth-Eaten" optically empty spaces on optical coherence tomography. *Ophthalmology.* 2016;123(8):1809-1816.

7. Pichi F, Massaro D, Serafino M, et al. Retinal astrocytic hamartoma: optical coherence tomography classification and correlation with tuberous sclerosis complex. *Retina*. 2016;36(6):1199-1208.

8. Shields CL, Roe R, Yannuzzi LA, Shields JA. Solitary circumscribed "pearl white" retinal mass (so-called retinal astrocytic proliferation) resides in deep retina or beneath retina: findings on multimodal imaging in 4 cases. *Retin Cases Brief Rep*. 2017;11(1):18-23.

9. Goldberg RA, Raja KM. Presumed solitary circumscribed retinal astrocytic proliferation in the fovea with OCT angiography: a misnomer. *Ophthalmic Surg Lasers Imaging Retina*. 2018;49(3):212-214.

10. Schwartz SG, Harbour JW. Multimodal imaging of astrocytic hamartomas associated with tuberous sclerosis. *Ophthalmic Surg Lasers Imaging Retina*. 2017;48(9):756-758.

11. Despreaux R, Mrejen S, Quentel G, Cohen SY. En face optical coherence tomography (OCT) and OCT angiography findings in retinal astrocytic hamartomas. *Retin Cases Brief Rep*. 2017;11(4):373-379.

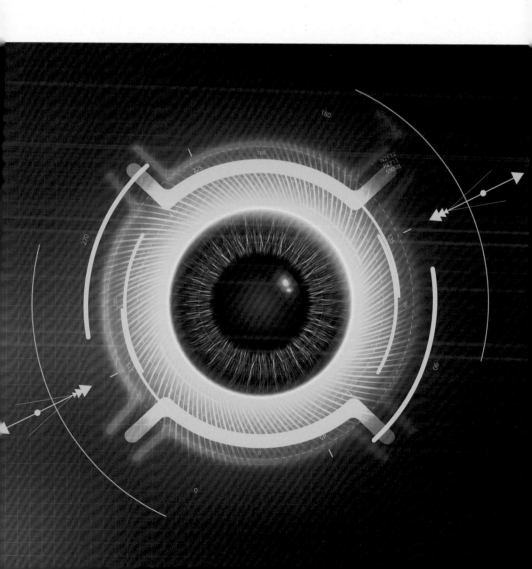

Part 8

Ocular Trauma

CHAPTER 80

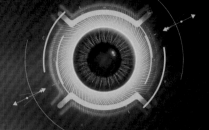

Commotio Retinae

SALIENT FEATURES

- Commotio retinae, also known as Berlin edema when involving the posterior pole, refers to the transient opacification of the retina secondary to blunt ocular trauma[1] (Figure 80.1).
- If macula is involved, it may lead to blurred vision and loss of central vision.
- Commotio retinae is typically self-limiting; there is no recommended treatment for it other than observation.[2]

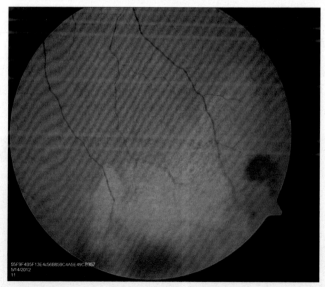

FIGURE 80.1 Color fundus photograph of peripheral commotio retinae with intraretinal hemorrhages in the left eye.

- Following injury, visual acuity usually resolves in about 4 weeks. However, complications such as retinal detachment, traumatic macular hole, retinal tears, choroidal rupture, or permanent photoreceptor/retinal pigment epitheium (RPE) atrophy may result in more permanent visual sequelae.[2]
- Optical coherence tomography (OCT) can confirm the diagnosis, evaluate persisting macular changes that may explain poor visual recovery, and identify concurrent injuries (eg, macular hole, choroidal rupture).[3]

OCT IMAGING

- The primary morphological feature of commotio retinae is disruption of photoreceptor outer segment (OS) layers (Figure 80.2).
- The hallmark feature of OCT imaging in commotio retinae is discontinuity of the ellipsoid zone (EZ, also known as IS/OS junction) as well as hyperreflectivity of the EZ with increased hyporeflectivity between EZ and and RPE. RPE layer disruption may also be present in more severe injury.[4]
- OCT imaging can be employed to evaluate injury severity of disrupted outer retina layers. More severe cases of commotio retinae, including defects of the external limiting membrane (ELM), EZ, and RPE are associated with worse visual acuity and anatomic outcomes over time (Figure 80.3).[5]
- Despite being referred to as Berlin edema, OCT imaging of commotio retinae does not illustrate any significant differences in foveal thickness and total macular volume.[4]

OCTA IMAGING

- The limited literature on optical coherence tomography angiography (OCTA) imaging in commotio retinae has not identified retinal vasculature changes or perfusion defects (Figure 80.4).[6,7]

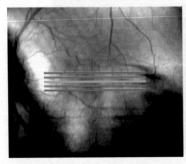
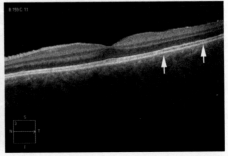

FIGURE 80.2 En-face and optical coherence tomography (OCT) B-scan of the same eye from Figure 80.1. Note the mild disruption of the ellipsoid zone temporally with increased hyporeflectivity cleft between ellipsoid zone and retinal pigment epitheium (RPE) (arrows).

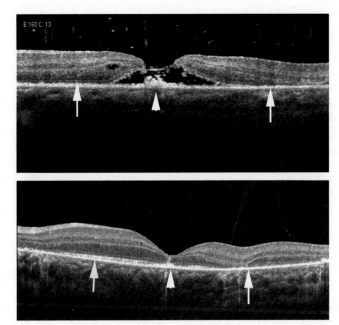

FIGURE 80.3 Optical coherence tomography (OCT) B-scan following blunt trauma to the eye. A, On the day of the injury, apparent "foveal rupture" is present with loss of foveal tissue and appearance of a macular hole (arrowhead, although the ILM appears to be bridging across the macular hole). Extensive ellipsoid zone loss is present (arrows) and hyperreflective foci are present in the vitreous, possibly from retinal disruption and/or vitreous hemorrhage). B, Two weeks following injury, the macular hole has spontaneously closed with subfoveal ellipsoid disruption but improvement (arrowhead). Outer retinal atrophy is present temporally (white arrow) and nasal ellipsoid zone reconstitution is noted (yellow arrow).

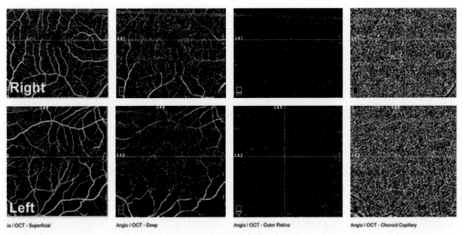

FIGURE 80.4 Optical coherence tomography angiography (OCTA) of traumatized right eye (top) and normal left eye (bottom) showing similar microvasculature in the superficial capillary plexus, deep capillary plexus, outer retina, and choriocapillaris. (Reprinted with permission from Mansour AM, Shields CL. Microvascular capillary plexus findings of commotio retinae on optical coherence tomography angiography. *Case Rep Ophthalmol.* 2018;9(3):473-478.)

References

1. Bradley JL, Shah SP, Manjunath V, Fujimoto JG, Duker JS, Reichel E. Ultra-high-resolution optical coherence tomographic findings in commotio retinae. *Arch Ophthalmol*. 2011;129(1):107-108. doi:10.1001/archophthalmol.2010.342.

2. Maiya AS, Zalaki B, Jayaram R, Ravi P, Noonthana S. Commotio retinae: report of 4 consecutive cases. *IOSR J Dental Med Sci*. 2015;14(10):45-48. doi:10.9790/0853-141044548.

3. Matri LE, Chebil A, Kort F, Bouraoui R, Largueche L, Mghaieth F. Optical coherence tomographic findings in Berlin's edema. *J Ophthalmic Vis Res*. 2010;5(2):127-129.

4. Park JY, Nam WH, Kim SH, Jang SY, Ohn YH, Park TK. Evaluation of the central macula in commotio retinae not associated with other types of traumatic retinopathy. *Korean J Ophthalmol*. 2011;25(4):262-267. doi:10.3341/kjo.2011.25.4.262.

5. Ahn SJ, Woo SJ, Kim KE, Jo DH, Ahn J, Park KH. Optical coherence tomography morphologic grading of macular commotio retinae and its association with anatomic and visual outcomes. *Am J Ophthalmol*. 2013;156(5):994-1001. doi:10.1016/j.ajo.2013.06.023.

6. Mansour AM, Shields CL. Microvascular capillary plexus findings of commotio retinae on optical coherence tomography angiography. *Case Rep Ophthalmol*. 2018;9(3):473-478. doi:10.1159/000494916.

7. Wangsathaporn K, Tsui I. Commotio retinae resulting from rubber band injury in two girls. *Ophthalmic Surg Lasers Imaging Retina*. 2019;50(5):309-313. doi:10.3928/23258160-20190503-08.

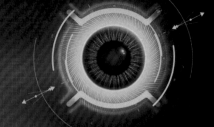

CHAPTER 81

Purtscher Retinopathy

SALIENT FEATURES

- Purtscher retinopathy is a rare retinopathy secondary to crushing chest or head injury.
- Purtscher-like retinopathy is used to describe similar findings in the setting of severe systemic insult such as acute pancreatitis, long bone fracture, renal failure, autoimmune disease, and others.
- The presentation is typically bilateral but may be asymmetric or unilateral.
- It is characterized by the presence of polygonal areas of retinal whitening between arterioles and venules (Purtscher flecken), cotton wool spots, and intraretinal hemorrhages in the posterior pole, generally peripapillary (Figure 81.1A).
- Purtscher flecken may be multiple, of variable size, and typically affect the superficial inner retina, with distribution generally limited to the macular and peripapillary regions.
- A pseudo–cherry red spot may be noted as a result of the contrast observed between the normal fovea and surrounding retinal whitening.
- Chronic signs commonly include optic disc pallor, retinal pigment epithelium (RPE) mottling, and retinal thinning.
- On fluorescein angiography, Purtscher and Purtscher-like retinopathy is characterized by areas of capillary nonperfusion, arteriolar occlusion, and late leakage of the optic disc and in areas of ischemia.

OCT IMAGING

- Cotton wool spots and Purtscher flecken manifest as hyperreflectivity and thickening of the nerve fiber layer and ganglion cell layer with posterior shadowing on optical coherence tomography (OCT) (Figures 81.1 and 81.2).

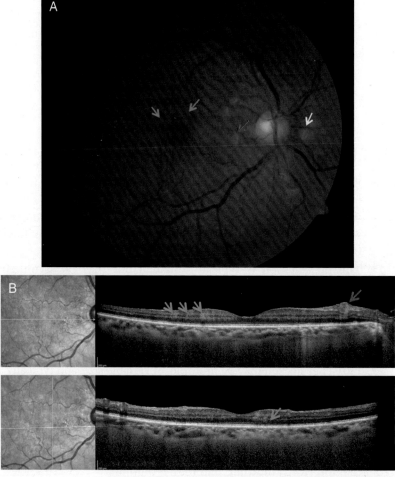

FIGURE 81.1 A, Color fundus photograph of a patient with Purtscher-like retinopathy in the subacute phase. The blue arrows demonstrate paracentral acute middle maculopathy lesions with subtle whitening on fundus photography and hyperreflectivity of the middle retinal layers on the corresponding optical coherence tomography (OCT) (B). The red arrow on fundus photography highlights a cotton wool spot which manifests as an area of hyperreflectivity of the retinal nerve fiber layer on OCT (B, red arrow). A larger polygonal area of retinal whitening is termed a Purtscher flecken (yellow arrow). B, Corresponding OCT image demonstrating hyperreflectivity in the nerve fiber layer (red arrow) with posterior shadowing consistent with a cotton wool spot, corresponding to an area of retinal whitening on fundus photo, and multiple areas of hyperreflectivity in the inner plexiform, inner nuclear, and outer plexiform layers (blue and green arrows).

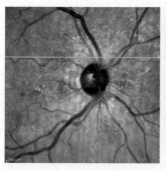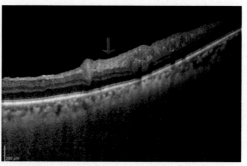

FIGURE 81.2 Optical coherence tomographic image through a Purtscher flecken demonstrates hyperreflectivity and thickening of the retinal nerve fiber layer (red arrow).

- Paracentral acute middle maculopathy lesions (bands of hyperreflectivity of the inner nuclear layer) may be identified with OCT, indicative of ischemia of the intermediate and deep capillary plexus (Figure 81.1, blue arrows).
- Subretinal and intraretinal fluid with retinal thickening may be present.
- In the chronic phase, there is inner retinal atrophy in prior areas of Purtshcer flecken and CWS, a finding which may carry prognostic value.

OCTA IMAGING

- Flow voids in both the superficial and deep capillary plexuses are seen on optical coherence tomography angiography (OCTA), often colocalizing to areas with cotton wool spots and Purtscher flecken.
- Nonperfusion regions may extend beyond clinically visible cotton wool spots.
- Revascularization, if it occurs, may correlate to visual improvement.

References

1. Agrawal A, McKibbin M. Purtscher's retinopathy: epidemiology, clinical features and outcome. *Br J Ophthalmol Lond.* 2007;91(11):1456.
2. Miguel AIM, Henriques F, Azevedo LFR, Loureiro AJR, Maberley DAL. Systematic review of Purtscher's and Purtscher-like retinopathies. *Eye Lond.* 2013;27(1):1-13.
3. Gil P, Pires J, Costa E, Matos R, Cardoso MS, Mariano M. Purtscher retinopathy: to treat or not to treat? *Eur J Ophthalmol.* 2015;25(6):e112-e115.
4. Hamoudi H, Nielsen MK, Sørensen TL. Optical coherence tomography angiography of Purtscher retinopathy after severe traffic accident in 16-year-old boy. *Case Rep Ophthalmol Med.* 2018;2018:4318354.
5. Xiao W, He L, Mao Y, Yang H. Multimodal imaging in Purtscher retinopathy. *Retina.* 2018;38(7):e59-e60.

6. Beckingsale AB, Rosenthal AR. Early fundus fluorescein angiographic findings and sequelae in traumatic retinopathy: case report. *Br J Ophthalmol.* 1983;67(2):119-123. doi:10.1136/bjo.67.2.119.

7. Holak HM, Holak S. Prognostic factors for visual outcome in Purtscher retinopathy. *Surv Ophthalmol.* 2007;52(1):117-118; author reply 118-9. doi:10.1016/j.survophthal.2006.10.012.

8. Gil P, Raimundo M, Marques JP, Póvoa J, Silva R. Optical coherence tomography angiography characterization of acute and late stage Purtscher retinopathy. *Eur J Ophthalmol.* 2018;28(4):NP1-NP6. doi:10.1177/1120672118769788.

9. Santamaría Álvarez JF, Serret Camps A, Aguayo Alvarez J, García García O. Optic coherence tomography angiography follow-up in a case of Purtscher-like retinopathy due to atypical hemolytic uremic syndrome. *Eur J Ophthalmol.* 2019;30(3):NP14-NP17. doi:10.1177/1120672119833277s.

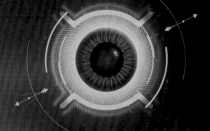

CHAPTER 82

Choroidal Rupture

SALIENT FEATURES[1]

- Choroidal rupture occurs most commonly as a result of nonperforating blunt ocular trauma.
- Although direct rupture can occur at the site of trauma, indirect rupture secondary to anteroposterior globe compression is most common. This compression causes shearing of the choroid in the horizontal plane and results in breaks in choroid, Bruch membrane, and retinal piment epithelium (RPE).
- On examination, choroidal rupture appears as a yellow/white, curvilinear, subretinal lesion and can be acutely accompanied by intra- or subretinal hemorrhage.
- Final visual outcomes are dependent on the location of the rupture site, concurrent injuries (eg, macular hole), and the occurrence of long-term complications (eg, development of choroidal neovascularization [CNV]).
- Poor-presenting visual acuity and rupture within the posterior pole are both associated with poorer final visual acuity.
- Risk factors associated with development of CNV include older age, posterior pole location, and increased length of rupture.
- Optical coherence tomography (OCT) imaging is routinely used in choroidal rupture to confirm Bruch membrane breaks and monitor for signs of CNV development at these sites.
- Optical coherence tomography angiography (OCTA) imaging can also be used to visualize CNV and gauge its response to treatment.

OCT IMAGING

- OCT can aid in assessing the extent, precise location, and severity of choroidal rupture (Figures 82.1 and 82.2).
- In addition, OCT provides additional information related to concurrent retinal injuries, such as full-thickness macular hole and commotion retinae (Figure 82.3).
- Rupture healing through fibrovascular proliferation and RPE hyperplasia can also be followed by OCT and typically appears as a new area of hyperreflectivity at rupture site (Figure 82.2)[2]; sites of severe tissue damage or choroidal/RPE discontinuity are less likely to exhibit signs of healing.[3]
- Long-term complications such as subretinal fibrosis and development of an exudative choroidal neovascular membrane (CNVM) can also be detected.[3]

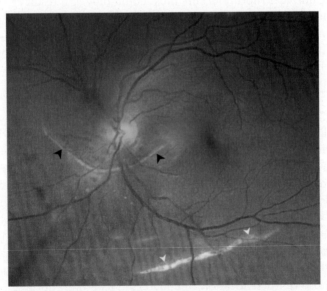

FIGURE 82.1 Fundus photo following blunt ocular trauma. Note the classic curvilinear pattern of the rupture just inferior to the optic nerve which extends both nasally and temporally into the macula (black arrowheads). A second linear choroidal rupture is found inferior to the inferotemporal arcade with visualization of the choroidal vessels (white arrowheads). Associated retinal hemorrhages are seen nasal to the ruptures and are common.

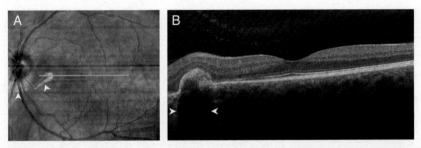

FIGURE 82.2 Optical coherence tomography (OCT) of choroidal rupture. A, Near-infrared imaging of the same patient in Figure 82.1 shows hyporeflectivity in the area of the choroidal rupture (white arrowheads). B, B-scan OCT demonstrates nasal choroidal rupture with disruption of the outer retinal layers and upward displacement the overlying inner retinal layers (red asterisk); a hyporeflective shadowing is also present below the lesion (white arrowheads).

OCTA IMAGING

- OCTA can be used to identify choroidal breaks which appear as a hypointense area within the choriocapillaris plexus.[4]
- Ruptures located within the macula are at highest risk for the development of CNVM.[3]
- OCTA imaging can be used to monitor for the development of CNV associated with rupture sites; sites of CNV appear as well-circumscribed, hyperintense vascular networks (Figure 82.4).[4,5]

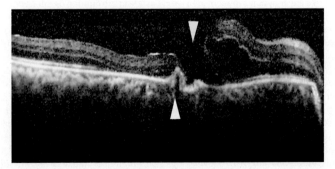

FIGURE 82.3 Choroidal rupture with associated full-thickness macular hole. Optical coherence tomography (OCT) B-scan demonstrating subfoveal choroidal rupture (white arrowhead), full-thickness macular hole (yellow arrowhead), and temporal outer retinal atrophy.

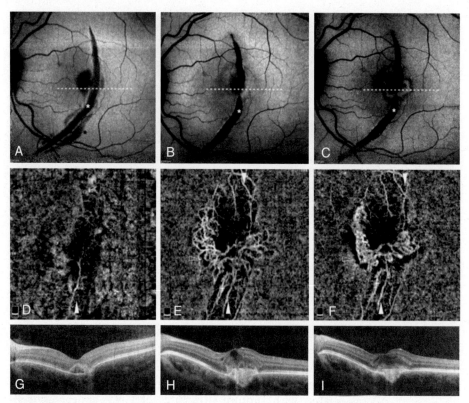

FIGURE 82.4 Imaging of development of choroidal neovascularization (CNV) secondary to choroidal rupture and following bevacizumab injection. Fundus autofluorescence (A-C), optical coherence tomography angiography (OCTA) (3 × 3 mm) (D-F), and optical coherence tomography (OCT) (G-I) at baseline (A, D, and G), at 6-month follow-up (B, E, and H), and 1 month after bevacizumab injection (C, F, and I). The white dotted line marks where the OCT section was taken. Fundus autofluorescence at baseline (A) shows the choroidal rupture with a linear hypofluorescent area (white asterisk) surrounded by intraretinal and subretinal hemorrhages corresponding to mild hypofluorescent areas (black asterisk). At serial follow-up (B and C), the hypofluorescent crescentic choroidal rupture (white asterisk) persists, with resolution of hemorrhages (B) and the CNV location visible by the appearance of a linear hypofluorescent area (white asterisk) with central hyperfluorescent area (black asterisk) (C). Baseline optical coherence tomography angiography (D) reveals the choroidal rupture as a line of severe choriocapillaris rarefaction with projection of superficial retinal vessels (white arrowhead). At 6-month post injection, the CNV is seen as a clear tangled network (white open arrowhead, E) associated with the site of choroidal rupture, improving post treatment as it appears smaller with clearly defined margins (white open arrowhead, F). Projections of superficial retinal vessels are present in OCTA scan (white arrowhead, E and F). Baseline optical coherence tomography scan (G) demonstrates the choroidal rupture as perturbation at multiple layers: retinal pigment epithelium, Bruch membrane, and choriocapillaris. On OCT, the CNV is marked by the presence of hyperreflective material and mild intraretinal fluid (H). Following injection, intraretinal fluid resolves with subfoveal hyperreflective material remaining (I). (Reprinted with permission from Preziosa C, Corvi F, Pellegrini M, et al. Optical coherence tomography angiography findings in a case of choroidal neovascularization secondary to traumatic choroidal rupture. *Retin Cases Brief Rep.* 2018;1-4.)

References

1. Ament CS, Zacks DN, Lane AM, et al. Predictors of visual outcome and choroidal neovascular membrane formation after traumatic choroidal rupture. *Arch Ophthalmol.* 2006;124:957-966.

2. Lavinsky D, Martins EN, Cardillo JA, Farah ME. Fundus autofluorescence in patients with blunt ocular trauma. *Acta Ophthalmol.* 2011;89:e89-e94.

3. Shin JY, Chung B, Na YH, et al. Retinal pigment epithelium wound healing after traumatic choroidal rupture. *Acta Ophthalmol.* 2017;95(7):e582-e586.

4. Lorusso M, Ferrari LM, Nikolopoulou E, Ferrari TM. Case report: optical coherence tomography angiography evolution of choroidal neovascular membrane in choroidal rupture managed by intravitreal bevacizumab. *Case Rep Ophthalmol Med.* 2019;2019:5241573. doi:10.1155/2019/5241573.

5. Preziosa C, Corvi F, Pellegrini M, Bochicchio S, Rosar AP, Staurenghi G. Optical coherence tomography angiography findings in a case of choroidal neovascularization secondary to traumatic choroidal rupture. *Retin Cases Brief Rep.* 2018. doi:10.1097/ICB.0000000000000704.

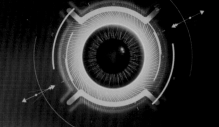

CHAPTER 83

Chorioretinitis Sclopetaria

SALIENT FEATURES

- Chorioretinitis sclopetaria involves the simultaneous rupture of the choroid and retina but not the sclera in the setting of trauma secondary to a high-speed missile, usually a bullet.
- Damage is believed to be from both direct deformation of the globe by the bullet and an indirect shockwave injury from the force of the bullet entering the orbit.[1]
- Acutely patients present with patches of choroidal and retinal hemorrhages (Figure 83.1). Within weeks, a full-thickness chorioretinal defect with white fibrous proliferation and surrounding pigmentary changes presents.[2] Rarely, patients will present with early retinal detachment.[3] Late retinal detachment is rare due to full-thickness choroidal and retinal scarring.
- Fluorescein angiography in chorioretinitis sclopetaria displays early hypofluorescence from both blocking from fibrous proliferation and focal loss of chorioretinal tissue. Late frames show hyperfluorescent staining at lesion edges and bed of sclera.
- Indocyanine green demonstrates a lack of choroidal flow within the lesion throughout the study.
- Fundus autofluorescence shows hypoautoflorescence of lesion due to lack of any chorioretinal structures.
- Computed tomography may reveal a retained orbital foreign body and/or bony defects.

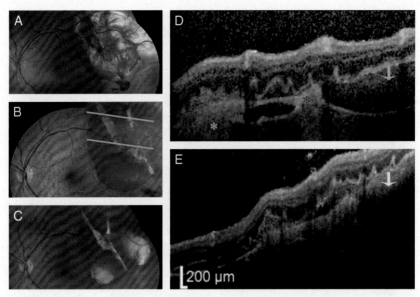

FIGURE 83.1 Fundus photos of 14-year-old male after firework injury to the left orbit at 1 day (A), 8 days (B), and 22 days (C) after presentation showing the evolution of pre-, intra-, and subretinal hemorrhages and temporal chorioretinal atrophy. Green arrows denote two spectral-domain optical coherence tomographies (SD-OCTs) cuts taken eight days after injury through the superior and inferior portions of the lesion (D and E) that demonstrate subretinal fibrosis (red asterisks), choroidal fibrosis (green asterisk), subretinal fluid (green arrow), and subretinal hemorrhage (yellow arrow).

OCT IMAGING

- Optical coherence tomography (OCT) can demonstrate full-thickness hyperreflectivity and disorganization consistent with chorioretinal disruption (Figure 83.1) and reparative gliotic proliferation (Figures 83.2B and 83.3).[4]
- Visual prognosis can be determined based on the degree of subfoveal hemorrhage and gliosis (Figure 83.4).
- The inner retina can become focally edematous (Figure 83.3), but outer retinal pathology is more common (Figures 83.2B, 83.3, and 83.4).

OCTA IMAGING

- Currently, optical coherence tomography angiography (OCTA) imaging holds no role in the diagnosis or management of chorioretinitis sclopetaria.

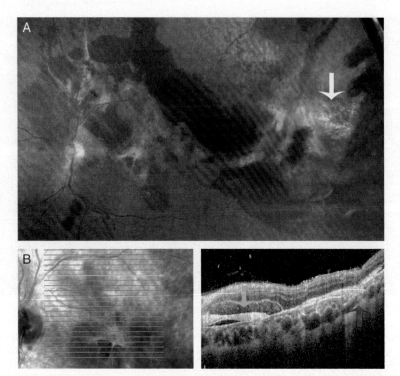

FIGURE 83.2 A, Fundus photo of 22-year-old female after gunshot wound to the left orbit showing full-thickness chorioretinal fibrosis temporal to the macula (white arrow). Subretinal, intraretinal, and preretinal hemorrhage are evident throughout the macula, especially superotemporally. B, Spectral-domain optical coherence tomography (SD-OCT) showing vitreous opacities consistent with hemorrhage and relative preservation of inner retina and mild thickening of the outer nuclear layer. Subretinal fluid, hemorrhage, and fibrosis are present (green arrow). Retinal pigment epithelium (RPE) and inner choroid are focally disrupted temporally, highlighted by increased shine through (red arrow).

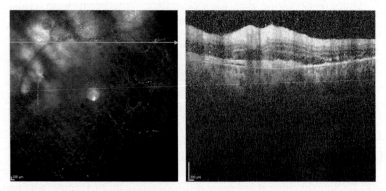

FIGURE 83.3 Spectral-domain optical coherence tomography (SD-OCT) of the superior macula of a 23-year-old male status post gunshot wound to the left orbit showing increased hyperreflectivity and thickening of the retinal nerve fiber layer, outer retinal lamination disruption, and subretinal fibrosis.

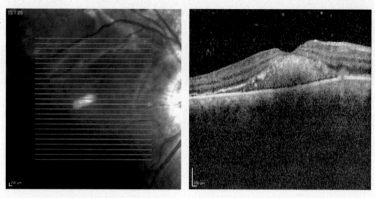

FIGURE 83.4 Spectral-domain optical coherence tomography (SD-OCT) of the right fovea of a 22-year-old male status post impalement of his right superior rectus complex by a metal-cutting diamond blade showing subretinal hemorrhage.

References

1. Richards RD, West CE, Meisels AA. Chorioretinitis sclopetaria. *Am J Ophthalmol.* 1968;66:852-860. Available at: http://www.ncbi.nlm.nih.gov/pubmed/5686914.

2. Martin DF, Awh CC, McCuen BW, et al. Treatment and pathogenesis of traumatic chorioretinal rupture (sclopetaria). *Am J Ophthalmol.* 1994;117:190-200. Available at: http://www.ncbi.nlm.nih.gov/pubmed/8116747.

3. Papakostas TD, Yonekawa Y, Wu D, et al. Retinal detachment associated with traumatic chorioretinal rupture. *Ophthalmic Surg Lasers Imaging Retina.* 2014;45:451-455. Available at: http://www.ncbi.nlm.nih.gov/pubmed/25153657.

4. Rayess N, Rahimy E, Ho AC. Spectral-domain optical coherence tomography features of bilateral chorioretinitis sclopetaria. *Ophthalmic Surg Lasers Imaging Retina.* 2015;46:253-255. Available at: http://www.ncbi.nlm.nih.gov/pubmed/25707053.

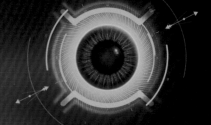

CHAPTER 84

Laser Maculopathy

SALIENT FEATURES

- Laser maculopathy most commonly occurs in teenagers but is reported in a wide range of ages.[1-3] It also has been associated with behavioral and mental disorders.[2,4]
- Patients present with decreased vision, some with profound vision loss and central scotoma.[1-7] Vision may improve over many years, but central scotoma may persist.[5]
- On fundus examination, streaky or focal yellow to white lesions are seen in the posterior pole. Pigmentary changes are commonly seen.[1-5] Retinal hemorrhage may be seen in the acute phase.[6]
- The lesion may evolve into lamellar or macular hole.[1,2]

OCT IMAGING

- Optical coherence tomography (OCT) may show ellipsoid zone (EZ) disruption, hyperreflective curvilinear lesion, hyporeflective cleft reminiscent of fluid, and macular hole (Figures 84.1 and 84.2). Near-infrared image can show streaky linear lesions (Figure 84.3).[1-7]
- With improvement in vision, improvement in OCT may be observed over time. Greater improvements are seen in the inner retina, while the outer retinal changes often do not fully resolve.[2,5]

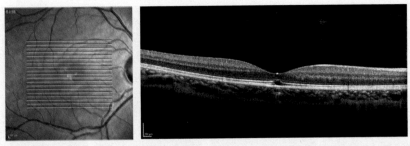

FIGURE 84.1 Self-inflicted laser maculopathy. Near-infrared image on the left shows multiple curvilinear lesions near the fovea. Optical coherence tomography (OCT) B-scan demonstrates disruption of ellipsoid zone (EZ) and interdigitation zone (IZ) with hyporeflective cleft centrally, corresponding to the lesion seen on near-infrared image. (Reprinted with permission from Riccardo Sacconi, MD, FEBO.)

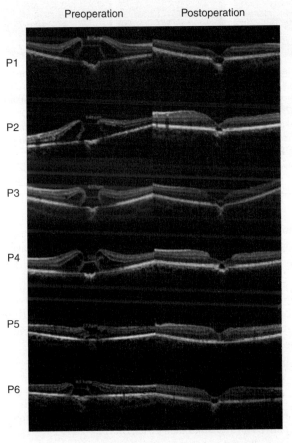

FIGURE 84.2 Macular spectral-domain optical coherence tomography (SD-OCT) of eyes with laser maculopathy–induced macular holes preoperatively and postsurgical repair. Subfoveal retinal pigment epithelium (RPE) disturbance is noted. (Reprinted with permission from Qi Y, Wang Y, You Q, Tsai F, Liu W. Surgical treatment and optical coherence tomographic evaluation for accidental laser-induced full-thickness macular holes. *Eye*. 2017;31(7):1078-1084.)

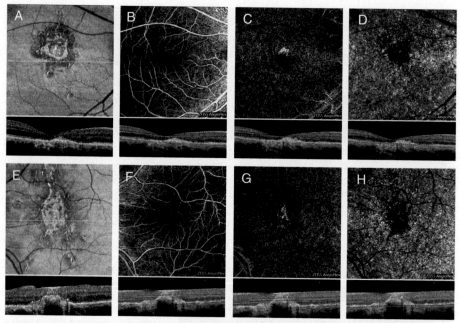

FIGURE 84.3 Near-infrared en-face image, structural optical coherence tomography (OCT), and optical coherence tomography angiography (OCTA) approximately 2 months after initial injury to right (top) and left eyes (bottom). Near-infrared en-face image shows coalesced lesion with associated radial marked change that matches ellipsoid zone (EZ) loss and disorganization seen in structural OCT (A and E). OCTA reveals vascular flow within the central areas of fibrosis (C and G) and an absent flow signal on the inner choroidal slab (D and H). The superficial capillary plexus did not show frank flow defect (B and F). (Reprinted with permission from Rabiolo A, Sacconi R, Giuffrè C, et al. Self-inflicted laser handheld laser-induced maculopathy: a novel ocular manifestation of factitious disorder. *Retin Cases Brief Rep.* 2018;12(suppl 1):S46-S50.)

OCTA IMAGING

- In the corresponding areas of changes in OCT, optical coherence tomography angiography (OCTA) shows hyperreflective material in the vascular pattern in the outer retina, resembling choroidal neovascularization.[3,4]

- In addition, there is an absence of flow signal in choriocapillaris layer. While this could be due to rarefaction of the choriocapillaris, this could also represent artifact due to hyperreflective changes overlying the choriocapillaris.[3,4,7]

- The superficial capillary plexus shows normal flow pattern.[3,4]

References

1. Bhavsar KV, Wilson D, Margolis R, et al. Multimodal imaging in handheld laser-induced maculopathy. *Am J Ophthalmol.* 2015;159:227-231.
2. Linton E, Walkden A, Steeples LR, et al. Retinal burns from laser pointers: a risk in children with behavioural problems. *Eye (Lond).* 2019;33(3):492-504.

3. Clemente-Tomás R, Bayo-Calduch P, Neira-Ibáñez P, Gargallo-Benedicto A, Duch-Samper AM. Bilateral maculopathy after exposure to a laser pointer: optical coherence tomography angiography findings. *Arch Soc Esp Oftalmol.* 2018;93(11):551-554.

4. Rabiolo A, Sacconi R, Giuffrè C, et al. Self-inflicted laser handheld laser-induced maculopathy: a novel ocular manifestation of factitious disorder. *Retin Cases Brief Rep.* 2018;12(suppl 1):S46-S50.

5. Chen X, Dajani OAW, Alibhai AY, Duker JS, Baumal CR. Long-term visual recovery in bilateral handheld laser pointer-induced maculopathy. *Retin Cases Brief Rep.* 2019.

6. Birtel JM, Harmening WU, Krohne TG, Holz F, Charbel Issa P, Herrmann P. Retinal injury following laser pointer exposure: a systematic review and case series. *Dtsch Arztebl Int.* 2017;114:831-837.

7. Tomasso L, Benatti L, La Spina C, et al. Optical coherence tomography angiography findings in laser maculopathy. *Eur J Ophthalmol.* 2017;27(1):e13-e15.

8. Qi Y, Wang Y, You Q, Tsai F, Liu W. Surgical treatment and optical coherence tomographic evaluation for accidental laser-induced full-thickness macular holes. *Eye.* 2017;31(7):1078-1084.

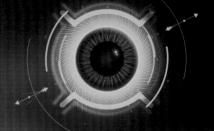

CHAPTER 85

Solar Retinopathy

SALIENT FEATURES

- Solar retinopathy occurs due to photochemical damage to the outer retinal layers, specifically, the external limiting membrane, photoreceptors, and the retinal pigment epithelium (RPE).[1-3]
- The wavelength of light mainly responsible for this damage is in the 400 to 500 nm range, and the mechanism of injury is largely due to free radical formation and oxidative damage.[2,4-6]
- Most cases are secondary to solar eclipse viewing, but retinopathy is also associated with sun gazing in the context of religious events, psychiatric conditions, and consumption of hallucinogens.[1,7]
- Fundus examination findings vary depending on the degree of damage and when the examination is performed.[7] Findings may be very minimal for mild damage and may include only slight grayish discoloration at the RPE level.[7] In cases of more significant damage, yellow spots at the foveola are seen acutely, and over time, they become reddish circular lesions at the foveola (Figure 85.1).[7]
- Fortunately, the prognosis of solar retinopathy is generally quite favorable as the majority of patients recover their baseline visual acuity at least partially, if not fully. A minority of patients have persistent central scotomas, metamorphopsia, and decreased visual acuity.[2,8]

OCT IMAGING

- Spectral-domain optical coherence tomography (SD-OCT) of retinal changes immediately after solar injury shows hyperreflectivity of all retinal layers at the center of the fovea, which is thought to suggest photoreceptor injury and disorganization in the hyperacute stage.[1,9]

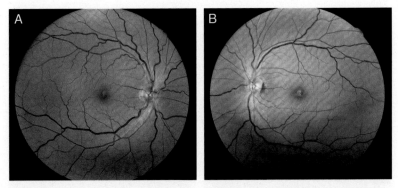

FIGURE 85.1 Fundus photos of a patient with solar retinopathy in both eyes. There is a well-circumscribed, yellow foveal lesion in both eyes, more prominent in the left eye (B) than the right eye (A). There is mild, symmetric vascular tortuosity in both eyes.

- Over time, the hyperreflectivity resolves and what remains are hyporeflective cavitations in the outer retina corresponding to EZ/interdigitation zone (IZ) loss (Figure 85.2).[1,9] There may also be RPE changes such as atrophy manifesting as hypertransmission light signaling (Figure 85.2) with or without reactive RPE hypertrophy.[1,9-12]

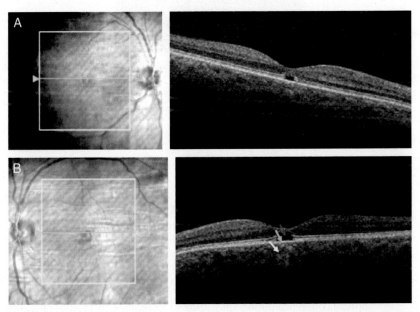

FIGURE 85.2 Spectral-domain optical coherence tomography (SD-OCT) of the right (A) and left (B) eyes of a patient with solar retinopathy. In the right eye, there is loss of the ellipsoid zone (EZ) and interdigitation zone (IZ) (red arrow). In the left eye, there is EZ/IZ loss (red arrow) as well as slight retinal pigment epithelium (RPE)/Bruch membrane complex attenuation (green arrow) with resulting signal hypertransmission (yellow arrow) to the choroid at the fovea.

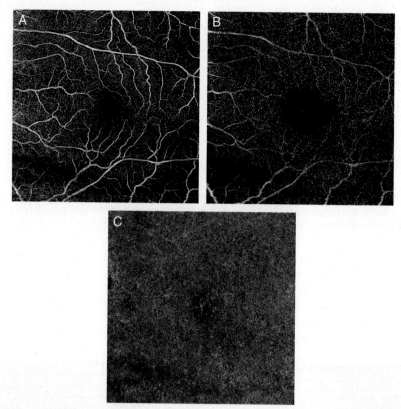

FIGURE 85.3 Swept-source optical coherence tomography angiography (SS-OCTA) of the left eye of the same patient in Figure 85.2. En-face SS-OCTA of the superficial capillary plexus (A) and deep capillary plexus (B) demonstrate normal vasculature. There is a focal flow void at the level of the choriocapillaris (C).

OCTA IMAGING

- OCT angiography (OCTA) is rarely utilized in this diagnosis. However, if the RPE is significantly affected, OCTA imaging at the level of the choriocapillaris may demonstrate flow voids (Figure 85.3, red arrow).

References

1. Wu CY, Jansen ME, Andrade J, et al. Acute solar retinopathy imaged with adaptive optics, optical coherence tomography angiography, and en face optical coherence tomography. *JAMA Ophthalmol.* 2018;136(1):82-85.
2. Begaj T, Schaal S. Sunlight and ultraviolet radiation-pertinent retinal implications and current management. *Surv Ophthalmol.* 2018;63(2):174-192.
3. Hope-Ross MW, Mahon GJ, Gardiner TA, Archer DB. Ultrastructural findings in solar retinopathy. *Eye (Lond).* 1993;7(pt 1):29-33.

4. Ham WT, Ruffolo JJ, Mueller HA, Clarke AM, Moon ME. Histologic analysis of photochemical lesions produced in rhesus retina by short-wave-length light. *Invest Ophthalmol Vis Sci*. 1978;17(10):1029-1035.

5. Okuno T. Hazards of solar blue light. *Appl Opt*. 2008;47(16):2988-2992.

6. Marshall J. Light in man's environment. *Eye (Lond)*. 2016;30(2):211-214.

7. Yannuzzi LA, Fisher YL, Slakter JS, Krueger A. Solar retinopathy. A photobiologic and geophysical analysis. *Retina*. 1989;9(1):28-43.

8. Atmaca LS, Idil A, Can D. Early and late visual prognosis in solar retinopathy. *Graefes Arch Clin Exp Ophthalmol*. 1995;233(12):801-804.

9. Merino-Suarez ML, Belmonte-Martin J, Rodrigo-Auria F, Perez-Cambrodi RJ, Pinero DP. Optical coherence tomography and autofluoresceingraphy changes in solar retinopathy. *Can J Ophthalmol*. 2017;52(2):e67-e71.

10. Goduni L, Mehta N, Tsui E, et al. Long-term multimodal imaging of solar retinopathy. *Ophthalmic Surg Lasers Imaging Retina*. 2019;50(6):388-392.

11. Chen KC, Jung JJ, Aizman A. High definition spectral domain optical coherence tomography findings in three patients with solar retinopathy and review of the literature. *Open Ophthalmol J*. 2012;6:29-35.

12. Jain A, Desai RU, Charalel RA, Quiram P, Yannuzzi L, Sarraf D. Solar retinopathy: comparison of optical coherence tomography (OCT) and fluorescein angiography (FA). *Retina*. 2009;29(9):1340-1345.

Part 9

Intraoperative and Postoperative Imaging

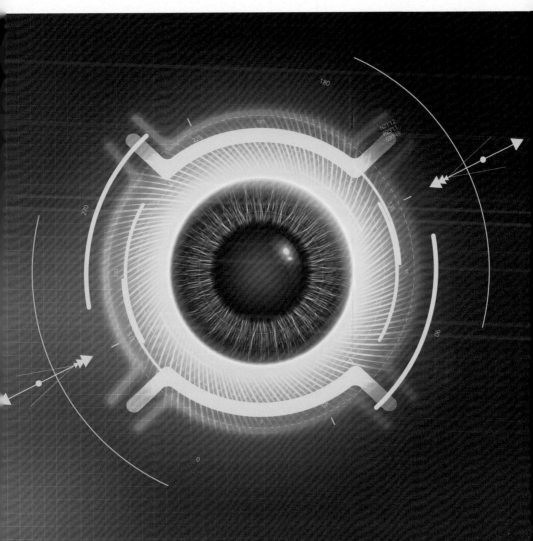

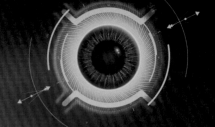

CHAPTER 86

Intraoperative Optical Coherence Tomography

SALIENT FEATURES

Evolution of Intraoperative OCT Devices

- The first commercial handheld ophthalmic optical coherence tomography (OCT) probe was developed in 2007 and in 2009 was first utilized for intraoperative OCT (iOCT).[1]
- Mounting systems that enabled attachment of portable probe to microscope head allowed for foot-pedal control and improved image reproducibility.
- Microscope-integrated OCT systems provided a more seamless platform for imaging during surgery and real-time visualization of instrument interactions with tissue without having to pause surgery for imaging.
- Heads-up display, enhanced targeting and tracking, tunable focus, and real-time volumetric visualization with high-speed swept-source iOCT systems have pushed the integration of OCT into the operating room forward.[2]

Clinical Utility

- iOCT has provided new insights to surgical pathology and demonstrated potential significant utility to surgical decision-making and intraoperative anatomic feedback for surgeons.[2-4]
- In posterior segment surgeries, iOCT has been shown to add surgeon-perceived valuable information in over 55% of cases and directly impact surgical decision in nearly 30% of cases.[3,4]

OCT IMAGING

Vitreoretinal Interface Conditions

- iOCT may be utilized during membrane peeling such as macular hole repair surgery, epiretinal membrane peel, and vitreomacular traction syndrome (Figures 86.1-86.4).
- iOCT provides key information about confirmation of adequate peel and presence of residual membranes.
- Instrument/retinal tissue interaction and anatomical changes such as increased distance between retinal pigment epithelium and ellipsoid zone following membrane peel can be visualized by iOCT.[3,4]

Retinal Detachment

- Occult subretinal and preretinal membranes, retinal breaks, persistent subretinal, and subclinical macular holes visualized by iOCT have potential impact on surgical decision-making (Figure 86.5).
- Intraoperative findings may be helpful in predicting postoperative functional outcomes.[3,4]

Proliferative Diabetic Retinopathy

- iOCT findings are particularly valuable in identifying surgical dissection planes, tractional membranes, retinal detachments, subclinical retinal breaks, and schisis for surgical proliferative diabetic retinopathy management.
- In cases with vitreous hemorrhage where preoperative assessment is limited, iOCT enables visualization of underlying pathology with high-level cross-sectional detail.

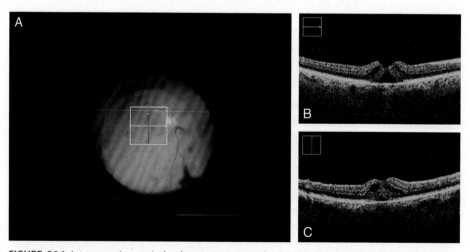

FIGURE 86.1 Intraoperative optical coherence tomography (iOCT) during macular hole (MH) repair. A, Intraoperative fundus photograph. Blue and pink lines show cross section of images in B and C, respectively. B and C, iOCT image of full-thickness MH with associated intraretinal cystic changes.

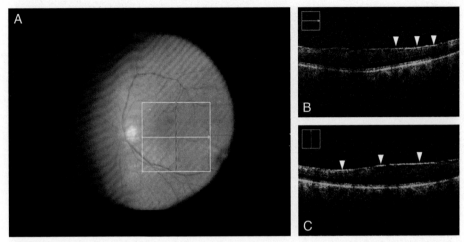

FIGURE 86.2 Intraoperative optical coherence tomography (iOCT) during epiretinal membrane surgery. A, Intraoperative fundoscopic fundus photograph prior to membrane peel following staining with indocyanine green (ICG). Blue and pink lines show cross section of images in B and C, respectively. B and C, iOCT image of epiretinal membrane represented by thin line of hyperreflectivity (arrowheads). Increased reflectivity and underlying retinal tissue shadowing are secondary to ICG staining and impact on OCT signal.

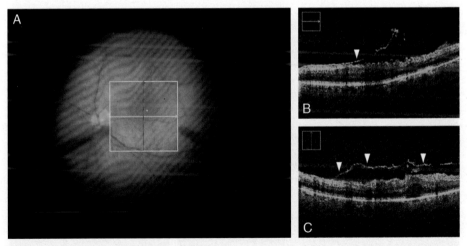

FIGURE 86.3 Intraoperative optical coherence tomography (iOCT) during epiretinal membrane peel. A, Intraoperative fundus photograph following partial membrane peel. Blue and pink lines show cross section of images in B and C, respectively. B and C, iOCT following membrane peeling demonstrates partial peel with membrane freely floating above foveal center (arrowheads). iOCT also identifies persistent nasal adherence of membrane.

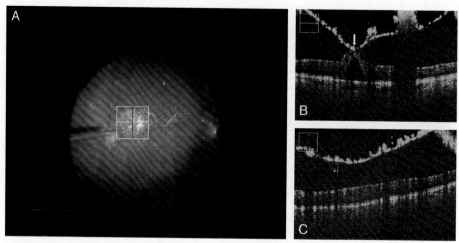

FIGURE 86.4 Intraoperative optical coherence tomography (OCT) demonstrating vitreomacular traction repair. A, Intraoperative fundus photograph prior to removal of the vitreous traction. Triamcinolone particles are visible in the vitreous. Blue and pink lines show cross section of images in B and C, respectively. B and C, Increased reflectivity is demonstrated at the posterior hyaloid secondary to triamcinolone, providing increased visualization of dissection planes. Foveal adhesion is well visualized (white arrow) with associated significant traction and subretinal fluid. Underlying shadowing of the retina is present due to the overlying triamcinolone particles.

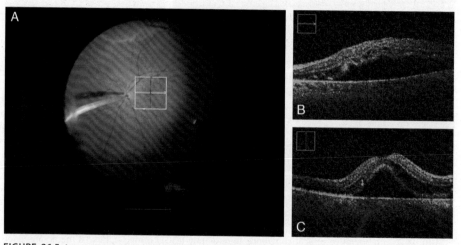

FIGURE 86.5 Intraoperative optical coherence tomography (iOCT) during retinal detachment repair. A, Intraoperative fundus photograph prior to perfluorocarbon liquid placement. Blue and pink lines show cross section of images in B and C, respectively. B and C, iOCT image demonstrates rhegmatogenous retinal detachment involving the macula with significant subretinal fluid and outer retinal undulations.

Other Retinal Pathologies

- Emerging areas of new surgical procedures may provide exciting opportunities for the application of iOCT technology.
- Retinal prosthesis placement, retinal biopsy, and delivery of targeted therapeutics such as gene and stem cell therapy are other interventions where iOCT may provide clinically useful information including tissue configurations, visualization of tissue-implant interface, and confirmation of location and volume of therapeutic delivery.

References

1. Dayani PN, Maldonado R, Farsiu S, Toth CA. Intraoperative use of handheld spectral domain optical coherence tomography imaging in macular surgery. *Retina*. 2009;29:1457-1468.
2. Khan M, Ehlers JP. Clinical utility of intraoperative optical coherence tomography. *Curr Opin Ophthalmol*. 2016;27:201-209.
3. Ehlers JP, Modi YS, Pecen PE, et al. The DISCOVER study 3-year results: feasibility and usefulness of microscope-integrated intraoperative OCT during ophthalmic surgery. *Ophthalmology*. 2018;125:1014-1027.
4. Ehlers JP, Dupps WJ, Kaiser PK, et al. The prospective intraoperative and perioperative ophthalmic ImagiNg with optical CoherEncE TomogRaphy (PIONEER) study: 2-year results. *Am J Ophthalmol*. 2014;158:999-1007.

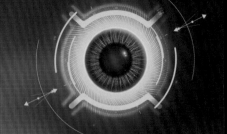

CHAPTER 87

Subretinal Perfluoron

SALIENT FEATURES

- Perfluorocarbon liquids (PFCLs) are used in a wide variety of vitreo-retinal surgeries but most commonly during repair of rhegmatogenous retinal detachments (RRDs), particularly when associated with proliferative vitreoretinopathy[1] or giant retinal tears (Figure 87.1).[1]
- PFCL properties include optical clarity, specific gravity higher than balanced saline solution, low viscosity, and surface tension.[2]

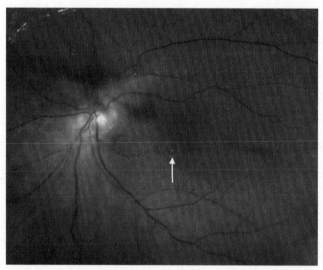

FIGURE 87.1 Optos image of initial presentation of a patient with chronic retained subfoveal perfluoro-carbon liquid (PFCL) after complex rhegmatogenous retinal detachment (RRD) repair (white arrow).

- The aforementioned properties permit flattening of the retina, unrolling of edges/folds with facilitation of subretinal fluid drainage, stabilization of the peripheral retina, maintenance of good visualization in complex cases, and straightforward injection and removal.
- Retained PFCL can lead to retinal toxicity with effects on the retinal pigment epithelium (RPE) and photoreceptors.[3]
- Retained subretinal PFCL can result in localized absolute scotoma and decreased visual acuity.[3]
- Surgical removal may be necessary, especially when located subfoveal.
- This is a challenging surgical situation with multiple approaches described. Recent use of intraoperative optical coherence tomography (OCT) can aid in this complicated surgery and in the identification of subretinal PFCL at the initial surgery.[4]

OCT IMAGING

- OCT is the modality of choice for imaging and confirming retained PFCL droplets as the diagnosis as it reveals characteristic features that help distinguish it from subretinal fluid or intraretinal cysts.
- Features of subretinal PFCL include homogenous hypoflective ovoid-shaped cystic structure. Larger bubbles appear to have significant displacement of overlying retinal tissue with significant thinning (Figure 87.2).

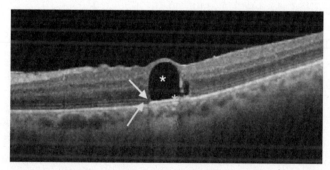

FIGURE 87.2 Optical coherence tomography (OCT) image of a patient after initial repair of rhegmatogenous retinal detachment (RRD) with retained perfluorocarbon liquid (PFCL). B-scan demonstrates subfoveal PFCL (white asterisk). Structural impact to the neurosensory retina is seen as disruption of the ellipsoid zone (blue arrow) and external limiting membrane (yellow arrow). Ovoidlike shape is demonstrated by the posterior edge width being more narrow (yellow arrow) than the central width of the PFCL bubble. Hyperreflectivity is noted at the interface of the RPE and PFCL with focal pseudoelevation of the RPE (green asterisk). The area below the PFCL bubble demonstrates increased choroidal signal with shadowing of the edges (red asterisk).

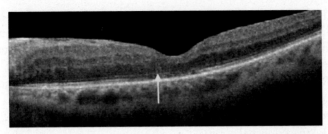

FIGURE 87.3 Optical coherence tomography (OCT) image of the same patient in Figure 87.2 after subretinal perfluorocarbon liquid (PFCL) removal. There is absence of PFCL bubble and return of more normal retinal thickness and some reconstitution of the retinal layers including the external limiting membrane (ELM) (yellow arrow).

- If PFCL is subfoveal, structural damages of the neurosensory, retina, and RPE have been demonstrated as RPE pigment disorganization, disruption of external limiting membrane (ELM) back-reflection line, and reflectivity of the photoreceptor inner and outer segment junction (Figure 87.2).[5]
- Hyperreflectivity at the base of the subfoveal PFCL bubble corresponds to the zone of damaged RPE/PFCL interface and increased signal with hypertransmission into the choroid (Figure 87.2). These findings may be due to decreased attenuation from reduced retinal tissue thickness.
- Slight pseudoelevation of the RPE and choroid may be noted at the base of the PFCL bubble, likely due to the refractive impact of the refractive properties of the bubble (Figure 87.2).
- The increased choroidal signal beneath the bubble is reversible once PFCL bubble is removed (Figure 87.3).

OCTA IMAGING

- Limited data are available on optical coherence tomography angiography (OCTA) of retained PFCL.
- Subfoveal PFCL has been associated with enlargement of the foveal avascular zone (FAZ) in both the superficial and deep layers with abnormal dark areas detectable in the choriocapillaris slab (Figures 87.4 and 87.5).
  - These changes resolved after surgical removal.

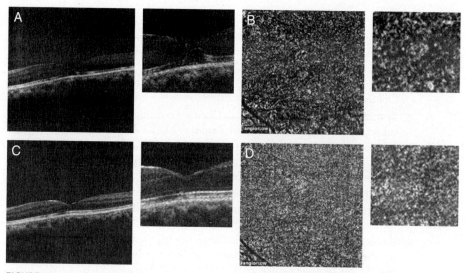

FIGURE 87.4 Optical coherence tomography (OCT) and choriocapillaris optical coherence tomography angiography (OCTA) with residual perfluorocarbon liquid (PFCL) (A) and resulting dark areas (*) detectable on choriocapillaris slab (B). OCT and OCTA postoperative showing resolution of defects (C and D). (Reprinted with permission from Wang H, Chen F, Cao H. Optical coherence tomography angiography characteristics of fovea in residual subfoveal perfluorocarbon liquid eye. *Ophthalmic Surg Lasers Imaging Retina.* 2016;47(11):1062-1066.)

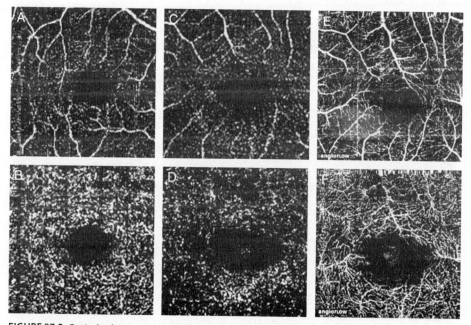

FIGURE 87.5 Optical coherence tomography angiography (OCTA) of the superficial (A) and deep (B) foveal avascular zones (FAZs) in a normal eye compared to perfluorocarbon liquid (PFCL) eye (C and D) showing increased FAZ that proceeded toward normalization postoperatively (E and F). (Reprinted with permission from Wang H, Chen F, Cao H. Optical coherence tomography angiography characteristics of fovea in residual subfoveal perfluorocarbon liquid eye. *Ophthalmic Surg Lasers Imaging Retina.* 2016;47(11):1062-1066.)

References

1. Chang S, Lincoff H, Zimmerman NJ, Fuchs W. Giant retinal tears. Surgical techniques and results using perfluorocarbon liquids. *Arch Ophthalmol.* 1989;107:761-766.
2. Chang S. Low viscosity liquid fluorochemicals in vitreous surgery. *Am J Ophthalmol.* 1987;103:38-43.
3. Tewari A, Eliott D, Singh CN, et al. Changes in retinal sensitivity from retained subretinal perfluorocarbon liquid. *Retina.* 2009;29:248-250.
4. Smith AG, Cost BM, Ehlers JP. Intraoperative OCT-assisted subretinal perfluorocarbon liquid removal in the DISCOVER Study. *Ophthalmic Surg Lasers Imaging Retina.* 2015;46:964-966.
5. Soheilian M, Nourinia R, Shoeibi N, Peyman GA. Three-dimensional OCT features of perfluorocarbon liquid trapped under the fovea. *Ophthalmic Surg Lasers Imaging.* 2010;(42):E1-E4.
6. Wang H, Chen F, Cao H. Optical coherence tomography angiography characteristics of fovea in residual subfoveal perfluorocarbon liquid eye. *Ophthalmic Surg Lasers Imaging Retina.* 2016;47(11):1062-1066.

CHAPTER 88

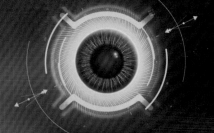

Disassociated Optic Nerve Fiber Layer

SALIENT FEATURES

- Disassociated optic nerve fiber layer (DONFL) appearance is a postoperative finding associated with internal membrane peeling (ILM).[1]
- DONFL was first described in 2001 after an ILM peel and characterized by a "moth-eaten" appearance with dark striae along nerve fibers in the retina.[2]
- These retinal changes are not seen in the acute postoperative period but typically develop in the first 6 months following surgery. Higher rates of occurrence have been reported in macular hole surgery compared to epiretinal membrane surgery (65.9% vs 13%).[1]
- DONFL appearance is generally thought to be secondary to inner retinal dimpling with possible associated nerve fiber layer atrophy instead of actual disassociation of the optic nerve fiber layer.[3]
- There are multiple hypothesizes for the pathophysiology behind the DOFNL appearance, including, but not limited to, Müller cell damage combined with inner retinal regeneration and healing, intraoperative use of dyes, ischemia, traction forces leading to retinal thinning, or deep inner retinal damage.[1,3,4]
- The long-term consequences of the DONFL appearance are uncertain. While final visual acuity does not seem to be impacted, there is some evidence for the development of paracentral scotomas.[4,5]

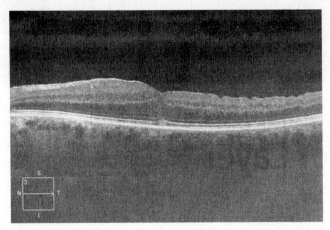

FIGURE 88.1 Optical coherence tomography (OCT) taken 3 months after epiretinal membrane peel in the left eye displaying dimpling of the inner retina, with slight thinning of the ganglion cell layer with relatively mild dissociated optic nerve fiber layer (DONFL).

OCT IMAGING

- Optical coherence tomography (OCT) is a key modality for identifying the DONFL appearance through *en-face* images, OCT thickness maps, and cross-sectional B-scan appearance[4] (Figures 88.1 and 88.2).
- *En-face* imaging can be used to track the development and progression of these inner retinal changes. There is some evidence that these findings increase in number through the first 3 months after surgery and, in some patients, up to 6 months following surgery[4] (Figure 88.3).
- Cross-sectional B-scans confirm focal thinning of both the nerve fiber layer and ganglion cell layer corresponding to areas of inner retinal dimpling or DONFL.[4]

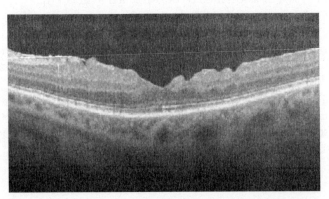

FIGURE 88.2 Optical coherence tomography (OCT) taken after epiretinal membrane peel in the left eye displaying moderate-severe dimpling of the inner retina consistent with dissociated optic nerve fiber layer (DONFL).

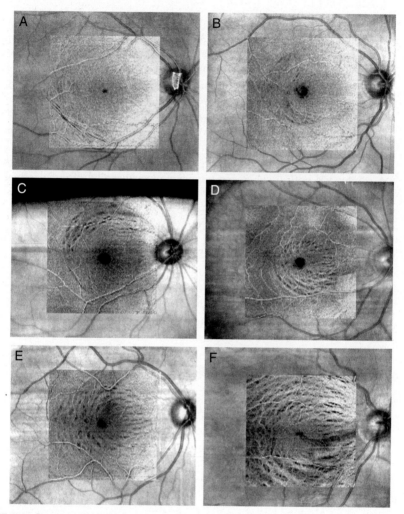

FIGURE 88.3 Postoperative en-face internal limiting membrane (ILM) optical coherence tomography (OCT) slabs demonstrating the characteristic, concentric dark striae with variable severity from no evidence of dissociated optic nerve fiber layer (A) to severe (F).

OCTA IMAGING

- En-face imaging with optical coherence tomography angiography (OCTA) also allows visualization of the DOFNL appearance.[4]
- OCTA has shown no change in vessel density at the level of the superficial vascular complex between preoperative measurements and 6-month postoperative period.[4]

References

1. Runkle AP, Srivastava SK, Yuan A, et al. Factors associated with development of dissociated optic nerve fiber layer appearance in the pioneer intraoperative optical coherence tomography study. *Retina.* 2018;38(suppl 1):S103-S109.

2. Tadayoni R, Paques M, Massin P, Mouki-Benani S, Mikol J, Gaudric A. Dissociated optic nerve fiber layer appearance of the fundus after idiopathic epiretinal membrane removal. *Ophthalmology.* 2001;108(12):2279-2283.

3. Spaide RF. "Dissociated optic nerve fiber layer appearance" after internal limiting membrane removal is inner retinal dimpling. *Retina.* 2012;32(9):1719-1726.

4. Navajas EV, Schuck N, Govetto A, et al. En face optical coherence tomography and optical coherence tomography angiography of inner retinal dimples after internal limiting membrane peeling for full-thickness macular holes. *Retina.* 2020;40:557-566.

5. Tadayoni R, Svorenova I, Erginay A, Gaudric A, Massin P. Decreased retinal sensitivity after internal limiting membrane peeling for macular hole surgery. *Br J Ophthalmol.* 2012;96(12):1513-1516.

Part 10
Drug Toxicities

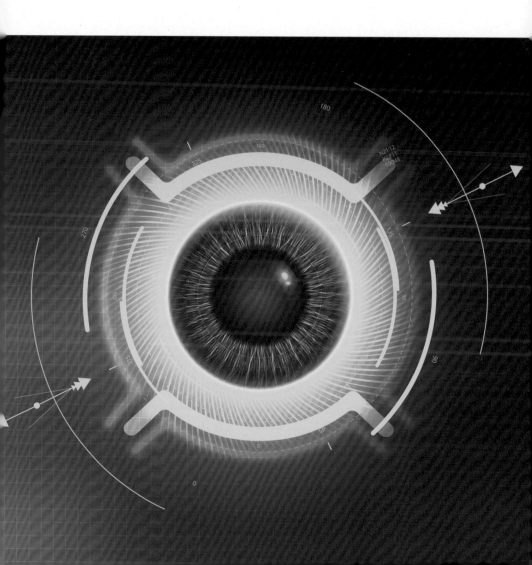

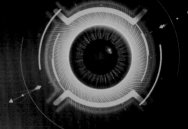

CHAPTER 89

Hydroxychloroquine Toxicity

SALIENT FEATURES

- Hydroxychloroquine (HCQ) is commonly used to treat rheumatoid arthritis, systemic lupus erythematosus, and many connective tissue diseases.[1-3]
- HCQ causes changes in the metabolism of retinal cells and binds to melanin in the retinal pigment epithelium (RPE), but it is not understood how these effects cause clinical toxicity.[1]
- The drug damages photoreceptor cells with subsequent degeneration of the RPE.[1]
- Until advanced stages, visual acuity can remain normal. With increasing damage, patients develop paracentral scotoma and decreased visual acuity.[1,2]
- Toxicity from HCQ is irreversible and can progress for 1 to 2 years after cessation of the drug.
- On fundoscopic examination, the retina may appear normal in the early stages but with advanced macular damage, a "bull's eye maculopathy" is seen due to photoreceptor damage and RPE atrophy.[1,2]
- Current screening recommendations (2016 AAO Guidelines) recommends Humphrey visual field (HVF) 10-2 and spectral-domain optical coherence tomography (SD-OCT). Multifocal electroretinography (ERG) may also be used for screening. Fundus autofluorescence demonstrates later toxicity and is thus an adjunct imaging modality. In patients of Asian descent, toxicity occurs outside of the parafoveal region and HVF 24-2 testing may be indicated.[1]

425

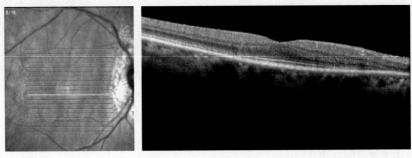

FIGURE 89.1 Spectral-domain optical coherence tomography (SD-OCT) macular scan of the right eye of a patient on hydroxychloroquine (HCQ) therapy. There is patchy attenuation of the ellipsoid zone (EZ) (red arrows) in the parafoveal region, but the center of the fovea is spared. This is consistent with mild toxicity.

OCT IMAGING

- Damage from HCQ primarily occurs in the outer retina: ELM, EZ, and RPE.[2,4,5] Initially, damage is localized to the parafoveal region and spares the center of the fovea. In severe toxicity, the entire macula is involved.[1,2,5]

- SD-OCT displays attenuation or loss of the ellipsoid zone (EZ) (Figures 89.1 and 89.2) and outer nuclear layer (ONL) thinning (Figure 89.2). In severe toxicity, the RPE is also involved (Figure 89.3). The progression of toxicity appears to be less severe if the drug is stopped prior to RPE involvement as opposed to after RPE damage has occurred.[4]

- External limiting membrane (ELM) thinning may also be seen in patients with HCQ toxicity (Figure 89.3).

- The status of the ELM at the time of diagnosis may have prognostic value. One study found that progression of HCQ toxicity was more common in patients with ELM loss at the time of diagnosis compared to patients with an intact ELM.[3]

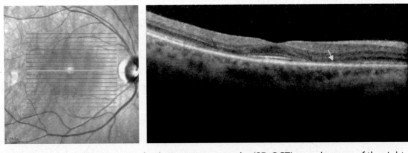

FIGURE 89.2 Spectral-domain optical coherence tomography (SD-OCT) macular scan of the right eye of a patient on hydroxychloroquine (HCQ) therapy. In this patient, there is greater loss of the ellipsoid zone (EZ) (red arrows) compared to the patient in Figure 89.1. The toxicity in this patient has also caused outer nuclear layer (ONL) thinning and attenuation of the external limiting membrane (ELM) (yellow arrow). The center of the fovea is spared. This is consistent with moderate toxicity. There is development on the near-infrared (NIR) image of an early hyporeflective bull's eye lesion.

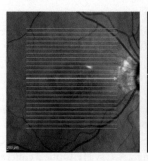
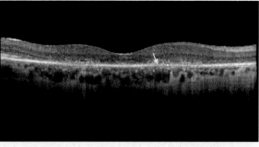

FIGURE 89.3 Spectral-domain optical coherence tomography (SD-OCT) macular scan of the right eye of a patient on hydroxychloroquine (HCQ) therapy. This patient has severe toxicity compared to the patients in Figures 89.1 and 89.2. There is ellipsoid zone (EZ), external limiting membrane (ELM), and outer nuclear layer (ONL) loss not only in the parafovea, but also in the center of the fovea as well. Additionally, there is retinal pigment epithelium (RPE) involvement with RPE thinning (yellow arrow), hyperplasia and migration (red arrows). This significant outer retinal loss allows hypertransmission of OCT signal to the choroid. In this severe state, the near-infrared (NIR) image clearly demonstrates a bull's eye lesion.

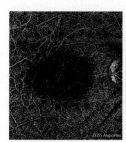
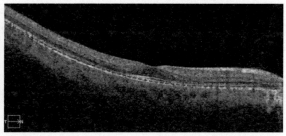

FIGURE 89.4 Optical coherence tomography angiography (OCTA) of the macula of the right eye in the same patient as in Figure 89.2. Deep plexus segmentation demonstrates mildly decreased parafoveal flow signal and a mildly enlarged foveal avascular zone.

OCTA IMAGING

- Decreased vascular density in all retinal layers and enlargement of the foveal avascular zone is noted in patients with more than 5 years of HCQ use (Figure 89.4).[6-8]
- The role of OCTA in HCQ screening and monitoring, however, has yet to be established.

References

1. Marmor MF, Kellner U, Lai TY, Melles RB, Mieler WF, American Academy of Ophthalmology. Recommendations on screening for chloroquine and hydroxychloroquine retinopathy (2016 revision). *Ophthalmology.* 2016;123(6):1386-1394.
2. Andreoli MT, Mittra RA, Mieler WF. Drug toxicity of the posterior segment. In: Schachat AP, Sadda SR, Hinton DR, Wilkinson CP, Wiedemann P, eds. *Ryan's Retina.* 6th ed. New York: Elsevier Inc.; 2018:1719-1745.

3. Scarinci F, Shaarawy A, Narala R, Jampol LM, Fawzi AA. Loss of external limiting membrane integrity predicts progression of hydroxychloroquine retinal toxicity after drug discontinuation. *Retina*. 2016;36(10):1951-1957.

4. Marmor MF, Hu J. Effect of disease stage on progression of hydroxychloroquine retinopathy. *JAMA Ophthalmol*. 2014;132(9):1105-1112.

5. de Sisternes L, Hu J, Rubin DL, Marmor MF. Localization of damage in progressive hydroxychloroquine retinopathy on and off the drug: inner versus outer retina, parafovea versus peripheral fovea. *Invest Ophthalmol Vis Sci*. 2015;56(5):3415-3426.

6. Bulut M, Akidan M, Gozkaya O, Erol MK, Cengiz A, Cay HF. Optical coherence tomography angiography for screening of hydroxychloroquine-induced retinal alterations. *Graefes Arch Clin Exp Ophthalmol*. 2018;256(11):2075-2081.

7. Ozek D, Onen M, Karaca EE, Omma A, Kemer OE, Coskun C. The optical coherence tomography angiography findings of rheumatoid arthritis patients taking hydroxychloroquine. *Eur J Ophthalmol*. 2019;29(5):532-537.

8. Goker YS, Ucgul Atilgan C, Tekin K, et al. The validity of optical coherence tomography angiography as a screening test for the early detection of retinal changes in patients with hydroxychloroquine therapy. *Curr Eye Res*. 2019;44(3):311-315.

9. Mehta N, Modi Y, Freund KB. ASRS X-files. *Retina Times*. 2017;35(71):66-67.

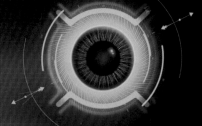

CHAPTER 90

Tamoxifen Toxicity

SALIENT FEATURES

- Tamoxifen citrate is an antiestrogen drug used in the treatment of estrogen-receptor–positive tumors such as advanced breast carcinoma (and in some estrogen-receptor–negative tumors such as hepatocellular carcinoma or glioblastoma) and as adjuvant therapy after surgical resection.
- Retinal toxicity is characterized by decreased visual acuity and color vision, while examination may demonstrate white intraretinal crystalline deposits (Figures 90.1A, B and 90.2A, B), macular edema, and/or punctate retinal pigmentary changes.
- Intraretinal deposits, which stain for glycosaminoglycans and may represent products of axonal degeneration, appear to reside in the inner retina and are most common in paramacular areas.
- While patients receiving high doses of the drug were initially thought to be at highest risk, chronic low-dose administration (10-20 mg/d) may also cause retinopathy.
- Visual function and edema may improve after discontinuation of tamoxifen, but the refractile deposits typically persist.

OCT IMAGING

- Optical coherence tomography (OCT) is a helpful diagnostic tool to confirm the diagnosis and to assess for cystoid macular edema (Figures 90.2C and D), if present, and possible response to treatment.[1]
- OCT imaging confirms the location of the crystalline deposits to the inner retina.

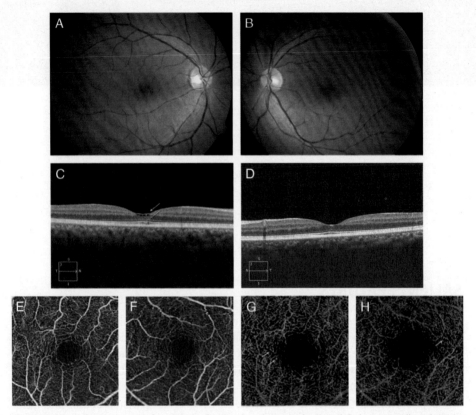

FIGURE 90.1 Early-stage tamoxifen retinopathy. Fundus photographs (A and B) show crystalline deposits and optical coherence tomography (OCT) images (C and D) show hyporeflective intraretinal foveal cavitation without macular thickening (yellow arrow) and a focal disruption of photoreceptors (red arrow). On en-face retinal segmentation slabs optical coherence tomography angiography (OCTA) images, saccular capillary telangiectasias (yellow arrow) are not seen in the superficial capillary plexus (E and F) but are seen in the deep capillary plexus (G and H).

- A characteristic finding of tamoxifen retinopathy on OCT is hyporeflective intraretinal foveal cavitation without macular thickening (Figures 90.1C and D); this can be seen in asymptomatic individuals but can also predispose to full-thickness macular holes.[2-4]

- In eyes with more severe toxicity on a higher dose of tamoxifen, cystoid macular edema and subretinal fluid can be seen with increased thickening.[3,4]

- Focal disruption of photoreceptors (ie, ellipsoid zone attenuation) can also be seen in approximately one-half of patients with known toxicity.

- Hyperreflective lesions, which may be reactive pigment epithelial proliferation, can also be seen with prominent thinning of the central macula.

- Both cavitations and crystalline retinopathy of tamoxifen toxicity are similar to those findings seen in idiopathic macular telangiectasia type 2 and may suggest a similar role of Müller cells in its pathogenesis.[2]

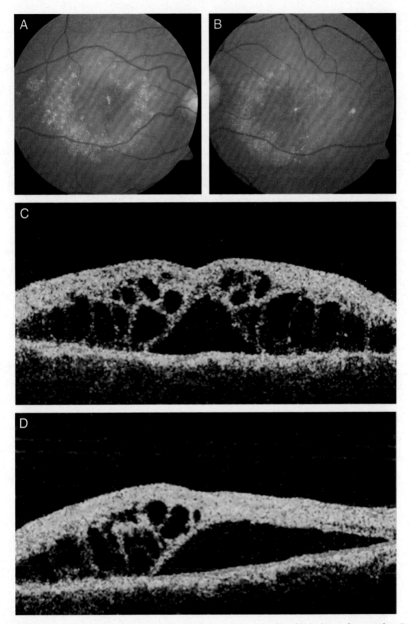

FIGURE 90.2 Severe tamoxifen retinopathy secondary to long-standing high dose of tamoxifen. Fundus photographs (A and B) show characteristic crystalline deposits and diffuse macular edema. Optical coherence tomography (OCT) images (C and D) show evidence of significant macular edema with intraretinal and subretinal fluid.

OCTA IMAGING

* On optical coherence tomography angiography (OCTA) imaging, prominent small dilated capillaries (relative to adjacent capillaries) may be seen in eyes with tamoxifen retinopathy.[3]
* These saccular capillary telangiectasias are seen mostly in the deep capillary plexus of the temporal juxtafoveal area but not in the superficial capillary plexus (Figures 90.1E-H).
* Less commonly, OCTA in tamoxifen retinopathy may demonstrate distinct forms of vessels differing from adjacent ones in terms of diameter and running direction; they appear to originate from a retinal vein and drop at right angles into the deeper retina.[3]
* Subretinal neovascular proliferation involving the retina is not characteristically seen.
* Vessel density for the parafoveal area at the superficial capillary plexus is significantly lower in eyes with tamoxifen retinopathy rather than in the control group.

References

1. Bourla DH, Sarraf D, Schwartz SD. Peripheral retinopathy and maculopathy in high-dose tamoxifen therapy. *Am J Ophthalmol.* 2007;144:126-128.
2. Doshi RR, Fortun JA, Kim BT, Dubovy SR, Rosenfeld PJ. Pseudocystic foveal cavitation in tamoxifen retinopathy. *Am J Ophthalmol.* 2014;157:1291-1298. e3.
3. Lee S, Kim H-A, Yoon Y. Optical coherence tomography angiographic findings of tamoxifen retinopathy: similarity with macular telangiectasia type 2. *Ophthalmol Retina.* 2019;3(8):681-689. doi:10.1016/j.oret.2019.03.014 .
4. Gualino V, Cohen SY, Delyfer MN, Sahel JA, Gaudric A. Optical coherence tomography findings in tamoxifen retinopathy. *Am J Ophthalmol.* 2005;140:757-758.

Part 11

Imaging of the Optic Nerve

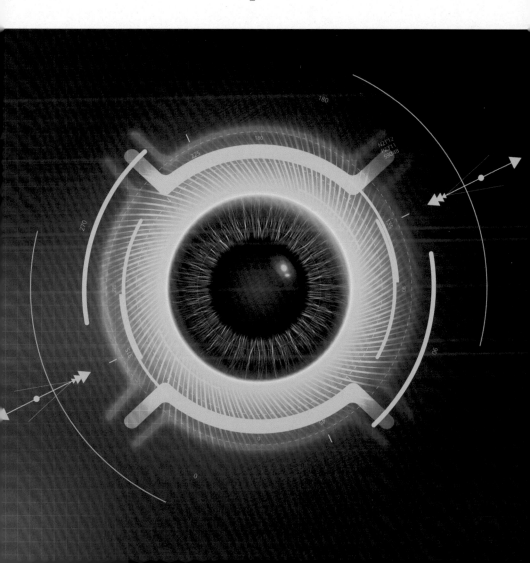

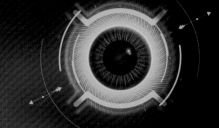

CHAPTER 91

OCT and OCTA Imaging in Glaucoma

SALIENT FEATURES

- Glaucoma is a group of optic neuropathies that share characteristic patterns of visual field loss due to degeneration of the optic nerve fibers.
- Glaucoma preferentially affects the ganglion cells and their axons that make up the inferior and superior retinal nerve fiber layer (RNFL).
- Characteristic visual field defects typically respect the horizontal midline due to the anatomic orientation of nerve fibers about the horizontal raphe. These include superior or inferior nasal steps, arcuate or Bjerrum scotomas, paracentral defects, altitudinal defects, or generalized depression sometimes sparing a central or temporal island of vision.
- Glaucomatous nerves on ophthalmoscopy generally appear to have a large optic cup, asymmetry of cupping, progressive enlargement of the cup, focal notching of the rim, vertical elongation of the cup, nerve fiber layer hemorrhage or loss, exposed lamina cribrosa, bayonetting or baring of the vessels, and peripapillary atrophy.
- Optic nerve head imaging along with intraocular pressure measurements and standard automated perimetry provide invaluable insights into the structural changes that occur throughout the course of the disease.

OCT IMAGING

- Optical coherence tomography (OCT) is a powerful tool in the diagnosis and monitoring of glaucoma that has greatly expanded our understanding of the effect of glaucoma on the eye.

435

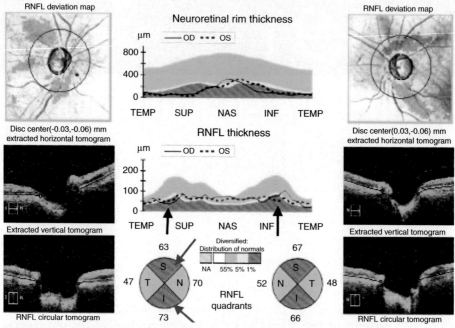

FIGURE 91.1 Optical coherence tomography (OCT) image of the optic nerve head and retinal nerve fiber layer (RNFL) analysis of a patient with advanced primary open angle glaucoma (POAG) in both eyes. Thinning of the superior and inferior neural rim is evident as red quadrants on the thickness map and quadrant thickness (blue arrows). Note the superior and inferior thinning on the RNFL deviation map which correlates with the lower peaks on the RNFL thickness line tracing (black arrows).

- The Cirrus RNFL OCT scan maps a 6 × 6mm cube, with a linear representation of A-scan data that represent the RNFL thickness 3.4 mm from the center of the optic disc.
- Algorithms developed to evaluate and follow patients include an RNFL thickness scan as well as a ganglion cell inner plexiform layer (GC-IPL) scan.
- The RNFL thickness measurements are compared against age-matched normative values. An area where the RNFL thickness is <5% compared to the normative database is flagged as yellow and <1% as red (OCT RNFL Analysis, Figure 91.1).
- Based on a longitudinal study, the age-related rate of reduction in RNFL thickness has been estimated to be −0.52 µm/y on average, −1.35 µm/y for the superior quadrant, and −1.25 µm/y for the inferior quadrant.[1]
- Glaucomatous eyes demonstrate thinning of the ganglion cell layer that can be measured and monitored on OCT ganglion cell analysis. This scan takes a segmentation of the ganglion cell layer and inner plexiform layer and compares the individual's data to a normative database (OCT Ganglion Cell Analysis, Figure 91.2).

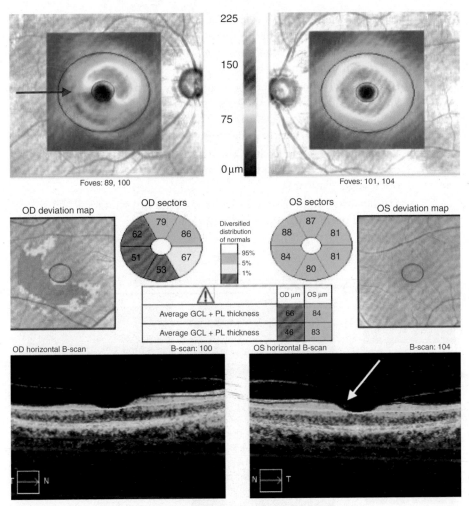

FIGURE 91.2 Optical coherence tomography (OCT) macular cube with ganglion cell analysis of a patient with advanced primary open angle glaucoma (POAG) in the right eye and mild POAG in the left eye. Note the area of inferior thinning in the ganglion cell layer forms a sharp horizontal line at the horizontal raphe (red arrow); this is characteristic of glaucomatous damage which would correlate with inferior notching of the optic nerve, and superior visual field loss. There is vitreomacular adhesion without traction (white arrow). In case of vitreomacular traction (not seen here), there may be artifactually thicker readings despite glaucomatous loss of macular ganglion cells, which may mask the true extent of disease.

OCTA IMAGING

- Ocular perfusion pressure is expressed as the difference between mean arterial pressure and intraocular pressure. Low ocular perfusion pressure has been implicated as a risk factor for glaucomatous optic neuropathy via ischemic damage to the optic nerve.

- Optical coherence tomography angiography (OCTA) imaging of the optic nerve head and the peripapillary retinal perfusion in the RNFL, as well as the superficial perifoveal macular vasculature are areas of interest in glaucoma.[2]
- Studies have shown there is a significant decrease in vessel density and flow indices within the optic nerve head and peripapillary retina in eyes with both preperimetric and perimetric primary open angle glaucoma[3] (OCTA Peripapillary Analysis, Figure 91.3).
- Peripapillary vessel density values have also been shown to be significantly decreased in pseudoexfoliation glaucoma compared to primary open angle glaucoma.[4]
- Studies have demonstrated conflicting data on whether RNFL thickness and peripapillary vessel density correlate.[5-7]

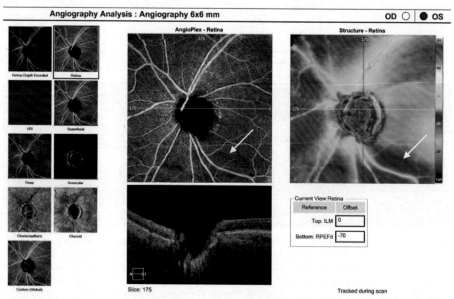

FIGURE 91.3 The microvasculature in the peripapillary region also undergoes changes as glaucoma progresses. Healthy eyes have dense microvascular networks, while preperimetric and glaucomatous eyes have been shown to have significantly diminished peripapillary microvascular density. The areas of decreased capillary densities on optical coherence tomography angiography (OCTA) (yellow arrow) correlate to areas of retinal nerve fiber layer (RNFL) thinning (white arrow).

References

1. Leung CK, Yu M, Weinreb RN, et al. Retinal nerve fiber layer imaging with spectral-domain optical coherence tomography: a prospective analysis of age-related loss. *Ophthalmology.* 2012;119:731-737.

2. Richter GM, Sylvester B, Chu Z, et al. Peripapillary microvasculature in the retinal nerve fiber layer in glaucoma by optical coherence tomography angiography: focal structural and functional correlations and diagnostic performance. *Clin Ophthalmol.* 2018;12:2285-2296.

3. Jia Y, Wie E, Wang X, et al. Optical coherence tomography angiography of optic disc perfusion in glaucoma. *Ophthalmology.* 2014;121(7):1322-1332. doi:10.1016/j.ophtha.2014.01.021.

4. Suwan Y, Geyman LS, Fard MA, et al. Peripapillary perfused capillary density in exfoliation syndrome and exfoliation glaucoma versus POAG and healthy controls: an OCTA study. *Asia Pac J Ophthalmol.* 2017;7:84-89.

5. Mansoori T, Sivaswamy J, Gamalapati JS, Balakrishna N. Topography and correlation of radial peripapillary capillary density network with retinal nerve fibre layer thickness. *Int Ophthamol.* 2018;38(3):967-974. doi:10.1007/s10792-017-0544.0.

6. Chen CL, Zhang A, Bojikian KD, et al. Peripapillary retinal nerve fiber layer vascular microcirculation in glaucoma using optical coherence tomography-based micro-angiography. *Invest Ophthalmol Vis Sci.* 2016;57:OCT475–OCT485. doi:10.1167/iovs.16-19420.

7. Liu L, Jia Y, Takusagawa HL, et al. Optical coherence tomography angiography of the peripapillary retina in glaucoma. *JAMA Ophthalmol.* 2015;133:1045-1052. doi:10.1001/jamaophthalmol.2015.2225.

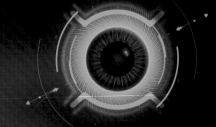

CHAPTER 92

Optic Disc Edema and Optic Neuropathies

SALIENT FEATURES

- Optic disc edema describes swelling of the optic nerve head anterior to the lamina cribosa.
- When disc edema is the result of elevated intracranial pressure, it is labeled papilledema.
- Optic nerves affected by optic neuropathies of various etiologies can appear swollen, flat, or pale/atrophic depending on etiology and duration of condition.
- A broad variety of pathology can result in optic neuropathy and optic disc edema:
  - Inflammation (optic neuritis)
  - Infection
  - Ischemia
  - Malignancy
    - Compressive lesions resulting in elevated intracranial pressure and axoplasmic stasis
    - Direct nerve infiltration
  - Idiopathic intracranial hypertension (IIH)
  - Nutritional deficiency and toxins
  - Compressive
  - Hereditary

- Optical coherence tomography (OCT) is widely used in clinical practice to monitor these conditions and can identify the more likely cause based on the pattern of peripapillary retinal nerve fiber layer (RNFL) and ganglion cell loss.
- OCT has become a routine outcome measure in clinical trials in conditions that affect the optic nerve.

OCT IMAGING

- The peripapillary RNFL is comprised of unmyelinated nerve axons, and, therefore, thinning as measured on circumpapillary RNFL measurements is thought to be representative of neuroaxonal degeneration.
- Retinal ganglion cell assessment by means of OCT ganglion cell analysis is a surrogate marker of optic nerve health.
- In inflammatory optic neuropathies, the RNFL thickness measurements may initially be elevated or in normal range. Over the course of 6 to 12 months, there will be axonal loss and thinning (Figure 92.1).
- In inflammatory optic neuropathies, the ganglion cell layer thickness will remain symmetric between the two eyes acutely but will decrease over the ensuing 6 to 12 months in the affected eye.
- Thinning of the RNFL over time in the absence of acute bouts of optic neuritis may suggest subclinical disease activity that correlates to brain atrophy in multiple sclerosis (MS).[1]
- In toxic and nutritional optic neuropathy, thinning of the macular ganglion cell layer on OCT may be seen early in the disease course.[2]
- OCT helps quantify the amount of optic disc edema with measures of RNFL thickness in papilledema. However, RNFL and ganglion cell layer thinning may be seen in cases of chronic papilledema even with a coexistent increase in intracranial pressure.
- On an OCT slice through the optic nerve, inward angulation of the adjacent retinal pigment epithelium/Bruch membrane complex toward the vitreous cavity suggests elevated intracranial pressure (papilledema) as the etiology for optic disc edema (Figure 92.2).[3]
- OCT technology with deeper penetration including enhanced-depth imaging and swept-source OCT may be used to differentiate optic disc edema from optic disc drusen.

OCTA IMAGING

- The role for optical coherence tomography angiography (OCTA) in clinical practice in managing optic neuropathy is currently being defined.
- On OCTA, all chronic optic neuropathies show a decrease in peripapillary vessel density that corresponds to RNFL thinning and visual field defects.[4]

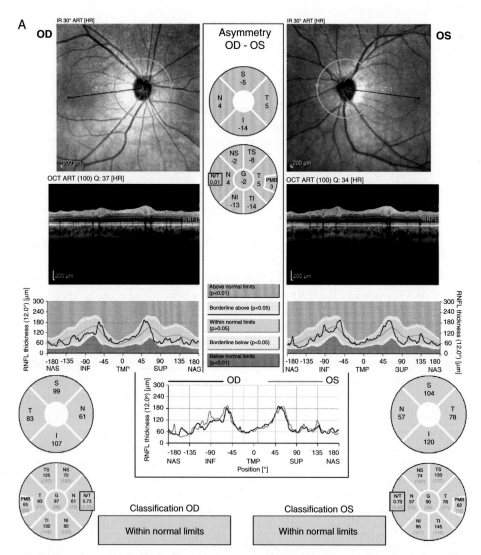

FIGURE 92.1 Optic nerve optical coherence tomography (OCT) image from a single patient with inflammatory optic neuritis of the left eye secondary to multiple sclerosis 4 weeks after (A) an acute episode with no apparent thinning of the retinal nerve fiber layer (RNFL) and (B) the same patient several months after the acute episode with progressive RNFL thinning. The right eye remains normal.

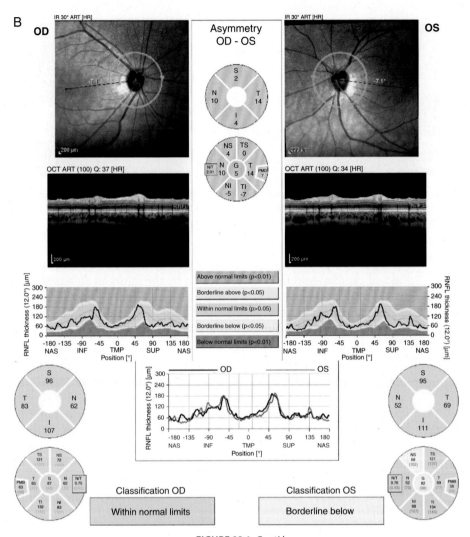

FIGURE 92.1 Cont'd

- It has been shown that there is decreased flow to the optic nerve head (OCT flow index) using OCTA in patients with MS, with or without a history of optic neuritis.[5]
- Patients with optic neuritis have been shown to have significant loss of the radial peripapillary capillaries, while those with papilledema from idiopathic intracranial hypertension have been shown to have an increased prominence of the optic nerve head and peripapillary retinal capillaries on OCTA.[5,6]

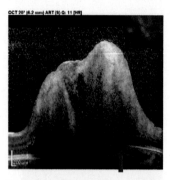 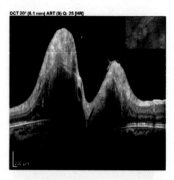

FIGURE 92.2 Optical coherence tomography (OCT) image from a patient with elevated intracranial pressure due to papilledema with Bruch membrane sloping inward toward the vitreous space of the right and left eyes (red arrows).

- In optic atrophy from various etiologies, OCTA often demonstrates loss of capillaries in the region affected by the injury in an anatomical distribution. For example, segmental or altitudinal optic nerve head capillary loss can be seen in anterior ischemic neuropathy and temporal or papillomacular bundle loss in dominant optic atrophy.[5,6]
- The role of OCTA in distinguishing papilledema from pseudopapilledema from optic disc drusen is still under investigation.[7]
- OCTA can identify subtle dilation of the peripapillary vessels in early cases of Leber hereditary optic neuropathy. OCTA also reveals peripapillary telangiectasias and capillary dilatation at the time of acute vision loss and reveals peripapillary attenuation in the chronic stages.[6,8,9]

References

1. Petzold A, Balcer LJ, Calabresi PA, et al. Retinal layer segmentation in multiple sclerosis: a systematic review and meta-analysis. *Lancet Neurol.* 2017;16:797-812.
2. Vieira LM, Silva NF, Dias dos Santos AM, et al. Retinal ganglion cell layer analysis by optical coherence tomography in toxic and nutritional optic neuropathy. *J Neuroophthalmol.* 2015;35:242-245.
3. Kupersmith MJ, Sibony P, Mandel G, Durbin M, Kardon RH. Optical coherence tomography of the swollen optic nerve head: deformation of the peripapillary retinal pigment epithelium layer in papilledema. *Invest Ophth Vis Sci.* 2011;52:6558-6564.
4. Chen JJ, AbouChehade JE, Iezzi R Jr, Leavitt JA, Kardon RH. Optical coherence angiographic demonstration of retinal changes from chronic optic neuropathies. *Neuroophthalmology.* 2017;41:76-83.
5. Spain RI, Liu L, Zhang X, et al. Optical coherence tomography angiography enhances the detection of optic nerve damage in multiple sclerosis. *Br J Ophthalmol.* 2018;102:520-524.

6. Spaide RF, Fujimoto JG, Waheed NK, Sadda SR, Staurenghi G. Optical coherence tomography angiography. *Prog Retin Eye Res.* 2017;64:1-55.
7. Chen JJ, Costello F. The role of optical coherence tomography in neuro-ophthalmology. *Ann Eye Sci.* 2018;3:35.
8. Asanad S, Meer E, Tian JJ, Fantini M, Nassisi M, Sadun AA. Leber's hereditary optic neuropathy: severe vascular pathology in a severe primary mutation. *Intractable Rare Dis Res.* 2019;8:52-55.
9. Gaier ED, Gittinger JW, Cestari DM, Miller JB. Peripapillary capillary dilation in Leber hereditary optic neuropathy revealed by optical coherence tomographic angiography. *JAMA Ophthalmol.* 2016;134:1332-1334.

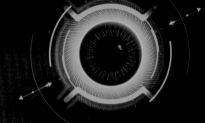

CHAPTER 93

Congenital and Acquired Optic Nerve Abnormalities

SALIENT FEATURES

- This chapter surveys a broad spectrum of malformations occasionally associated with significant visual impairment.
- Strabismus, nystagmus, and amblyopia may be associated with the congenital defects and should be addressed as best as possible.
- Associated systemic abnormalities (namely, neurologic, endocrinologic, and musculoskeletal) can be associated with the various pathologies.[1,2]
- Optic nerve hypoplasia (ONH)
  - This is a sporadic, nonprogressive, unilateral or bilateral, congenital defect with minimal to profound visual loss that does not correlate with the size of the optic disc. Afferent pupillary defect may be present. It is suggested that a supranormal regression of axons during the development of the optic nerve is a driving pathology.
  - ONH accounts for 15% to 20% of children with significant congenital visual loss.[1]
  - A variable fundus presentation includes a small optic disc, peripapillary "double-ring" sign, and vascular tortuosity.
  - The outer ring of the "double-ring" sign is the result of a normal junction between the sclera and the lamina cribrosa, and the inner ring is a manifestation of an abnormal extension of the retina and pigment epithelium (RPE) over the outer portion of the lamina cribrosa (inner ring) approaching the hypoplastic optic nerve head.

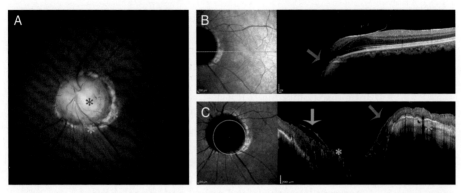

FIGURE 93.1 Disc photography (A), linear spectral-domain optical coherence tomography (SD-OCT) (B), and circular SD-OCT (C) of a cavitary optic nerve with morning glory features (red asterisk in A). Multiple straightened radial vessels emanate from the optic disc, and these can be seen as small circular hyperreflective lesions with clear lumens on the circular OCT (teal asterisk). Annular chorioretinal pigmentary changes can be seen on photography (green asterisk) which manifest as disorganized hyperreflective retinal and choroidal changes on the circular OCT (green asterisk). The excavation is poorly visualized on the macular OCT (B), but laminated retina can be seen extending outward into the excavated area (red arrows in B and C). Vitreous prepapillary bands can be seen (green arrow). There is no readily identifiable central glial tuft on photography or OCT.

- ONH is associated with a variety of systemic defects including hypoplastic optic chiasm, agenesis of the septum pellucidum (septo-optic dysplasia), and posterior pituitary ectopia; thus, neuroimaging and hormonal workup are indicated.
- Superior segmental ONH with inferior field defects is associated with maternal insulin-dependent diabetes.
- The three most common congenital cavitary optic nerve anomalies are morning glory disc anomaly, optic disc coloboma, and optic disc pit.
  - Morning glory disc anomaly or syndrome (MGS)
    - MGS is characterized by a unilateral funnel-shaped excavation of the posterior fundus involving the optic nerve which is filled with glial tissue and surrounded by chorioretinal pigmentation. An increased number of straightened cilioretinal vessels radiate from the edge of the disc (Figures 93.1A and 93.2A).

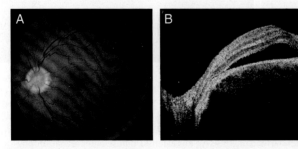

FIGURE 93.2 Patient with morning glory disc anomaly seen on fundus photograph (A) and associated serous macular detachment on optical coherence tomography (OCT) (B).

- Visual acuity is generally poor. MGS can be associated with transsphenoidal encephalocele, hypopituitarism, moyamoya disease, and other ocular, facial, and neurologic abnormalities.
- Retinal detachments may occur, typically with a small retinal break at the disc margin.
- Optic disc coloboma (ODC)
  - An ODC is a large, sharply demarcated excavation of the inferior edge of the optic disc thought to result from failure of fusion of the optic fissure.
  - *PAX2* gene mutations have been identified.
  - ODC can be associated with peripapillary retinal detachment, peripapillary schisis, and retinal and iris colobomas.
- Optic disc pit
  - This supposed less severe variant of ODC features a round; focal; gray, white, or yellow excavation of the optic nerve head (Figures 93.3A, and 93.4A and C), perhaps due to a more focal defect in the lamina cribrosa. Histological studies have shown dysplastic retinal tissue herniating into a collagen-line pocked extending posterior to a defect in the lamina cribrosa.

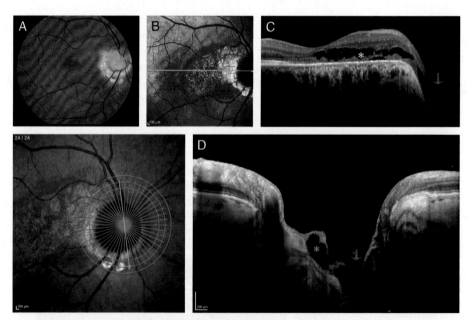

FIGURE 93.3 Disc photography (A) of a patient with an optic disc pit. There is a circular, yellow excavation at the inferonasal rim of the optic disc (teal arrow). This patient had undergone previous laser photocoagulation and pars plana vitrectomy with posterior hyaloid separation to address chronic optic pit maculopathy. B, False color near-infrared image reveals mottling extending from the temporal papillary to the fovea. C, Spectral-domain optical coherence tomography (SD-OCT) through the macula and nasal optic nerve reveals chronic intraretinal fluid or schisis (yellow asterisk), diffuse outer retinal atrophy (green arrows), and (D) a steep excavation of the optic nerve with continuation of the retina into the optic disc pit (red arrow). (Reprinted with permission from Dr. Tahira Scholle, MD.)

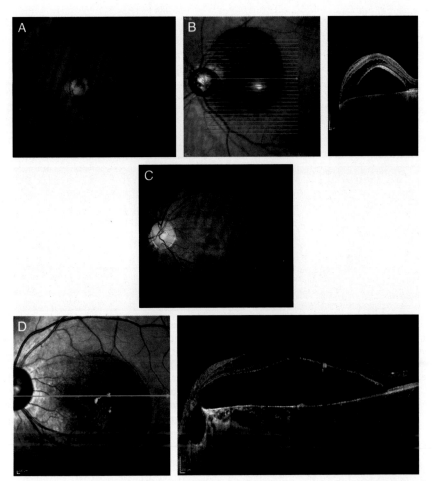

FIGURE 93.4 Two patients with optic pits and serous retinal detachments on fundus photographs (A and C) and optical coherence tomography (OCT) (B and D). OCT images show characteristic cystic outer retinal edema with schisis cavity and a serious retinal detachment.

- These may be acquired in patients with glaucoma or pathologic myopia.
- Patients are generally asymptomatic; although serous macular detachments and intraretinal cystoid spaces may occur, most commonly in the third or fourth decade of life. The nature of the subretinal fluid is debated, with some studies suggesting the presence of a connection to the subarachnoid space and other suggesting liquefied vitreous may pass through an opening created by the pit.
- Another even rarer cavitary optic disc abnormality is peripapillary staphyloma, a sporadic, isolated, unilateral deep excavation of the area of the fundus surrounding the optic disc.

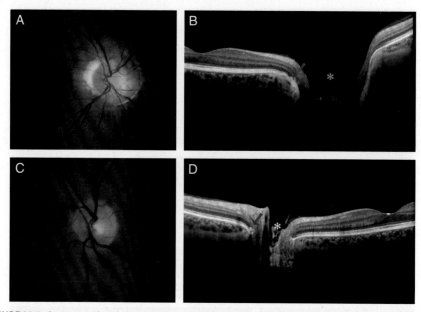

FIGURE 93.5 Optic nerve head photo (A) from a patient with a unilateral megalopapilla. Note the enlarged optic disc with relatively normal features. There is mild peripapillary atrophy. B, Spectral-domain optical coherence tomography (SD-OCT) through the fovea and optic nerve reveals an enlarged disc diameter, cup depth, and cup width (green asterisk). However, morphology of the optic disc and surrounding tissues appears relatively normal. Retinal laminations and the RPE terminate at the intersection with the peripapillary sclera (red arrows), there are no peripapillary schisislike changes, and the cup depth is relatively uniform. Compare to the patient's contralateral normal optic nerve disc (C) and SD-OCT (D) in which overall morphology is similar but smaller. There is a small vitreous plug (yellow asterisk).

- Megalopapilla, an enlarged optic disc with normal disc morphology without visual significance, is not considered a cavitary optic nerve anomaly (Figure 93.5A).
- Optic disc drusen (ODD)
  - This is an acquired optic disc abnormality with deposition of calcified axonal debris buried within the optic disc. Fundus examination reveals focal nodular elevation of the optic nerve head (Figure 93.6A and B). Patients are usually asymptomatic, but, in some cases, drusen can cause visual field defects. Decreased visual acuity from disc drusen is not typical, although disc drusen predispose to retinal vascular occlusion and ischemic optic neuropathy.
  - Ultrasound through ODD demonstrates a focal hyperechoic lesion at the optic nerve head with posterior shadowing.
  - On fundus autofluorescence, a focal area of marked hyperautofluorescence may be seen within the optic nerve head (Figure 93.6E and F).

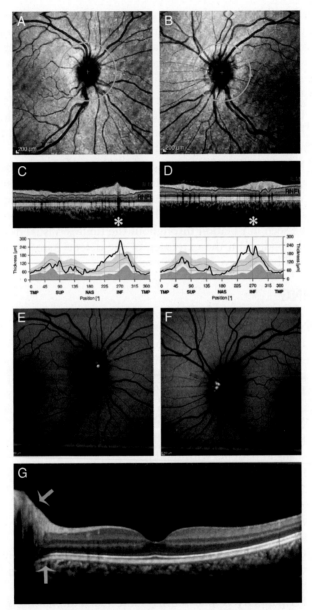

FIGURE 93.6 Multimodal imaging of optic disc drusen. A and B, False color images with green circles demonstrate the retinal nerve fiber layer thickness measurement locations. C and D, Retinal nerve fiber layer (RNFL) thickness measurements and normative data overlay demonstrates focal thickening of the RNFL (yellow asterisk). E and F, Fundus autofluorescence (FAF) imaging reveals focal areas of hyperauto-fluorescent signal (red arrows) consistent with the diagnosis of optic disc drusen. Further calcific deposits may be present deeper within the nerve which may not show on FAF imaging. G, Spectral-domain optical coherence tomography (SD-OCT) through the nerve and macula of the left eye demonstrates a normal macula and large round hyperreflective lesion within the optic nerve (green arrow). The retinal pigment epithelium (RPE) line remains without inward bowing (teal arrow), suggesting that the elevation of the disc is less likely due to high intracranial pressure (papilledema). The retina overall appears normal.

- Peripapillary choroidal neovascular membranes can occasionally occur in patients with congenital or acquired optic nerve abnormalities and can cause significant subretinal fluid and hemorrhage, leading to vision loss. Peripapillary hemorrhage, retinal thickening, and exudates may be seen on examination (Figure 93.7A and C).
- Titled disc syndrome (TDS)
  - Isolated, unilateral, or bilateral oblique insertion of the optic nerve head is the hallmark feature of TDS (Figures 93.8 and 93.9).
- Myelinated nerve fiber layer (MNFL)
  - MNFL is a common congenital anomaly where aberrant retinal nerve fiber axon myelination results in the appearance of bright white or yellow streaks usually extending from the upper or lower borders of the nerve fiber layer (Figure 93.10). However, they may be seen in isolation throughout the fundus. Visual defects can exist depending on the extension of the defect. Associated myopia and amblyopia have been reported.

OCT IMAGING

- ONH
  - Decreased cup depth, cup diameter, and disc diameter (measured from nasal edge to the temporal edge of the RPE) can be seen on horizontal raster through center of the hypoplastic optic nerve.
  - Peripapillary retinal nerve fiber layer (RNFL) thickness is decreased, and the degree of thinning is associated with optic disc size.
  - Macular thinning, with thinner RNFL and ganglion cell layer (GLC), is noted on macular optical coherence tomography (OCT) scans in patients with ONH.
  - Continuation of the inner retinal layers may be seen through the central macula (fovea plana), resembling the features of foveal hypoplasia.[3,4]
- Cavitary disc abnormalities
  - All cavitary disc anomalies demonstrate some degree of excavation of the optic disc and surrounding tissues on OCT.
  - Continuation of the RPE and the laminated retina into the excavated optic discs can be seen in the cavity disc abnormalities (Figure 93.1B and C, red arrows).[5]
  - Peripapillary retinal schisis, subretinal fluid, and vitreous traction can also be seen to some degree in all cavitary disc anomalies (Figure 93.1C, green arrow, Figures 93.2B, 93.3C, and 93.4B and D).
  - Peripapillary RNFL thickness measurements may demonstrate variable derangements in the cavitary optic disc abnormalities, and measurement zones may need to be manually edited to account for the larger disc areas.[6]
    - In contrast, RNFL thickness measurements are often normal in megalopapilla.

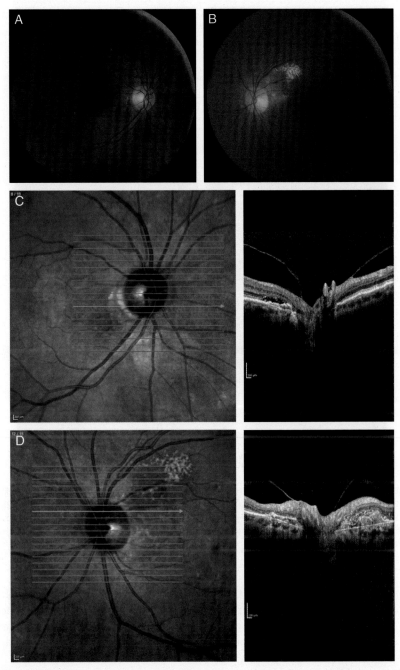

FIGURE 93.7 Patient with bilateral peripapillary choroidal neovascular membranes. Fundus photographs (A and B) show peripapillary hemorrhage, thickening, and exudates. Optical coherence tomography (OCT) images (C and D) show subretinal choroidal neovascular membranes, subretinal fluid, and exudates.

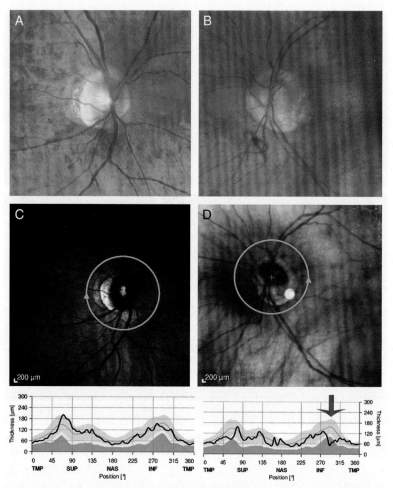

FIGURE 93.8 Fundus photographs of the right (A) and left (B) eye from a patient with unilateral tilted disc of the left eye. Note the inferonasal approach of insertion. There is perpipapillary atrophy in both eyes, but more pronounced inferiorly in the left eye. C and D, Right and left nerve false color image and retinal nerve fiber layer (RNFL) thickness measurements demonstrate focal thinning of the inferotemporal region of the left eye only.

- MGS
  - Straight rasters through the optic nerve demonstrate excavation of the posterior pole involving all retinal layers and choroid approaching an optic nerve that contains an overlying central hyperreflective tuft. The hyperreflective tuft can help distinguish MGS from other cavitary disc abnormalities.
- ODC
  - OCT demonstrates a deeply excavated optic nerve with retinal tissue herniating into the excavated space. Underlying scleral tissue has been reported to be sparse and disorganized with multiple linear hyperreflective lines with hyporeflective gap spaces.[7]

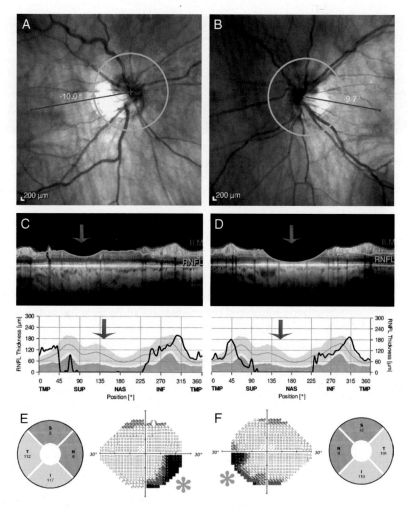

FIGURE 93.9 A and B, Near-infrared reference images for retinal nerve fiber layer (RNFL) thickness measurements from the right (A) and left (B) eyes of a patient with bilateral tilted discs. The nerves insert in an inferotemporal direction in each eye. Note the artifactual RNFL thinning in the superonasal quadrant in each eye (red arrows), which corresponds to the point of greatest anterior-posterior protrusion of the nerves. The patient has bilateral inferonasal depressions on a 24-2 standard perimetry (E and F, teal asterisks) that do not correspond to the RNFL thickness maps.

- Optic disc pit
  - A focal excavation of the optic disc can be seen on dedicated vertical or horizontal scans through the round gray or black lesion seen on fundus examination (Figure 93.3D, red arrow, Figure 93.4D).

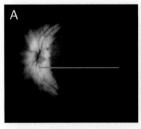 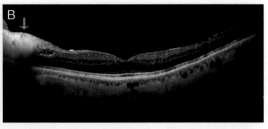

FIGURE 93.10 A, Fundus photograph through the right eye of a patient with myelinated retinal nerve fiber layer (MLF) with characteristic yellow streaks following the path of the retinal nerve fiber layer (RNFL) and extending outward from the optic nerve head. Spectral-domain optical coherence tomography (SD-OCT) (B) through the macula demonstrates thickened bright RNFL (green arrow) corresponding to the lesion on fundus photography.

- En-face OCT through the optic nerve head can readily highlight the hyporeflective area associated with the excavation.[8]
- A thin rim of moderately hyperreflective tissue, suspected to be dysplastic herniated retinal tissue, can be seen lining the walls of the optic pit (Figure 93.3D, green asterisk).
- Retinal scans may demonstrate peripapillary intraretinal and/or subretinal fluid that can extend to the fovea, causing what has been termed optic pit maculopathy (Figures 93.3C, and 93.4B and D). Swept-source OCT occasionally demonstrates a small pocket of fluid just posterior to the base of the optic pit suspected to be the subarachnoid space which may be the source of the exudate.[7]

- OCT through a peripapillary staphyloma reveals a deeply seated, relatively normal optic disc sitting adjacent to an atrophic staphyloma of the peripapillary retina and choroid.[9]

- ODD appears as hyperreflective round bodies above the edges of the RPE on spectral-domain (SD)-OCT (Figure 93.6G).

- Peripapillary choroidal neovascularization will manifest on SD-OCT as peripapillary retinal pigment epithelial detachments with associated intraretinal fluid, subretinal fluid, and hyperreflective dots (Figure 93.7C and D).

- In the tilted disc syndrome, RNFL thinning can often be seen in the quadrant of the greatest protrusion of the optic nerve head (directly opposite the orientation of the nerve insertion). However, the thinning does not always correlate to the location of visual field defects (Figures 93.8 and 93.9).[10]

- In MNFL, a thickened hyperreflective RNFL can be seen on SD-OCT (Figure 93.10B, green arrow).

OCTA IMAGING

- The radial peripapillary microvascular network has been demonstrated to be diminished or absent in both optic disc coloboma and optic disc pit using optical coherence tomography angiography (OCTA).[11] In contrast, this plexus is present, if not increased in MGS.[12,13]
- The radial peripapillary microvascular network has been noted to be normal in a patient with superior segmental ONH.[14]

References

1. Dutton GN. Congenital disorders of the optic nerve: excavations and hypoplasia. *Eye.* 2004;18:1038-1048.
2. Amador-Patarroyo MJ, Pérez-Rueda MA, Tellez CH. Congenital anomalies of the optic nerve. *Saudi J Ophthalmol.* 2015;29:32-38.
3. Pilat A, Sibley D, McLean RJ, et al. High-resolution imaging of the optic nerve and retina in optic nerve hypoplasia. *Ophthalmology.* 2015;122:1330-1339.
4. Jeng-Miller KW, Cestari DM, Gaier ED. Congenital anomalies of the optic disc: insights from optical coherence tomography imaging. *Curr Opin Ophthalmol.* 2017;28:579-586.
5. Munk MR, Simjanoski E, Fingert JH, Jampol LM. Enhanced depth imaging optical coherence tomography of congenital cavitary optic disc anomaly (CODA). *Br J Ophthalmol.* 2015;99:549-555.
6. Wu YK, Wu TEJ, Peng PH, Cheng CK. Quantitative optical coherence tomography findings in a 4-year-old boy with typical morning glory disk anomaly. *J AAPOS.* 2008;12:621-622.
7. Ohno-Matsui K, Hirakata A, Inoue M, et al. Evaluation of congenital optic disc pits and optic disc colobomas by swept-source optical coherence tomography. *Invest Ophthalmol Vis Sci.* 2013;54:7769-7778.
8. Maertz J, Kolb JP, Klein T, et al. Combined in-depth, 3D, en face imaging of the optic disc, optic disc pits and optic disc pit maculopathy using swept-source megahertz OCT at 1050 nm. *Graefes Arch Clin Exp Ophthalmol.* 2018;256:289-298.
9. Woo SJ, Hwang JM. Spectral-domain optical coherence tomography of peripapillary staphyloma. *Graefes Arch Clin Exp Ophthalmol.* 2009;247:1573-1574.
10. Brito PN, Vieira MP, Falcão MS, et al. Optical coherence tomography study of peripapillary retinal nerve fiber layer and choroidal thickness in eyes with tilted optic disc. *J Glaucoma.* 2015;24:45-50.
11. Jiang S, Turco B, Choudhry N. Vascular perfusion density mapping using optical coherence tomography angiography comparing normal and optic disk pit eyes. *Retin Cases Brief Rep.* 2019;00:1-7.
12. Cennamo G, Rossi C, Ruggiero P, et al. Study of the radial peripapillary capillary network in congenital optic disc anomalies with optical coherence tomography angiography. *Am J Ophthalmol.* 2017;176:1-8.

13. Romano F, Giuffrè C, Arrigo A, et al. Case report: optical coherence tomography angiography in morning glory disc anomaly. *Optom Vis Sci.* 2018;95:550-552.

14. Shin JH, Jung JH. Optical coherence tomography angiography findings in superior segmental optic nerve hypoplasia. *J Neuroophthalmology.* 2019;39:103-104.

INDEX

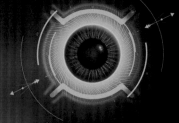